Acquired Brain Injury

Jean Elbaum   Deborah M. Benson

Editors

Acquired Brain Injury

An Integrative Neuro-Rehabilitation Approach

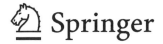 Springer

Jean Elbaum
Transitions of Long Island®
North Shore-Long Island
  Jewish Health System
1554 Northern Boulevard
Manhasset, NY 11030
USA
jelbaum@nshs.edu

Deborah M. Benson
Transitions of Long Island®
North Shore-Long Island
  Jewish Health System
1554 Northern Boulevard
Manhasset, NY 11030
USA
dbenson@lij.edu

Library of Congress Control Number: 2006939129

ISBN-10: 0-387-37574-0   e-ISBN-10: 0-387-37575-9
ISBN-13: 978-0-387-37574-8   e-ISBN-13: 978-0-387-37575-5

Printed on acid-free paper.

9 8 7 6 5 4 3 2 1

springer.com

Contents

Contributors

Jennifer Anderson, MOTR/L
Department of Occupational Therapy, Transitions of Long Island®,
North Shore-Long Island Jewish Health System

Anthony Aprile, R.N.
Department of Nursing, Southside Hospital, North Shore-Long Island
Jewish Health System

Gopal H. Badlani, M.D.
Department of Urology, Chief–Division of Neurourology,
North Shore-Long Island Jewish Health System

Mihai D. Dimancescu, M.D., F.A.C.S.
Department of Neurosurgery, Winthrop University South Nassau
Hospital System, Chairman Emeritus – Coma Recovery Association

Robert Duarte, M.D
Department of Neurology, North Shore-Long Island Jewish Health System

Olga Fishman, M.D.
Resident, Department of Neurology, North Shore-Long Island
Jewish Health System

M.H. Esther Han, O.D., FCOVD
Department of Clinical Sciences, SUNY State College of Optometry

Matthew E. Karlovsky, M.D.
Neurourology – Private Practice, Phoenix, Arizona

Tricia Kearney, OTR/L
Department of Occupational Therapy, Transitions of Long Island®,
North Shore-Long Island Jewish Health System

Peggy Kramer, M.S., CCC-SLP
Department of Speech–Language Pathology, Transitions of Long Island®,
North Shore-Long Island Jewish Health System

Tami McGowan, M.S., OTR/L
Department of Occupational Therapy, Transitions of Long Island®,
North Shore-Long Island Jewish Health System

James Megna, P.T., M.S., NCS
Department of Physical Medicine and Rehabilitation, Southside Hospital,
North Shore-Long Island Jewish Health System

Jennifer Napolitano, M.A., CCC-SLP
Department of Speech-Language Pathology, Transitions of Long Island®,
North Shore-Long Island Jewish Health System

Manisha Patel, M.D.
Resident, Department of Psysical Medicine and Rehabilitation,
North Shore-Long Island Jewish Health System

Marykay Pavol, Ph.D., ABPP
Department of Rehabilitation Medicine, Staten Island University Hospital,
North Shore-Long Island Jewish Health System

Kelly Reilly, R.N.
Department of Education and Research, Southside Hospital,
North Shore-Long Island Jewish Health System

Craig Rosenberg, M.D.
Department of Physical Medicine and Rehabilitation, Southside Hospital,
North Shore-Long Island Jewish Health System

Angela Scicutella, M.D., Ph.D.
Department of Psychiatry, North Shore-Long Island Jewish Health System

Deena Shein, M.A., CCC-SLP
Department of Speech-Language Pathology, Transitions of Long Island®,
North Shore-Long Island Jewish Health System

Jessie Simantov, M.D.
Resident, Department of Physical Medicine and Rehabilitation,
North Shore-Long Island Jewish Health System

Deborah Strosahl, M.S., OTR/L
Monefiore Medical Center, Jack D. Weiler Division

Robin Tovell-Toubal, M.Ed., CRC
Department of Obstetrics and Gynecology, Columbia University Medical Center

1
Introduction

JEAN ELBAUM AND DEBORAH M. BENSON

Crimmins (2000) marveled at the greatness of the "three pound-blob" that is our brain and control system. As seasoned clinicians in the field of neuro-rehabilitation, we still marvel each day at the resilience of the brain and at the exciting recoveries that we attempt to facilitate in survivors of acquired brain injuries (ABIs). We observe the survivor who used to have frequent and severe behavioral outbursts each hour now remain calm and focused throughout the day. We note the survivor who once was a major safety risk due to lack of insight now act as our ally motivating other survivors by his experiences. We see survivors who were admitted to our rehabilitation program with a multitude of challenges, broken and vulnerable, discharged each week to productive, meaningful activities, competent and compensating for their residual weaknesses.

On the other hand, we've encountered a disillusioning number of situations in which distraught survivors and family members find themselves in crisis, sometimes years after the injury. The survivor with a preexisting psychiatric illness, that goes undiagnosed and untreated after his brain injury, resulting in psychiatric hospitalization for a suicide attempt a few years after discharge from acute rehabilitation. The woman with chronic pain that prevents her from returning to work, despite the significant gains she demonstrated in physical and cognitive functioning during her rehabilitation stay. The bright college student whose mild brain injury went unrecognized, who never received rehabilitative services, and whose premature return to school resulted in failure, depression, and the onset of substance abuse.

From both the successes and failures of our rehabilitation efforts, we have learned that the best way to achieve positive outcomes for our clients and families is by ensuring a comprehensive, integrated approach; one which spans the continuum of care, allowing us to support our survivors and families from the earliest stages of recovery, throughout their rehabilitation and beyond.

We have become highly aware of the value of, and need for, such a team approach to neuro-rehabilitation; including both highly trained specialists (e.g., the neuro-urologist, neuro-optometrist), as well as holistically oriented coordinators (e.g., case managers, discharge planners), who will assume very different, yet interwoven, roles in the rehabilitation of the individual post-ABI. While the benefits of this comprehensive approach may be apparent, the challenges of ensuring co-ordination and integration of care across each of these components/specialists are significant. The survivor and family must know that their care is being coordinated as well as the purpose and function of each of their care providers. Equally impor-tant, all rehabilitation team members must be knowledgeable about the different roles of their interdisciplinary colleagues, and maintain open communication that crosses multidisciplinary borders.

Thus, the goal of this text is to provide an introduction to many of the key members of the neuro-rehabilitation team, including their roles, approaches to evaluation, and treatment. The book was written for interdisciplinary students of neuro-rehabilitation as well as practicing clinicians interested in developing their knowledge of other discipline areas. It may also be of interest to survivors, care-givers, and advocates for persons with acquired brain injury, to help explain and unravel the mysteries and complexities of the rehabilitation maze. Case examples were included in each chapter to help illustrate real life challenges. Dimancescu (Chapter 2) describes the role of the neurosurgeon in treating clients post acquired brain injuries and highlights the importance of providing educational information to families to help reduce feelings of confusion and powerlessness. Rosenberg, Simantov, and Patel (Chapter 3) and Duarte and Fishman (Chapter 4) describe the central roles of physiatry and neurology in diagnosing and treating clients post ABI. They highlight the importance of team collaboration and discuss topics such as neu-roplasticity, spasticity management, medical complications, headaches, seizures, and sleep disorders. Aprile and Reilly (Chapter 9) review the specific challenges of the neuro-rehabilitation nurse in addressing the needs of the individual recovering from brain injury. Kearney et al. (Chapter 12) and Kramer, Shein and Napoli-tano (Chapter 13) discuss the essential roles of the occupational therapist, and the speech/language pathologist on the neuro-rehabilitation team. Megna (Chap-ter 11) reviews the importance of conducting vestibular evaluations for clients with dizziness and balance difficulties post-ABI, so that appropriate treatment can be rendered. Karlovsky and Badlani's chapter on neuro-urology (Chapter 5) involves a review of the common urological and sexual difficulties post-ABI as well as treatment strategies. Han (Chapter 8) describes common visual difficulties post-ABI and the role of the neuro-optometrist. Scicutella (Chapter 6), Benson and Pavol (Chapter 7), and Elbaum (Chapter 14) discuss the emotional, behavioral, and cognitive challenges of clients post-ABI and the importance of addressing these difficulties through an integration of counseling, neuro-cognitive intervention, and proper medication management. The specific challenges of families and ways to meet their needs effectively through appropriate interventions are reviewed in a separate chapter (Chapter 15). Finally, Tovell (Chapter 10) reviews the key role of the case manager in coordinating the complex and varied aspects of treatment for individuals with ABI. The text ends with a discussion of life after neuro-rehabilitation, including long-term challenges for clients and factors that influence outcome.

We wish to thank, above all, the many survivors and families, whose hard work, perseverance, and resilience serves as a continual source of inspiration to us, as well as a reminder of how we must continue to strive to improve our services and supports, not only as rehabilitation professionals, but as a community and society, for survivors of brain injury and their families. We also would like to thank our professional colleagues, whose passion, enthusiasm, and devotion to the field of neuro-rehabilitation allow us to continue to push ourselves as a team, and raise the bar in order to provide the best care we can offer. And we offer thanks to our administrative support staff, who rarely get the credit for our successes and achievements, but whose "behind the scenes" efforts are the glue that holds the complex structure of our programs together.

Reference

Crimmins, C. (2000) *Where is the Mango Princess?* New York: Vintage Books.

2
Neurosurgery and Acquired Brain Injury
An Educational Primer

MIHAI D. DIMANCESCU

Introduction

Injuries of the nervous system are particularly frightening to clients and families because of the many unknowns that still revolve around nervous system function, and because of the potential for resulting life-long disabilities or functional deficits. Recovery from brain injury is best achieved with the full participation of the patient and/or his or her family. To this end, each patient and involved family member needs to have an understanding of basic brain anatomy, physiology and pathology, as well as recuperative abilities, expressed as clearly as possible in understandable language. Because the organization of the brain is extremely complex and since an understanding of the brain and types of possible injuries is not part of our elementary, high-school, or even college education, teaching the patient and family is an ongoing process throughout treatment and rehabilitation. It behooves the neurosurgeon to provide as much of that education as possible during the acute care period of time, and to prepare the patient and family for the rehabilitation process during which the therapists will continue to provide education. The latter phase should also include preparation for re-integration into the community or for long-term care.

The nervous system consists of the brain, the spinal cord, and the peripheral nerves. While the neurosurgeon is usually involved in the care of any part of the nervous system, this chapter will address only injuries of the brain. The basic information required by an injured individual and/or his family to understand the injury, its implications and its treatment will be introduced in the following pages.

Anatomy

The **brain** is a soft mass weighing about two and a half pounds, fairly tightly packed in a three-layered skin known as the **meninges** (Truex & Carpenter, 1971). The inner or **pial** layer is translucent and is firmly adherent to the brain. Over the pia, the middle or **arachnoid** layer is extremely thin and is separated from the pia by a narrow space containing a clear colorless fluid called **cerebrospinal fluid**

(CSF). The outermost layer is the **dura mater**, thick and tough, easily separable from the arachnoid, with several folds to be identified later (Truex & Carpenter, 1971). The brain and its coverings are contained in a hard, closed box, the **skull**. The only opening out of the skull is at the skull base where the brain connects with the spinal cord through the **foramen magnum** (large opening) (Truex & Carpenter, 1971). If a brain is removed from the skull and the outer layer of meninges—the dura—is peeled off, the brain surface is noted to have multiple folds or **convolutions** and grooves or **sulci** coming together in a large mushroom like structure sitting on a narrow stalk—**the brain stem**. The large mushroom-like portion has **two halves**, the left brain and the right brain, separated by a deep groove at the bottom of which is a bridge of brain connecting the two halves. A fold of the dura extends down the groove and is called the **falx**. The main body of the brain is separated from a lower smaller portion of the brain—**the cerebellum**—located just behind the brain stem. Another fold of the dura called the **tentorium** separates the two parts of the brain (Brodal, 1969; Standing, 2005; Truex & Carpenter, 1971). The brain shares its space inside the skull with blood vessels—**arteries and veins**—and with the cerebrospinal fluid (CSF). A normal brain contains 140 to 170 cc (4.7 to 5.7 oz) of CSF manufactured in four almost slit-like cavities in the brain called **ventricles**. The brain produces approximately one cupful of fluid every 24 hours. The entire structure—brain, meninges, blood vessels, cerebrospinal fluid, and skull—is perched at the very top of the spinal column (Rouviere et al., 1962; Standing, 2005; Watson, 1995).

The basic anatomical functional unit of the brain is the **neuron**. Billions of neurons are located in several layers near the surface of the brain. This is the **gray matter**. Other neurons are packed in clusters deep in the brain, called **basal ganglia**. Each active neuron has about 80,000 connections with neurons around it. The connections occur at microscopic contact points known as **synapses**. Longer connections between the neurons and deeper parts of the brain travel in bundles through the **white matter** (Dimancescu, 2000; Standing, 2005; Truex & Carpenter, 1971). At the subcellular level, each neuron contains multiple structures that manufacture chemicals and provide energy. Around the neurons are trillions of smaller support cells—the **glial cells** (Brodal, 1969). With special staining techniques in the laboratory, these structures can be seen under a microscope and constitute the cellular anatomy of the brain.

Physiology

The brain has autonomic, sensory, motor, and cognitive functions. In very simple terms, autonomic functions are located deep in the brain, in the **midbrain** and in the **brain stem**; sensory functions in the back parts of the brain, **occipital**, **parietal**, and **posterior temporal** lobes; motor function in the **frontal** lobes; and cognitive functions, including memory, concentration, and emotions are more diffusely represented, requiring integration of both sensory and motor functions of the brain (Dimancescu, 1986, 2000; Rouviere et al., 1962). The cerebellum, or hindbrain, is mainly involved in coordination and modulation of movement as well as balance. The right brain controls the left side of the body and the left brain controls the right side. Right-handed individuals are left-brain dominant. Speech centers are mostly in the left brain.

To function smoothly, **sensory** information has to be provided to the brain. Sensations include smell, vision, taste, hearing, and tactile senses. The tactile senses include light touch, pressure, temperature, vibration, and pain. Other sensations are sent to the brain from sensors providing information related to joint positions or to the various organs in the body. The sensations travel to the brain along sensory nerves, into the spinal cord and up to the brain (Victor & Roper, 2001; Wilkins & Rengachay, 1996). To avoid a chaotic bombardment of information into the brain, a wonderful apparatus exists in the brain stem called the **reticular system**. Its function is to filter sensory information as it enters the brain and to allow through only that information required by the brain at any given moment (Rouviere et al., 1962; Wilkins & Rengachay, 1996).

The neurons receiving sensory information integrate the data and initiate transmission of information to the **motor** parts of the brain that trigger an appropriate movement or series of movements. Such movements may be very gross, including movements of the trunk, shoulder or hips or may be very fine movements such as writing, playing a musical instrument, eye movements, or talking. The smoothness or accuracy of each movement is dependent on the quality of the sensory information received (if there is no feeling in a hand and the eyes are blindfolded, it will be impossible to write or to find an object on a table) and on appropriate modulation by the cerebellum to avoid over- or undershooting. Certain parts of the brain are able to learn patterns of movement such as picking up glass and pouring water from a pitcher, complex athletic movements, and playing musical instruments. Thus, a command can be given for a complex patterned movement without having to break the movement down into its components (Andrews, 2005; Victor & Roper, 2001; Wilkins & Rengachay, 1996). The healthy brain has the capacity to process enormous amounts of sensory information and to provide a very large variety of motor responses or activities.

Autonomic functions of the brain emanate from deep brain and brain stem areas. Classified in this category are blood pressure, heart rate, breathing and digestive functions. Their deep location makes them the best protected of the many brain functions (Brodal, 1969; Rouviere et al., 1962; Wilkins & Rengachay, 1996).

The most complex function of the brain and the one that distinguishes humans from all other living creatures is **cognitive function**. Cognition is the ability to be aware of oneself and of one's condition, to concentrate, to analyze and to synthesize information consciously, to imagine and to create, to remember and to retrieve memories. Memories are stored throughout the brain in many neurons and are thus visual or olfactory, tactile or auditory, motor or emotional, or different combinations. Memories can be simple, such as a single smell, or complex, such as a whole series of events. One memory can trigger another. While it is recognized that memory is stored in neurons in the form of proteins, and that some memories are for short-term periods and other memories are long term, the process of memory retrieval still remains mysterious. How the brain is able to use given information to create new information or ideas is also unknown (Brodal, 1969; Truex & Carpenter, 1971; Victor & Roper, 2001).

Most of us are familiar with computers and in many ways the brain functions like a computer—a very complex computer that human inventiveness has not yet been able to match. Each neuron is like a computer microchip, with all the microchips able to communicate with each other, but without any input into the computer, there is no output. Furthermore, the input has to be appropriate: wrong information in, equals wrong information out. The output is triggered by an event—with computers the event is the touch of a key or of several keys. However, a computer functions electronically. The brain functions through a combination of chemical reactions and electrical impulses triggered by chemical changes, too complex for further explanation here (Dimancescu, 1986, 2000; Guyton & Hall, 2006).

For a computer to function, a source of energy is needed—electricity. Energy for the brain comes from oxygen. Oxygen is the brain's fuel, brought to the neurons by the flow of blood. No oxygen is stored in the brain; consequently a good flow of blood is required for the brain to receive the needed oxygen to provoke the appropriate chemical reactions. In addition good nutrition is necessary to supply the building blocks of the tissues and to supply the basic chemicals that allow the various chemical reactions to take place. An appropriate balance of proteins, fats, sugars, minerals, and vitamins is needed to assure a healthy functioning brain (Dimancescu, 1986, 2000; Guyton & Hall, 2006).

The anatomical and physiological overview described represents a summary of the extremely complex brain anatomy and physiology. It is hoped that the information provided is sufficient to understand some of the basics of what happens to the brain when an injury occurs.

Injuries to the Brain

The two most common mechanisms of injury to the brain are the application of a mechanical force or the interruption of a normal supply of oxygen. Occasionally the two mechanisms occur together.

Mechanical Force Injuries

Blows to the head are the type of force most commonly associated with brain injury. The simplest of these may be a simple bump on the head on an overhead cabinet, or a punch to the head, accidentally or intentionally. Other times the blow may be forceful, as in a fall striking the head against the ground, or hitting one's head against a tree while skiing, falling off a bicycle, a skateboard or rollerblades, or being struck by a falling object such as a tree branch, a brick, or an overhead fixture. Greater forces are transmitted to the brain in hammer, crowbar, poolstick, or lead-pipe attacks, or in automobile, motorcycle, or motorboat accidents or any accident where speed is involved and a rapid deceleration occurs. All of these types of injuries may occur in the home, the workplace or during travel and may be commonplace or recognized work hazards. Some are criminal in nature, others are related to negligence or carelessness and still others are unavoidable (Dimancescu, 1979, 1995, 2000). Yet another type of mechanical force injury includes penetrating injuries such as a bullet wound, shards of metal, axe or pick wounds, harpoon injuries, imbedded bone fragments or wounds caused by any other hard object that penetrates the brain (Dimancescu, 2000; Rowland, 2005a).

Occasionally mechanical force is applied to the brain from within, without any external blows being exerted against the head. Such forces occur with spontaneous hemorrhages (bleeding) into or around the brain. Such hemorrhages may result from a ruptured aneurysm, a weak spot on an artery around the base of the brain, or from a ruptured arterio-venous malformation—an abnormal tangle of weak arteries and veins. Other times bleeding may occur into a brain tumor or may result from the use of blood-thinning medications (aspirin, warfarin, plavix) that can also worsen any bleeding resulting from a blow to the head. Bleeding into the brain as a result of high blood pressure is not uncommon (Dimancescu, 1995).

The type of injury suffered by the brain after a blow to the head or following a spontaneous hemorrhage depends in part on the degree of injury, the location or locations of the injuries, and the site and size of the hemorrhage. Associated factors intervene as well in determining the effect of the injury, such as age, coexisting disease or illness, nutritional state, fitness, medications, illicit drugs, and injuries to other parts of the body such as might occur in a serious motor vehicle accident or in a fall from a great height.

The least serious injury to the brain resulting from a blow to the head is a **concussion**, defined as a brief period of loss of consciousness lasting a few minutes following which there may or may not be a period of memory loss (amnesia), and with no brain abnormalities noted on any diagnostic testing (Rowland, 2005a,b; Victor & Roper, 2001). A more serious injury is the **cerebral contusion** or hemorrhagic contusion, usually associated with a brief loss of consciousness, frequently accompanied by some weakness of an arm or a leg on one side of the body or by mental changes such as poor attention span and sometimes speech difficulties, all of which are usually, though not always, temporary. Diagnostic tests show areas of bruising of the brain (Rowland, 2005a,b; Victor & Roper, 2001). Some injuries to the brain consist of brain swelling or **edema** without any noted bruises or hemorrhages. The edema may be short-lived or prolonged, very focal or diffuse, and associated with minimal deficits or with serious brain dysfunction such as coma. More serious brain injuries cause bleeding or hemorrhages that may occur in different locations defined by the anatomy and the relationship of the hemorrhages to the three layers of the meninges covering of the brain.

Working from the surface down into the depths of the brain, the most superficial hemorrhage is an **epidural hematoma**, located between the skull and the dura or outermost meningeal layer. An epidural hematoma results from a ruptured vein or artery. The latter are usually more serious because the higher blood pressure in an artery causes more bleeding and a larger clot. Epidural hematomas in the temporal region (just above and in front of the ear) can be lethal, causing sudden death, one to two hours after an injury (Rowland, 2005a). A hemorrhage between the next two layers is a **subdural hematoma**, in the space between the dura and the arachnoid. Acute subdural hematomas have a very high mortality rate, usually because of the size of the blood clot that covers a large surface, compressing the brain and accompanying underlying injury of the brain itself. Occasionally an *acute subdural hematoma* may be silent, without any clinical signs, but over a period of one to two months, liquefies, increases in size and becomes a *chronic subdural hematoma* with mild to severe signs and symptoms. Occasionally subdural hematomas occur without any known blow to the head in individuals taking blood-thinning medications (Rowland, 2005a). Bleeding into the third space of the meninges, under the arachnoid layer, is a **subarachnoid hemorrhage**. In this type of bleeding, the blood spreads through the cerebrospinal fluid and insinuates into the grooves of the brain. The most serious of these types of hemorrhages are not from blows to the head, but from a spontaneous rupture of a weak spot *(aneurysm)* on a blood vessel. They may or may not be serious and may or may not have devastating consequences, but all spontaneous subarachnoid hemorrhages are potentially lethal (Rowland, 2005a). Any hemorrhage into the meat of the brain is known as an **intracerebral** or **intraparenchymal hemorrhage**. These blood clots may be deep or superficial, may be large or small, may be near or removed from vital structures, may be relatively inconsequential or devastating, frequently leaving an individual with long-term signs and symptoms. They may result from blows to the head or may result from hypertension *(high blood pressure)* (Rowland, 2005a). The final location of a hemorrhage may be in one or more of the ventricles, the narrow cavities of the brain that manufacture cerebrospinal fluid. These are **intra-ventricular hemorrhages**, represented by a few drops of blood in the CSF or by massive bleeding, casting the ventricles and impeding the flow of CSF (Rowland, 2005a). Each of the described injuries may occur in isolation or in combination.

Interruption of Oxygen Supply

The brain does not store any oxygen, yet it is totally dependent on oxygen to function. If the brain is totally deprived of oxygen for two minutes, the brain dies. Many situations occur where oxygen is deprived to parts of the brain *(focal anoxia)* or where the oxygen supply is diminished but not totally cut off *(hypoxia)*. Focal anoxia or hypoxia may occur without mechanical blows to the head but are frequently associated with mechanical force injuries. Conversely, spontaneous occurrences also frequently result in internal mechanical force injuries (Dimancescu, 1996). Spontaneous situations accompany arteriosclerosis (hardening of the arteries) with narrowing of the arterial openings and decreased blood flow to areas of the brain *(ischemic stroke)*. Atheromatous plaques on the carotid artery sometimes result in formation of clots that travel into the arteries of the brain and shut down the blood supply and oxygen supply to a specific area of the brain. That is commonly known as a **stroke** (or *embolic stroke*) (Dimancescu, 1996). Clots forming on abnormal heart valves may also travel into the arteries of the brain causing embolic strokes. Heart attacks requiring prolonged resuscitation efforts result in very weak blood flow to the brain during the resuscitation process, seriously decreasing the amount of oxygen delivered to the brain. The net result is a diffuse decrease in oxygen supply affecting the entire brain *(diffuse hypoxia)* (Dimancescu, 1996). Strangulation, suffocation, near drowning, and smoke inhalation all deprive the lungs of breathed-in oxygen, thereby decreasing the amount of oxygen in the blood and causing a diffuse hypoxia (Rowland, 2005a; Truex & Carpenter, 1971). Focal hypoxia and diffuse hypoxia result in chemical changes that in turn result in edema or brain swelling. Swelling compresses brain cells and small blood vessels feeding the brain, adding a mechanical compressive component to the hypoxic or anoxic component of the injury (Rowland, 2005a; Truex & Carpenter, 1971). Conversely, primary mechanical injuries to the brain cause compression of blood vessels surrounding the blood clot or hemorrhage, resulting in a focal decrease of blood supply or oxygen to that area of the brain. A vicious cycle is frequently initiated compounding the initial effect of the injury and explaining why some individuals progressively worsen during the days following a blow to the head. As bleeding or swelling increases, pressure in the skull increases (Dimancescu, 2000). Ischemic and embolic strokes are not traditionally associated with brain injuries but the end result is the same—the brain is injured and its functions are impaired.

Signs and Symptoms of Brain Injury

Brain injury causes signs and symptoms related to levels of consciousness, breathing, vital signs, pupillary function, motor function, sensory function, and autonomic function.

1. *Levels of consciousness* change with increasing degrees of brain injury or with increasing pressure within the skull. A normal individual is considered to be alert, but as consciousness becomes impaired, the individual becomes *lethargic,* then *obtunded*, then *stuporous,* and finally *comatose,* in a light, moderate, or deep coma (Dimancescu, 2000; Victor & Roper, 2001).
2. *Breathing* also changes with increasing intracranial pressure. One of the first signs of increased intracranial pressure is *hyperventilation,* a rapid breathing rate representing the brain's effort to blow off CO_2 and thereby cause constriction of blood vessels and a decrease in the volume of blood in the head. As the condition worsens, the breathing pattern changes to one of regularly increasing amplitude of each breath followed by a progressively decreasing amplitude in repeating cycles; this is known as *Cheyne–Stokes breathing.* The next phase, called *Kussmaul breathing,* is ominous, indicating impairment of brain stem function and consists of an inspiration followed by a pause then an expiration followed by a pause and this cycle repeats itself. An even more ominous respiratory pattern is *agonal breathing*, in which very irregular breaths are followed by pauses of varying lengths (Rowland, 2005a; Victor & Roper, 2001).
3. *Vital signs* consisting of blood pressure and heart rate are modified by increased intracranial pressure, with a decreasing heart rate and an increasing blood pressure

noted. This is known as the *Cushing response* (Rowland, 2005a,b; Victor & Roper, 2001).

4. *The pupils* of the eyes are always examined following brain injury. *Dilatation* of one pupil that does not constrict when a bright light is shined in the eye is an indication of increased pressure on the same side of the brain as the dilated pupil. When both pupils are dilated and fixed to light stimulation, increased intracranial pressure is bilateral, secondary to bleeding or to swelling affecting both right and left hemispheres of the brain (Rowland, 2005a,b; Victor & Roper, 2001).

5. *Changes in motor function* follow a similar progression reflecting a worsening condition, starting with weakness, then paralysis on one side of the body, opposite the side of the brain injury. Weakness or paralysis of both sides reflects bilateral brain injury. As pressure in the skull increases, abnormal reflexive movements develop, known as *decorticate* or *decerebrate* posturing. In the former, either spontaneously or to stimulation, the arm flexes over the chest and the hand turns inward. In the latter the arm extends stiffly by the side, inwardly rotated. In both conditions, the leg extends stiffly with the foot and toes pointing downward. In some patients, seizures or convulsions represent an irritation of the surface of the brain as a result of the injury sustained (Rowland, 2005c; Victor & Roper, 2001).

6. *Sensory function* is the least reliable parameter to observe since it can only be fully assessed in an alert and cooperative individual; therefore, other than responses to pain in an injured person with an altered level of consciousness, sensory function is not very helpful in determining the degree of injury to the brain (Rowland, 2005c; Victor & Roper, 2001).

7. *Autonomic function* impairment is usually manifested by a rapid heart rate and profuse sweating (Rowland, 2005a,c; Victor & Roper, 2001).

8. *The Glasgow Coma Scale* is a rapid bedside assessment tool developed 30 years ago by two neurosurgeons (see Table 2.1). The score provides a measure of the severity of the brain injury and enables the nurses and physicians to follow the patient's progress over the days following the injury (Dimancescu, 2000). The

TABLE 2.1. Glasgow Coma Scale*

Best Eye Response (4)	Best Verbal Response (5)	Best Motor Response (6)
1. No eye opening	1. No verbal response	1. No motor response
2. Eye opening to pain	2. Incomprehensible sounds	2. Extension to pain
3. Eye opening to verbal commands	3. Inappropriate words	3. Flexion to pain
4. Eyes open spontaneously	4. Confused	4. Withdrawal from pain
	5. Oriented	5. Localizing pain
		6. Obeys commands

*The GCS is scored between 3 and 15, with 3 being the worst and 15 the best. It is composed of three parameters : Best Eye Response, Best Verbal Response, Best Motor Response, as shown above. Note that the phrase "GCS of 11" is essentially meaningless, and it is important to break the figure down into its components, such as E3V3M5 = GCS 11. A Coma Score of 13 or higher correlates with a mild brain injury, 9 to 12 is a moderate injury, and 8 or less a severe brain injury.

Source: Teasdale G., Jennett B., *Lancet* (ii) 81–83, 1974.

score measures the ability to open the eyes, to vocalize or to speak, and to move the limbs. The scores range from 1 to 4 for eye opening, 1 to 5 for vocalization and speech, and 1 to 6 for the best motor movement, with 1 representing the worst score, i.e., absence of activity. The lowest possible total score is a 3, indicating extremely severe brain injury. The highest score of 15 is near normal. A score of 8 or less indicates coma.

Testing

The initial testing when a brain-injured individual first comes to the emergency room is a bedside examination to assess the ability to breathe and to measure the blood pressure, which indicates adequacy of blood circulation and can detect possible blood loss from associated injuries. Once a good airway has been established (sometimes requiring insertion of a tube and placement on a respirator), blood loss has been controlled (sometimes requiring a transfusion), and blood pressure has been stabilized, a CT scan is performed. This computerized image of the skull and the brain will show whether any contusions or hemorrhages have occurred and where they are located, may show skull fractures if any are present, and will indicate the existence of edema of the brain. Any foreign bodies in the brain will also be visualized. Sometimes, after testing is complete, an intracranial pressure monitor will be inserted by the neurosurgeon through a tiny opening in the skull. If there is clinical, CT scan or intracranial pressure monitoring evidence of increased intracranial pressure, intravenous medications will be started emergently in an attempt to reduce swelling and pressure (Rowland, 2005a; Victor & Roper, 2001; Wilkins & Rengachay, 1996).

Treatment

The role of the neurosurgeon following brain injury is to do everything reasonably possible to *assure the survival* of the individual and to try to minimize the long-term effects of the injury. The neurosurgeon's intervention starts in the emergency room. Based on the bedside examination and the CT scan results, the neurosurgeon will decide if an intracranial pressure monitor needs to be inserted, and what intravenous medications need to be administered to attempt to reduce swelling. In addition, if the individual needs to be on a respirator to support the breathing mechanism, the neurosurgeon may request that the respirator rate be set faster than the normal rate of breathing to blow off CO_2 and further reduce intracranial pressure. Every effort is made from the onset to *decrease pressure in the skull*. If the pressure increases too much, the brain becomes more compressed, causing further injury, and with high intracranial pressure, blood flow to the brain is impaired, the normal blood pressure being insufficient to overcome the increased intracranial pressure. A certain amount of pressure inside the skull is normal for everyone, but if the intracranial volume increases because of a blood clot or because of swelling, or both, as the volume increases the pressure increases slowly until it reaches a critical point at which a very tiny increase in volume causes a massive increase in intracranial pressure (Dimancescu, 1999; Wilkins & Rengachay, 1996).

Immediately after the emergency CT scan of the head is performed, the neurosurgeon needs to decide whether a surgery is needed to remove a blood clot to decrease intracranial pressure, whether the blood clot—depending on its location—can be safely removed or not, and whether the emergency operating team has to be alerted for immediate surgery or whether the surgery can safely be performed a few hours later (Dimancescu, 2000). Epidural hematomas in the temporal region (above and in front of the ear) and intracerebral hemorrages behind the brain stem usually require an immediate, emergent operation because of their potentially rapidly lethal effect if untreated surgically. Any injury in which there is communication between the brain and the outside environment through a scalp laceration also requires emergent surgical intervention, as do penetrating injuries of the brain (Dimancescu, 2000; Wilkins & Rengachay, 1996). The rapidity with which other hematomas that need surgery have to be evacuated depends on the individual's clinical condition, stability or instability, and the neurosurgeon's judgment (Victor & Roper, 2001; Wilkins & Rengachay, 1996).

With or without surgery, brain-injured patients require a period of observation and treatment in an intensive care unit setting to prevent and treat brain edema which may last for several days after an injury before subsiding, to treat seizures if they develop, and to monitor serial CT scans for possible re-bleeding or extension of contusions and the possible need for delayed surgery or re-operation (Dimancescu, 1979, 1999; Wilkins & Rengachay, 1996).

J.S. was an 18-year-old female who was brought to the emergency room unresponsive after a severe motor vehicle accident in which she was the driver, broadsided by another vehicle. Her breathing was labored, requiring immediate intubation while the staff checked her vital signs and examined her body for external signs of injury. After placement of an intravenous line and a Foley catheter a portable X-ray was taken to check the placement of the endotracheal tube, she was sent for an emergency CT scan of the head. A call was immediately placed to the neurosurgeon. The neurosurgeon noted a hemorrhagic contusion of the brain stem on the scan. Vital signs showed an elevated blood pressure and a slow heart rate. The patient remained unresponsive with dilated fixed pupils, bilateral posturing, and a Glasgow Coma Score of 4. Immediately upon transfer to the ICU, the neurosurgeon inserted an intracranial pressure monitor through the skull and discussed the ventilator settings with the respiratory therapist. He discussed the patient's care with the other specialists called in to help with her management and reviewed the plan of care with the nursing staff. While ordering the appropriate medications, the neurosurgeon also requested a physical therapy consult. As the patient's condition stabilized the neurosurgeon continued to communicate regularly with the physical therapist to allow increased bedside activity and with the other surgeons for eventual placement of a tracheostomy tube and a gastrostomy tube. From the time of admission on, the neurosurgeon discussed the patient's condition with the family on a regular basis, describing progress, prognosis, and treatment options with detailed explanations to educate the family regarding brain injury and potential for recovery. After 8 weeks in the hospital the patient was ready for transfer to a brain-injury rehabilitation unit. During the course of rehabilitation the neurosurgeon maintained an open line of communication with the family and therapists at the rehabilitation facility, and at the time of eventual discharge home, helped assure continuity of treatment in the home setting. After 2 years of supervised home therapies, this patient made a remarkable recovery, went on to obtain BS and RN degrees, and today is the clinical director of a traumatic brain injury rehabilitation facility.

D.L., 49 years old, was rushed to the emergency room after collapsing following the sudden onset of a severe headache. His previous health had been good. The neurosurgeon was called at the same time as the patient was sent to the CT unit with an elevated blood pressure but with normal respiration and heart rates. He was unresponsive and flaccid on the right side, but able to withdraw to pain on the left side. Because of the CT scan evidence of a massive subarachnoid hemorrhage the neurosurgeon ordered an emergency cerebral angiogram to identify a likely ruptured aneurysm. The angiogram confirmed the suspicion of an aneurysm, located on the left middle cerebral artery, requiring surgery. The neurosurgeon consulted with the internist, who was called in to help stabilize the patient for surgery, and held a lengthy discussion with the family to educate them regarding the patient's condition, prognosis, planned treatment, and potential outcome as well as the likely need for prolonged therapy. Following the craniotomy and clipping of the aneurysm, the patient began to recover slowly—he was initially unresponsive but within 2 days began to awaken and to move better, but with aphasia and a definite right-sided weakness. Daily discussions with the ICU staff and with the therapists helped to prepare the patient for discharge to a rehabilitation facility 1 week postoperatively. After 6 weeks in the rehabilitation facility, the patient was ready for discharge to his home, where he received continued outpatient therapies coordinated by the neurosurgeon, with a team of therapists, nurses, and the family. Eight months later, the patient was able to communicate effectively and to function independently despite some residual right-sided weakness and spasticity.

Outcomes

With or without surgery, the outcome for any one individual following brain injury cannot be readily predicted. Some injuries that appear devastating at the onset result in full or near full recoveries. Others, appearing relatively minor initially (e.g., concussion), can result in long-term deficits requiring prolonged rehabilitation that may not relieve all the functional limitations.

Rehabilitation

Some individuals with minor brain injuries, even those that require surgery, recover fully while still in the hospital and are able to go home without any further treatment (Dimancescu, 1984, 1995). Some injuries as minor as a concussion, however, can result in delayed symptoms characterized by short attention span, learning difficulties, and memory problems requiring cognitive rehabilitation (Dimancescu, 1984, 1995). Many individuals with acquired brain injuries require extensive rehabilitation to deal with a multiplicity of problems (Andrews, 1996; DeYoung & Grass, 1984; Dimancescu, 1978, 1984, 1988). An old myth that prolonged coma lasting several days to several weeks was an irreversible condition no longer holds true. The author of this chapter has spent over 25 years treating prolonged coma with many successful outcomes, motivating the development of coma arousal (or stimulation) programs in many traumatic brain injury rehabilitation facilities and providing educational workshops on coma arousal techniques (Andrews, 1996, 2005; DeYoung & Grass, 1984; Dimancescu, 1979, 1984, 1986, 1995).

The brain has remarkable recuperative powers and regeneration of connections between brain cells (synaptic connections) has been well demonstrated. Evidence also exists demonstrating takeover of destroyed areas of the brain by other unin-jured, healthy, previously unused portions of the brain. While this may not occur for all individuals, it can occur for many (DeYoung & Grass, 1984; Dimancescu, 1978, 1984, 1996).

For rehabilitation to be successful, it must start in the intensive care unit setting as soon as the individual is reasonably stable, and each family has to be prepared early for the possibility of long-term care lasting months to years (Andrews, 1996, 2005; DeYoung & Grass, 1984; Dimancescu, 1984, 1994). The most successful outcomes occur when family members are intimately involved in patient care and are well educated with respect to the injury and the recovery process (Dimancescu, 1978; 1984).

Conclusion

Education of the patient and family starts on the day of the injury. Families equipped with all the information provided in this chapter can become effective care providers. Family education can significantly reduce feelings of helplessness and confusion. The role of the neurosurgeon in initiating the educational process cannot be underestimated.

The neurosurgeon is the individual best qualified to start the educational pro-cess. When the patient is transferred to a rehabilitation unit, the education continues with the treating physicians (e.g., neurologist, physiatrist) and therapists and when indicated, the rehabilitation team is encouraged to communicate with the neuro-surgeon on an ongoing basis. Maintaining an open line of communication between the neurosurgeon, other members of the team caring for the patient, and the family assures good continuity of care, which is critical in ensuring a favorable outcome. Family participation is essential not only during hospitalization and inpatient re-habilitation, but even more so after the patient returns home and needs to continue outpatient or home-based therapies. Professionals enter the patient's life for a short, finite period of time, whereas family members are with the patient for the rest of his or her life.

References

Andrews, K. (1996) International working party on the management of the vegetative state: Summary report. *Brain Injury* 10:797–806.
Andrews, K. (2005) Rehabilitation practice following profound brain damage. *Neuropsy-chological Rehabilitation* 15(3–4):461–472.

Brodal, A. (1969) *Neurological Anatomy*, 2nd ed. London: Oxford University Press, pp. 661–680.

DeYoung, S., Grass, R.B. (1984) Coma recovery program. *Rehabilitation Nursing* 12(3):121–124.

Dimancescu, M.D. (1978, Nov.) Human neurological development: Past, present and future. *US Department of Commerce, National Technical Information Service* N79-15887–15897.

Dimancescu, M.D. (1979, June) Outcome of severe head injuries: 194 cases. *Medical Society of the State of New York* (Presentation).

Dimancescu, M.D. (1984, Jan.). Controversies in rehabilitation. *University of Miami* (Presentation).

Dimancescu, M.D. (1986) What is coma? *CRA Quarterly Report.*

Dimancescu, M.D. (1988) Stress factors and their effects. *CRA Quarterly Report.*

Dimancescu, M.D. (1994) The spine and the long bones in prolonged coma. *CRA Quarterly Report.*

Dimancescu, M.D. (1995) Intracranial hemorrhages. *South Nassau Communities Hospital* (Lecture).

Dimancescu, M.D. (1996) Oxygen radicals in brain injury: Innovative treatment techniques for traumatic brain injury survivors. *CRA Symposium*, NY: Uniondale.

Dimancescu, M.D. (1999) Seizures, significance and treatment. *CRA Quarterly Report.*

Dimancescu, M.D. (2000) What you want to know about traumatic brain injury? *CRA Quarterly Report.*

Guyton, C, Hall, J.E. (2006) *Textbook of Medical Physiology*, 11th ed. New York: Elsevier, pp. 555–747.

Rouviere, H., Cordier, G., Delmas, A. (1962) In Masson et al. (eds.): *Human Anatomy*, 9th ed. Paris: Librairies de l'Academie de Medecine, pp. 31–35, see also pp. 469–475, 517–518, 673–683.

Rowland, L.P. (ed.) (2005a) *Merritt's Neurology*, 11th ed. New York: Lippincott, Williams and Wilkins, pp. 67–126.

Rowland, L.P. (ed.) (2005b) *Merritt's Neurology*, 11th ed. New York: Lippincott, Williams and Wilkins, pp. 483–501.

Rowland, L.P. (ed.) (2005c). *Merritt's Neurology*, 11th ed. New York: Lippincott, Williams and Wilkins, p. 1195.

Standing, S. (ed. in chief) (2005) *Gray's Anatomy*, 39th ed. New York: Elsevier, pp. 43–50, see also pp. 227–235, 275–285, 387–410, 419–430.

Truex, R.C., Carpenter, M.B. (1971) *Human Neuroanatomy*, 6th ed. Baltimore: Williams and Wilkins Company, pp. 12–20, see also pp. 44–57, 148.

Victor, M., Roper, A. (2001) *Principles of Neurology*, 7th ed. New York: McGraw Hill, pp. 925–951.

Victor, M., Roper, A. (2001) *Principles of Neurology*, 7th ed. New York: McGraw Hill, pp. 933–942.

Victor, M., Roper, A. (2001) *Principles of Neurology*, 7th ed. New York: McGraw Hill, pp. 947–950.

Watson, C. (1995) *Basic Human Neuroanatomy*, 5th ed. Boston: Little, Brown and Company, pp. 44–69.

Wilkins, R., Rengachay, S.S. (1996) *Neurosurgery*, 2nd ed. New York: McGraw Hill, pp. 2611–2666.

Wilkins, R., Rengachay, S.S. (1996) *Neurosurgery*, 2nd ed. New York: McGraw Hill, pp. 275–294.

Wilkins, R., Rengachay, S.S. (1996) *Neurosurgery*, 2nd ed. New York: McGraw Hill, pp. 2717–2846.

Wilkins, R., Rengachay, S.S. (1996) *Neurosurgery*, 2nd ed. New York: McGraw Hill, pp. 305–514, see also pp. 2699–2708.

3
Physiatry and Acquired Brain Injury

CRAIG H. ROSENBERG, JESSIE SIMANTOV, AND MANISHA PATEL

Introduction

Physiatrists are specialists who focus not only on the disease process but also on the secondary effects that may occur as a result of the disease process. We utilize a biopsychosocial model that is unlike conventional medicine, which tends to focus on the diagnosis and treatment specifically geared toward the disease process (biomedical model) (Stiens, 2002). The underlying principle is based on treating each patient as a "whole." Rehabilitation medicine takes physical, emotional, and social needs into account when formulating a treatment plan. The physiatrist utilizes therapeutic exercises and physical agents in addition to medications to treat patients. The role of the physiatrist is to restore a patient's overall quality of life. Our emphasis is on maximizing a patient's functional capabilities.

Historical Perspective

Rehabilitation medicine dates back as far as World War I. It was during this era that physicians began to incorporate physical agents to help rehabilitate injured and disabled soldiers in what was known as "reconstruction hospitals." In 1926, Dr. John Stanley Coulter made it possible for physical medicine to be a part of formal education in medical school. Dr. Coulter joined the faculty of Northwestern University Medical School as the first academic physician in physical medicine and was the first to initiate a training program for physicians (Association of Academic Physiatrists, 1999).

In 1936, Dr. Frank Krusen established the first 3-year residency training program in physical medicine at Mayo Clinic. Dr. Krusen was the first to coin the word "physiatrist" to describe the physicians who applied physical medicine to treat various neurological and musculoskeletal ailments.

In 1942, Dr. Howard A. Rusk, as Chief of Army Air Forces Convalescent Training Program, demonstrated how rehabilitation allowed injured soldiers to be reinstated to duty and disabled soldiers to return back home at a functional level. He believed in an aggressive approach to rehabilitation medicine and advocated early ambulation, physical therapy, and activities of progressive intensity supplemented with psychological support (Association of Academic Physiatrists, 1999). After World War II, the daunting task of helping the thousands of disabled soldiers return to their previous way of life led to a realization and the eventual recognition of the importance of rehabilitation medicine. This led to a surge in the development of this field of medicine.

In 1947, the Advisory Board of Medical Specialties declared Physical Medicine and Rehabilitation (PM&R) as a specialty of medicine. Since then it has been a rapidly growing specialty. PM&R residency entails one year of internship (medicine or surgery) and three years of training in the field of PM&R. Today there are up to 80 ACGME accredited residency training programs in the field of rehabilitation medicine.

The Role of the Physiatrist

It is the physiatrist's role to identify a patient's physical deficits as well as the functional impact of these deficits in order to better highlight a patient's impairment, disability and handicap. The World Health Organization defines impairment as "any loss or abnormality of psychological, physiological or anatomical structure or function"; disability as "any restriction or lack of ability, resulting from an impairment, to perform an activity in the manner or within the range considered normal"; and handicap as "a disadvantage for a given individual, resulting from an impairment or a disability, that limits or prevents the fulfillment of a role that is normal for that individual in the community." By identifying these three components of functional assessment, the physiatrist can construct a treatment plan that can help to minimize the impact of the impairments in day-to-day life.

This holistic way of treating patients requires an interdisciplinary approach. The multifaceted nature of the clinical consequences of acquired brain injuries make the interdisciplinary team approach the most appropriate strategy for treatment (Roth & Harvey, 2000). The rehabilitation team typically consists of the physiatrist, physical therapist, occupational therapist, recreational therapist, a rehabilitation nurse, speech therapist, neuropsychologist, dietitian, and social worker. In an interdisciplinary team approach, the patient's progress with each discipline is communicated through team meetings which are led by the physiatrist. Team meetings are scheduled on a regular basis. These meetings allow the members of the rehabilitation team to establish goals in order to provide patients with a unified, coordinated treatment plan. The team will determine the most appropriate disposition (home versus an alternate living facility), establish a discharge date and identify services the patient may need upon discharge. Good communication skills among the members of the team are required to construct a rehabilitation program that is individualized for each patient. The overall goal of comprehensive rehabilitation is to optimize a patient's quality of life and achieve maximal independent functioning.

The Physiatrist's Role in the Acute Care Hospital

A study done by Wagner et al. (2003) showed that "early physical medicine and rehabilitation consultation positively impacts upon functional status and length of stay for patients with traumatic brain injury during acute hospitalization". Rehabilitation should begin as early as possible to provide stimulation and prevent further complications.

Physiatrists will often be consulted during the patient's acute hospitalization. Early intervention is crucial. Clinical trials have shown that early initiation of therapy results in a more favorable outcome (Brandstater, 1998). Early rehabilitation consultation provides an opportunity to educate other members of the health care team about rehabilitation issues.

Mr. Smith, a 39-year-old with no significant past medical history, was an unrestrained driver involved in a motor vehicle accident. He sustained loss of consciousness for about 30 minutes. Upon regaining consciousness he had a Glasgow coma score of 11 on the field. On admission to the hospital, imaging was positive for a left subdural hematoma. He was placed on phenytoin (Dilantin) for seizure prophylaxis and haloperidol (Haldol) for agitation by the medical team. Three days later, physiatry was consulted. The evaluation involved assessing the severity of the brain injury and prognosis as well as the patient's impairments and functional status. Mr. Smith was found to have both motor and cognitive deficits, but he was able to follow commands. As per the initial GCS score, Mr. Smith's injury was classified as a moderate traumatic brain injury. Based on the evaluation, he was deemed to be a candidate for acute inpatient rehabilitation in the brain injury unit.

The initial consultation provides an opportunity for the physiatrist to structure the rehabilitation program while the patient is on the acute medical floor. Therapists must be apprised of any precautions the patient may have. This can include cardiac, pulmonary, fall, and sensory precautions. The consultation should include a thorough physiatric history and physical exam including a thorough functional assessment. Recommendations are made by the physiatrist, which focus on minimizing the patient's impairment or disability (Stiens, 2002). As a consultant, the physiatrist helps to identify, treat, and prevent problems such as contractures, pressure sores/ulcers, bowel and bladder dysfunction, heterotopic ossification, and spasticity.

Some concern about massed practice in the first few days after stroke has been raised after the experimental finding in rats that the size of the infarct increased or perhaps more neurons were damaged secondary to early overuse of an affected, paretic limb (Dobkin, 2004). However, the author noted that "the level of exercise of a rat running on a rotating wheel is much greater than that a patient could possibly experience" (Dobkin, 2004). Generally, exercise by rats that was initiated several days after an induced stroke had positive effects on mechanisms of plasticity, such as production of brain-derived neurotrophic factor (BDNF) (Dobkin, 2004).

The preventative aspect of the rehabilitation consult should emphasize issues such as lifestyle changes and medical treatment for secondary stroke prophylaxis as well as prophylaxis for deep venous thrombosis. Encouraging early range of motion while the patient is on the medical floor helps to prevent contractures. Nurses should be made aware of the importance of weight shifting and frequent position changing to prevent pressure sores. Staff should also be educated on aspiration precautions in the presence of dysphagia and techniques that should be used when assisting the patient with meals.

Rehabilitation of the Patient with Acquired Brain Injury

Acquired brain injury (ABI) is a diagnostic category that includes traumatic brain injury, anoxia, stroke, infection, toxic-metabolic injury, and brain tumors. Many patients share a similar clinical course regardless of the etiology of the brain injury. The clinical course, which begins with global impairment of brain function, goes through a period of functional recovery and ends in a stable level of functioning with no further deterioration, is the basis for treating patients with different etiologies of injury in the same rehabilitation program.

ABI affects all age groups and poses a unique challenge to the rehabilitation professional. The effective management of ABI patients requires an understanding of the physical and cognitive impairments that may be seen. ABI can be divided into primary injuries, occurring at the moment of impact, and secondary injuries, which begin after the trauma and continue indefinitely. Secondary injuries occur as a result of the injuring event (Elovic et al., 2004). The injury may be further classified as focal (for example, contusions) or diffuse (diffuse axonal injury or DAI). Issues specifically related to stroke (CVA) and the rehabilitation of stroke survivors will be covered later in this chapter.

Common ABI-Related Impairments

The patient with ABI may be left with a combination of physical and neurobehavioral impairments. These interact to produce a broad array of handicaps and disabilities that may persist long after the injury. The pattern of deficits seen in ABI varies greatly from person to person, based on the severity of injury, location and nature of the brain injury, and medical complications (Whyte et al., 1998). However, deficits in cognition are nearly ubiquitous after moderate or severe ABI (Whyte et al., 1998). Changes in behavior, mood, and personality are frequently seen. Other common impairments that must be addressed after ABI include cranial nerve injuries; sensory deficits; increased muscle tone and contractures; motor disturbances; vestibular dysfunction; visual impairments, including oculomotor and accommodative dysfunction as well as visual field loss; dysphagia; dysarthria; aphasia; apraxia; and bladder and bowel dysfunction.

Upon admission to the brain injury unit, Mr. Smith was noted to have impaired speech, moderate to severe cognitive deficits, dysphagia, and dense right-sided weakness. He was at a cognitive functioning level of IV on the Ranchos Los Amigos Scale. His functional assessment on admission revealed that he had limited active range of motion on the right side of his body. He required maximum assistance with transfers and he was unable to ambulate. Mr. Smith was started on a comprehensive rehabilitation program that included rehabilitation nursing, dietary evaluation, physical therapy, occupational therapy, speech therapy, recreational therapy, and neuropsychological therapy.

During the initial team conference, an appropriate rehabilitation program was constructed in an interdisciplinary manner by all the members of the team under the guidance of the physiatrist to address Mr. Smith's impairments. Initial functional independent measure scores were recorded by each discipline. Based on the initial evaluation, goals were set by each discipline.

A bedside swallowing evaluation performed by the physiatrist on admission revealed signs of dysphagia. A full evaluation was completed by the speech pathologist. The modified barium swallow test revealed penetration of thin liquids. As a result, Mr. Smith was placed on a soft diet with thickened liquids.

While on the medical floor, Mr. Smith had developed a Stage I decubitus ulcer in the buttock region and right heel. On the brain injury unit, nurses were instructed regarding weight shifting and placement of pressure relief ankle foot orthoses while in bed. A gel-filled cushion for Mr. Smith's wheelchair was ordered by the occupational therapist to ensure pressure relief as well.

Predictors of Outcome Post ABI

Brain injuries are classified as mild, moderate, or severe based on the Glasgow Coma Scale score (see Chapter 2, Table 2.1). The GCS score is one of the best indicators of the severity of brain injury and it is a good predictor of outcome post-ABI. The duration of post-traumatic amnesia (PTA) has also been used as an index of injury severity and predictor of outcome (Russell, 1932). PTA is described as the time when patients are out of coma but are disoriented and amnesic for day-to-day events. There is little to no carryover from one day to the next while a patient is said to be in PTA, which typically lasts four times the length of coma. The duration of PTA is measured from the onset of ABI to the resumption of ongoing memory, so the duration of coma is included. The Galveston Orientation and Amnesia Test (GOAT), developed by Harvey Levin and colleagues, is a standard technique for assessing PTA. It is both reliable and objective. GOAT scores range from 0 to 100, with a score greater than 75 defined as normal, a score of 66 to 75 defined as borderline, and a score less than 65 defined as impaired. The period of PTA has ended when a patient achieves a score greater than 75 for 2 consecutive days.

Other early predictors of severity and outcome include age, pupillary and motor response (both are components of GCS), and the presence or absence of intracerebral lesions (Watanabe et al., 2003). Generally, these are better at predicting survival than eventual outcome. Patients that experienced a compromise in hemodynamic stability, oxygenation, or maintenance of adequate cerebral perfusion pressure, typically have a poorer functional outcome.

Stages of Recovery Following ABI

The stages of neurobehavioral recovery from anoxic brain injury, anterior communicating artery aneurysm rupture, and many other nontraumatic brain injuries are similar to those of ABI (Boake et al., 2000). The Levels of Cognitive Functioning scale was developed at Rancho Los Amigos Medical Center (Malkmus et al., 1980) to describe the sequence of neurobehavioral recovery from ABI and to provide a rationale for cognitive rehabilitation at each recovery stage. In reality, recovery from ABI is much more variable, but the scale is still useful for distinguishing major stages of recovery and determining appropriate rehabilitation strategies.

Neuroplasticity and the Rehabilitation Process

The main goal of neuro-rehabilitation is to promote recovery in patients with acquired brain injury through various therapeutic interventions involving retraining and facilitating neuroplasticity. Patients improve after brain injury by several different means. Adaptation and training may help patients compensate for their deficits and reduce disability even in the absence of neurological recovery. Pharmacotherapeutic agents that affect certain central neurotransmitters may modulate recovery. Natural spontaneous neurological recovery may lead to a decrease in the extent of neurological impairment. This may be explained by resolution of local edema, resorption of local toxins, improved local circulation, and recovery of partially damaged ischemic neurons (Roth & Harvey, 2000).

Neuroplasticity is a concept that refers to the potential ability of the CNS to modify its structural and functional organization. It is another explanation for recovery after brain injury. According to Flanagan et al. (2003), "a growing body of evidence has emerged demonstrating that the brain remains highly dynamic throughout adulthood, and remains capable of changing in response to experience and injury."

Neural plasticity is influenced by the environment and stimulation, repetition of tasks, and motivation. It occurs through neuronal regeneration or collateral sprouting, and the unmasking of previously latent functional pathways. Following cerebral injury, surviving neurons retain the ability to form new synapses. Research shows that "animals housed as adults in complex environments with access to various toys and activities develop more dendritic branching and more synapses per neuron and have higher gene expression for trophic factors than animals housed individually or in small groups in standard cages" (Johansson, 2000).

According to Cotman and Berchtold (2002), "exercise induces the expression of genes associated with plasticity, such as that encoding brain-derived neurotrophic factor (BDNF), and in addition promotes brain vascularization, neurogenesis, functional changes in neuronal structure and neuronal resistance to injury." Physical activity initiates a cascade of changes in gene expression in the hippocampus, a brain region critical for learning and memory (Cotman & Engesser-Cesar, 2002). This suggests that exercise initiates modifications in molecular mechanisms supporting the health and enhancing the plasticity of the brain (Cotman & Engesser-Cesar, 2002).

Pharmacological Augmentation of Recovery

Even with optimized neuro-rehabilitation, pharmacological manipulation may be necessary during the process of brain injury recovery. Many of the medications that a physiatrist may prescribe are reviewed by Scicutella (Chapter 6). The current emphasis will be on particular examples of pharmacology as related to patient care from the physiatrist's perspective.

Physicians must be aware of potential negative effects of several commonly prescribed medications and substitute agents that may be more appropriate for patients with acquired brain injury. One example of this is metoclopramide, which is a commonly prescribed antiemetic, which pharmacologically is a neuroleptic. There is some evidence that neuroleptic medications may impact negatively on cognition, and thus replacing metoclopramide with erythromycin, an antimicrobial that increases gastrointestinal motility without the sedating and negative effects of the neuroleptics, may be an option. In addition, if a patient is being prescribed a neuroleptic for a behavioral problem, it is best to minimize the number of agents from the same class to avoid the possibility of additive side effects. The antiepileptic medications are another example of this principle, some of which can have more cognitive and mood side effects than others. Phenytoin, which may cause confusion and drowsiness, may be substituted with carbamazepine (Tegretol), valproic acid (Depakote), gabapentin (Neurontin), or lamotrigine (Lamictal).

In contrast, other medications can help to enhance recovery by augmenting certain neurotransmitter systems which are known to be damaged in brain injury. For example, it has been demonstrated by Meythaler et al. (2002) that in the first few hours after ABI, catecholamine levels are increased in the cerebrospinal fluid (CSF), whereas later, catecholamine production is decreased and CSF levels drop (Bakay et al., 1986). Animal studies have shown that amphetamine increased the rate of motor recovery in experimentally injured rats as compared to controls and norepinephrine has a beneficial effect on recovery, while depletion completely blocks improvement of functional skills (Flanagan et al., 2003; Hovda & Feeney, 1984; Kline et al., 1994; Schmanke & Barth, 1997; Kikuchi et al., 2000; Hovda et al., 1989). Clinically this has had application for those with acquired brain injuries through the use of psychostimulants which cause the release of catecholamines such as dopamine and norepinephrine from presynaptic neurons. A recent study by Walker-Batson et al. (2001) suggested that dextroamphetamine administration resulted in a significant improvement in language skills in a group of patients with stroke-induced aphasia when paired with speech-language therapy as compared to controls.

Medications that enhance the dopaminergic pathway have been successful in improving levels of awareness and alertness in patients with moderate to severe ABI (Meythaler et al., 2002). Dopaminergic fibers are involved in stimulating the reticular activating system, which modulates arousal. Dopaminergic receptors are found in areas of the brain linked to movement, learning, and memory (McElligott et al., 2003). Amantadine facilitates the release of dopamine and delays its re-uptake by neural cells. Amantadine may have NMDA receptor antagonist effects as well, and this action may contribute to its neuroprotective effects early after injury (Zafonte et al., 2001). In addition, dopamine agonists have also been used with some success for the treatment of neglect. Mukand et al. (2001) administered levodopa and carbidopa (Sinemet) to four patients with left neglect. In this small case series, three of the four patients had substantial improvements on a modi-fied version of the Behavioral Inattention Test and their functional status on the Functional Independence Measure (FIM) assessment.

Upon review of his medications, phenytoin was discontinued since Mr. Smith had been seizure free for an entire week on the medical floor. In addition, the haloperidol was imme-diately discontinued because of its negative impact on recovery. Future episodes of agitation were managed successfully with nonpharmacologic interventions, which included behav-ioral and environmental strategies. On the third day following admission to the brain injury unit, staff expressed their concerns regarding Mr. Smith's inability to concentrate and follow through with commands. Mr. Smith's neurobehavioral deficits involving attention, cognitive efficiency, memory, reasoning, and judgment proved to be very challenging due to their ef-fects on all aspects of rehabilitation. He was started on a trial of methylphenidate (Ritalin) and donepezil (Aricept), which proved to have a remarkable effect on his attention and memory as well motor recovery.

Spasticity

Spasticity is defined as "a motor disorder characterized by a velocity-dependent increase in tonic stretch reflexes with exaggerated tendon jerks, resulting from hyperexcitability of the stretch reflex, as one component of the upper motor neuron syndrome" (Katz et al., 2000). It is the increase in resistance that is felt while passively moving the patient's limb at a particular joint.

Spasticity is commonly found in patients with acquired brain injury. At the bedside, spasticity is graded using the modified Ashworth Scale. Complications secondary to spasticity include contractures, heterotopic ossification, pressure ul-cers, and respiratory infections.

When considering treatment for spasticity, it is important to determine if the spasticity is causing functional impairment. This should be done by observing the patient's functional activities, including gait and the synergy patterns. Functional goals of treatment are to improve hygiene, decrease pain, decrease deformity, im-prove orthotic fit, improve gait, decrease energy expenditure of gait, and facilitate motor control (Boake et al., 2000). In some patients, spasticity may be required to carry out certain functional activities. For example, extensor spasticity in the lower extremities may help some patients to stand or ambulate.

The first step in treating spasticity is to avoid exposure to noxious stimuli (i.e., pressure ulcers, urinary tract infection, constipation, ingrown toe nails). Proper positioning, stretching, and range of motion are essential components of the treatment process. This can be accompanied by modalities, serial casting, and/or dynamic splinting.

Cryotherapy has been shown to decrease muscle stretch reflex excitability and increase range of motion (Katz et al., 2000). Other modalities that can be used are biofeedback and electrical stimulation. Electrical stimulation has been shown to decrease tone in antagonistic muscle groups in hemiplegic and quadriplegic patients (Katz et al., 2000). Serial casting involves placing casts on the spastic limb to increase joint range of motion progressively. Skin should be monitored when placing and removing the casts. Skin breakdown can be a noxious stimulus and worsen the spasticity. Similarly, splinting is another option to help stretch the spastic limb.

Oral medications can also be used in conjunction with these methods. There is a long list of anti-spasticity medications. Unfortunately many of them, such as diazepam, cause cognitive impairments as previously described. In the setting of acquired brain injury, the recommended medication is dantrolene sodium. Dantrolene is the only antispasticity medication that acts peripherally, thereby sparing any central side effects. The mechanism of action involved is depolarization-induced calcium efflux into the sarcoplasmic reticulum (Boake et al., 2000). The side effects of this medication include lethargy and generalized weakness. Due to its hepatotoxic effects, liver function tests should be performed periodically for patients on this medication. Patients usually start at 25 mg/day.

Other treatment options include phenol or botulinum toxin injections for local treatment and intrathecal baclofen pump placement for generalized spasticity management. The mechanism of action for phenol injections involves chemical neurolysis. The effects of this type of injection may last close to a year although more typically it lasts approximately 3 months. A common side effect is dysesthesias occurring as a result of blocking sensory nerves. Botulinum toxin prevents acetylcholine vesicles from binding with proteins needed for fusion to surface membranes. This decreases the number of presynaptic transmitter vesicles preventing neuromuscular transmission. In essence, this produces a weakening of the muscle. The effects of the botulinum toxin injections typically last up to 3 months.

The intrathecal baclofen pump allows baclofen to be administered directly into the intrathecal space. It has been shown to be more efficacious for lower extremity spasticity. A patient who is considering the baclofen pump can undergo a trial in which the baclofen is injected intrathecally and the patient's response is monitored. Surgical procedures for spasticity are less frequently used. These include tendon lengthening and transfers and rhizotomies.

Mr. Smith exhibited spasticity in the right upper and lower extremity muscles. The extensor tone in the right lower extremity enabled him to stand up and walk. However, in occupational therapy, it was noted that functional use of the right upper extremity was limited because of pain secondary to increased tone. The physiatrist performed a selective botulinum toxin injection in the biceps brachii muscle to relieve flexor tone. Stretching was also performed by the therapists to work in conjunction with the effects of the botulinum toxin injection.

Fall Prevention

Most patients on the rehabilitation unit are at a high risk for falling. Therefore, fall prevention is a major initiative on most rehabilitation units. Urinary incontinence, neglect, and visuospatial deficits, as well as the use of sedatives increase the risk for falls after stroke. Additional risk factors for falls include impulsivity, bilateral strokes, confusion, male gender, and poor activities of daily living performance. Right hemispheric strokes confer a greater risk due to the association with neglect, visuospatial deficits, and impulsivity. Preventive measures must be in place to minimize falls. These may include adequate staff supervision of patients, fall prevention education, balance training, bed and chair alarms, timed voiding, minimizing the use of sedatives and diuretics, and restraints when absolutely necessary. One option includes issuing "ambulation orders" based on the patient's evaluation and performance, without which patients are not permitted to ambulate independently on the rehabilitation unit. These orders are brought to the attention of the patient and the entire rehabilitation team, including aides, as well as the patient's family and visitors. Ambulation orders are frequently updated as the patient progresses through rehabilitation.

Medical Complications Commonly Encountered on the Neuro-Rehabilitation Unit

All members of the rehabilitation team should be vigilant in monitoring for signs of complications. Up to 75% of patients admitted to a rehabilitation unit may experience medical complications following a stroke (Moroz et al., 2004).

Deep Venous Thrombosis (DVT)

Venous thromboembolic disease (VTE), including DVT and pulmonary embolus (PE), are among the most significant complications seen in both stroke and ABI survivors. VTE is related to increased mortality in the rehabilitation setting. The incidence of DVT in neurorehabilitation admissions ranges from 10% to 18% (Elovic et al., 2004), and in the stroke population occurs in 20% to 75% of survivors. Stroke patients remain at high risk for PE for up to 3 months post-stroke. Clinicians must have a high index of suspicion for DVT among these patients with frequent motor weakness and ambulation difficulties. DVT occurs most frequently in the lower limbs and is classically associated with venous stasis, endothelial vessel damage, and hypercoagulable states. It is also associated with prolonged immobility, paresis, fractures, soft tissue injuries, and age over 40 (Elovic et al., 2004). Most patients admitted to the rehabilitation unit are on a prophylactic regimen for DVT prevention. Commonly used agents for anticoagulation include low-dose unfractionated heparin (5,000 units q8 to 12 hours), low molecular weight heparin, and warfarin. An inferior vena cava (IVC) filter can be placed in patients who have contraindications to anticoagulation use, for example acute cerebral hemorrhage, although a filter should not be used as the sole method for prophylaxis. Intermittent pneumatic compression devices are also used in conjunction with another method of prophylaxis.

The diagnosis of DVT requires a high index of suspicion. Noninvasive techniques include ultrasonography, impedance plethysmography, contrast venography, and D-dimer serum assays. Contrast venography remains the gold standard for the diagnosis of clinically suspected DVT. Pulmonary angiography remains the gold standard for diagnosing PE. Treatment of DVT usually involves anticoagulation for 3–6 months.

Dopplers of the lower extremities on admission were negative for DVT. Given the history of SDH, anticoagulation was contraindicated for deep venous thrombosis (DVT) prophylaxis. As a result, Mr. Smith was placed on intermittent pneumatic compression devices. Range of motion was performed by the therapists on a daily basis to prevent contractures and to minimize the risk of formation of heterotopic ossification.

Heterotopic Ossification (HO)

HO is the formation of bone in abnormal, ectopic locations such as soft tissue. HO occurs primarily in the proximal joints of the upper and lower extremities in 11% to 76% of severely injured patients. Risk factors for HO in brain-injured patients include prolonged coma (greater than 2 weeks), spasticity, long-bone fractures, and decreased range of motion. Joints most frequently affected in brain-injured patients are hips, elbows, shoulders, knees. HO may present with pain, warmth, swelling, and contracture formation, but may be occult as well. The earliest method for detecting HO is the triple phase bone scan. HO may be seen within the first 2–4 weeks in Phase I and Phase II (blood-flow and blood-pool phases) of a triple phase bone scan. Phase III (static phase) will detect HO after 4–8 weeks. HO may not be evident on plain X-rays for 3 weeks to 2 months. Serum alkaline phosphatase levels are increased but this finding is nonspecific.

Prophylaxis for HO includes ROM exercises, control of muscle tone, nonsteroidal anti-inflammatory drugs (NSAIDS) such as indomethacin, and radiation, although use of radiation in younger patients is controversial. The treatment for HO is diphosphonates (etidronate) and NSAIDS (indomethacin). Salicylates may also be used. Etidronate will decrease the ongoing formation of HO. ROM exercises play an important role in both the prophylaxis and treatment of HO. ROM exercises are crucial in preventing ankylosis. Surgical resection of HO may only be performed after bony maturation, typically 12–18 months after the onset of HO. At the point of maturation, serum alkaline phosphatase levels return to normal.

Post-Traumatic Hydrocephalus (PTH)

Ventriculomegaly, due to cerebral atrophy and focal infarction of brain tissue, or hydrocephalus ex vacuo, is commonly seen in patients after ABI. The reported incidence is 40% to 72% of severe ABI patients (Elovic et al., 2004). True hydrocephalus is not as common, with the incidence being 3.9% to 8%. Hydrocephalus in ABI patients is most commonly the communicating type, specifically, normal pressure hydrocephalus. Unfortunately, the classic trial of incontinence, ataxia, and dementia is not always seen and is of little help in severely disabled patients. Initial manifestations of hydrocephalus can include headache, vomiting, confusion, and drowsiness. The physician must have a high index of suspicion and team members must report subtle behavioral or functional deteriorations. Failure to improve or deterioration of cognitive or behavioral function should prompt assessment with a CT scan (Whyte et al., 1998). The "tap test," the withdrawal of cerebrospinal fluid via lumbar puncture, may be both diagnostic and therapeutic. Patients may require surgical shunt placement.

Patients that already have ventricular shunts may experience shunt failure. Therefore, CT scanning and shunt flow study or pressure measurements should be performed if clinical deterioration is noted.

Autonomic Dysfunction and Post-Traumatic Hypertension

ABI patients may suffer from central dysautonomia. This may present with alterations in blood pressure and pulse and impaired temperature regulation. Hypertension and tachycardia may be secondary to a hyperadrenergic state. It may be caused by injuries to the hypothalamus and is usually self-limited. HTN may also be iatrogenic (methylphenidate).

Hyperthermia or "central fever" may be due to a lesion in the hypothalamus or can be an indication of decerebration. Temperatures may reach higher than 104° F. Central fever is always a diagnosis of exclusion and other causes for the fever must be ruled out. Treatment involves cooling the patient with indomethacin or dopamine agonists and dantrolene. Hypothermia may be secondary to a lesion in the posterior hypothalamus.

Post-traumatic hypertension is associated with intracerebral hemorrhage and DAI. Hypertension, tachycardia, and increased cardiac output in the acute post-injury period may result from the increased levels of circulating catecholamines (Whyte et al., 1998). Beta blockers may be useful for treatment. The use of highly polar beta blockers which only minimally cross the blood-brain barrier is suggested. These include atenolol and nadolol. Sustained hypertension is infrequent in ABI, unless it was a premorbid medical condition. When long-term therapy is needed, angiotensin-converting enzyme (ACE) inhibitors, calcium channel blockers, and some diuretics are least likely to cause cognitive impairment.

Endocrine Complications

Individuals who have had a brain injury may be subject to associated neuroendocrine problems due to injury to the hypothalamus or pituitary gland. During stressful episodes such as trauma, release of antidiuretic hormone (ADH) from the hypothalamus is increased. Elevated ICP may further contribute to release of this hormone. The most commonly seen syndromes are cerebral salt-wasting (CSW) syndrome and the syndrome of inappropriate antidiuretic hormone secretion (SIADH). CSW and SIADH both result in hyponatremia; however, patients with CSW syndrome are in fact volume depleted, whereas in SIADH, patients are euvolemic. CSW is presumed to occur because of direct neural effect on renal tubular function.

The treatment for CSW is hydration/fluid replacement and serum electrolyte correction. Remember these patients are volume-depleted. In SIADH, the treatment usually begins with fluid restriction to ~1 L/day with or without use of a loop diuretic. Serum sodium levels should be checked daily and weight changes should be closely monitored. Hypertonic saline is administered in patients with symptoms such as confusion, convulsions, or coma. Profound hyponatremia can be fatal but serum sodium must be corrected gradually to avoid central pontine myelinolysis.

Diabetes insipidus (DI) is a less common disorder of the pituitary gland and is often associated with basal skull fractures. A fracture in or near the sella turcica may tear the stalk of the pituitary gland. This can result in DI due to disruption of ADH secretion from the posterior lobe of the pituitary. It is characterized by polyuria, polydipsia, and hypernatremia. The hallmark is excessive excretion of dilute urine (urine osm <290 mmol/kg, SG 1.010). The decrease in intravascular volume can lead to hypotension and decreased cerebral perfusion pressure.

Treatment for DI is hormone replacement with desmopressin acetate, an analog of antidiuretic hormone. The medication chlorpropamide potentiates the effects of ADH on the renal tubules and is used in patients with partial ADH deficiency. If the patient is experiencing significant mental status changes, intravenous hypotonic fluid replacement must be administered.

Other endocrine problems may occur as well. Menstrual irregularities are common following severe head trauma and it may take several months to resume a normal menstrual cycle. Gynecomastia and galactorrhea may occur from elevations in prolactin levels. Sexual dysfunction is commonly attributed to psychosocial issues but may be partially accounted for by endocrine dysfunction. If a patient appears to show a premature plateau or decline in function and recovery, a complete endocrine profile should be assessed including thyroid and adrenal gland function.

Common Stroke-Related Impairments

Disability in stroke is a result of CNS injury by which physical, cognitive, and psychological functioning become impaired. Specific impairments appear when focal regions and neural systems within the brain are damaged by vascular compromise (Roth & Harvey, 2000). Common impairments caused by stroke include: motor weakness (90%), deficits in higher mental function, ataxia (20%), hemianopsia (25%), visuoperceptual deficits (30%), aphasia (35%), cranial nerve impairments, dysarthria (50%), apraxia, neglect syndrome, dysphagia, spasticity, sensory impairment, balance, coordination and posture impairments, and bladder and bowel dysfunction.

Rehabilitation of Stroke Survivors

A stroke is a nontraumatic, acquired brain injury caused by the occlusion or rupture of cerebral blood vessels resulting in the sudden development of a persisting neurological deficit (Roth & Harvey, 2000). The focal brain lesions encountered in patients with stroke produce a wide array of neurologic deficits. Roth (1992) listed five major functions of stroke rehabilitation:

1. Prevention, recognition, management, and minimizing the impact of preexisting medical conditions, ongoing general health functions, and secondary medical complications.
2. Training for maximal functional independence.
3. Facilitating optimal psychosocial adaptation and coping by both the patient and family.
4. Promoting community reintegration, resumption of prior life roles, and the return to home, family, recreational, and vocational activities.
5. Enhancing quality of life.

Predictors of Outcome Post Stroke

The most reliable and consistent predictor of functional outcome is the person's functional ability at admission. An admission FIM score of 60 or greater is associated with a higher likelihood of functional improvement. Other noted predictors of functional outcome include age, previous stroke, urinary incontinence, consciousness at onset, severity of paralysis, sitting balance, visuospatial deficits, unilateral hemineglect, and level of social support. Unilateral visual neglect may adversely affect functional outcome and is associated with poor safety awareness, disrupted daily activities, and decreased likelihood of returning to work or driving (Mukand et al., 2001). Wade and associates (1983) studied 83 stroke patients and found the best predictors of function after 6 months were sitting balance, age, hemianopsia, urinary incontinence, and motor deficit in the arm. The mortality from all strokes ranges from 17% to 34% in the first 30 days (O'Neill et al., 2004). The rate in hemorrhagic strokes may be as high as 48%, but this may be related to stroke severity, and not necessarily the type of stroke. Patients with intracerebral hemorrhage are more likely to have higher stroke severity and poorer outcome (Jorgensen et al., 1995).

Stages of Motor Recovery after Stroke

Up to 88% of acute stroke patients have hemiparesis (Zorowitz et al., 2004). Hemiparesis and motor recovery have been the most studied of all stroke impairments. Motor recovery following stroke has been described by Twitchell (1951) and Brunnstrom (1970). Twitchell described the pattern of motor recovery following a stroke. The pattern he described is most consistent with recovery in patients with a CVA in the middle cerebral artery (MCA) distribution. Total loss of voluntary movement and loss or decrease of tendon reflexes occurs at the onset of hemiplegia, typically involving the arm more than the leg. Tone and "tight coupling of movement at adjacent joints" (later termed synergy by Brunnstrom) developed before isolated voluntary movement returned. As spasticity increased, clonus appeared (Zorowitz et al., 2004). He also noted that motor function typically returned proximally before distally and lower extremity function recovered earlier and more completely than upper extremity function. The majority of recovery occurred in the first 12 weeks, with only minor additional recovery after 6 months.

Brunnstrom divided the recovery process into seven different stages. Initial loss of voluntary motion is accompanied by limb flaccidity. This stage is followed by an increase in reflexes, spasticity and weak basic synergy patterns. Stage 3 is delineated by prominent spasticity with patient regaining some voluntary control over synergy patterns. This is followed by some voluntary, selective activation of muscles outside of synergy patterns with some reduction in spasticity. Stage 5 is marked by further decrease in spasticity with most limb movement independent of synergy. Stage 6 is resolution of spasticity with near normal coordination and isolated movements. Normal function is restored in the seventh and final stage.

Major Theories of Rehabilitation Training Post-Stroke

Traditional approaches for improving motor control and coordination emphasize the need for repetition of specific movements for learning, the importance of sensation for the control of movement, and the need to develop basic movements and postures. Several neurophysiological theories of rehabilitation for motor deficits have been developed. No single approach has been proven to be more effective and therapists typically incorporate aspects from several theories when formulating a treatment plan.

Proprioceptive neuromuscular facilitation (PNF)-based rehabilitation uses diagonal and spiral pattern techniques to facilitate movement patterns. It uses mechanisms such as maximum resistance, quick stretch, and spiral diagonal patterns to facilitate normal movement by "irradiation" of impulses to other parts of the body associated with the primary movement.

The Bobath/neurodevelopmental treatment (NDT) approach emphasizes suppressing abnormal muscle patterns and avoiding mass synergies, because these may reinforce spasticity and increased reflexes. The goal of NDT is to normalize tone, inhibit primitive patterns of movement, and to facilitate automatic, voluntary reactions and subsequent normal movement patterns (Zorowitz et al., 2004).

In contrast to NDT, the Brunnstrom approach (Choi et al., 2003) utilizes primitive postural reactions and synergies to facilitate motor function. Patients are encouraged to learn to control and use the synergistic motor patterns available at each particular phase of recovery.

The Rood or sensorimotor approach employs cutaneous sensorimotor stimulation such as brushing, stroking, tendon tapping, vibration, icing, and quick stretch to activate motor function and inhibit spastic antagonists.

Carr and Shepherd's motor relearning program (Roth, 2002) is based on a theory of cognitive motor relearning and emphasizes functional training, practice, and repetition in the performance of specific tasks, and carryover of those skills into functional activities.

Electrical neuromuscular stimulation may also elicit motor and functional gains. According to Dobkin (2004), "functional electrical stimulation is also used to activate paretic muscles timed to a movement, such as contraction of the tibialis anterior muscle to clear the foot during the swing phase of walking."

Body weight-supported (BWS) treadmill training is geared specifically to the recovery of walking ability. BWS has been shown to restore gait faster in non-ambulatory patients when compared with nonambulatory patients who received conventional therapy (Wernig & Muller, 1992). Gait retraining in this approach consists of walking a patient on a treadmill at his/her maximum comfortable speed, whereas a percentage of his/her body weight is supported centrally at the trunk by an overhead harness. The amount of body weight that is supported typically ranges from 0% to 40% (Bogey et al., 2004). BWS treadmill walking is typically well tolerated after stroke. In a trial with acute-stroke patients, Malouin et al. (1992) demonstrated good compliance. Patients were able to withstand up to 45 minutes of treadmill walking. However, no trials have been done studying the efficacy of BWS walking therapy in the acute stroke rehabilitation setting. The optimal timing for intervention with BWS walking has not been determined and there is some evidence supporting this type of training even 2 years post-stroke (Malouin et al., 1992). An approach such as BWS treadmill training is not meant to be an exclusive method of training and must be complemented by other treatment approaches.

In the past, functional gains were incorrectly said to plateau by 3–6 months post injury. However, many patients retain latent sensorimotor potential that may be nurtured and released any time after injury with a course of goal-directed therapy.

Constraint-Induced Movement Therapy

Constraint induced movement therapy (CIMT) is based on the observation that some of the disability in stroke patients resulted from lack of use of the affected limb. Learned nonuse of the affected arm is common because of pain, slow and increased effort, and energy requirements to use the affected limb, and ease of use of the unaffected limb. In this "use it or lose it" forced-use intervention, the unaffected limb is restrained in an attempt to force use of the affected limb. Research has shown that CIMT is both feasible and tolerated, and associated with less short-term arm impairment than traditional therapy (Dromerick et al., 2000). According to Dobkin (2004), "traditionally CIMT is performed for approximately 6 hours per day for 2 weeks, but less intensity may work as well, and may be effective even when initiated 2 years post stroke." The patient must have a minimum of 20 degrees of voluntary wrist extension and 10 degrees of extension in two fingers at the metacarpophalangeal or interphalangeal joints of the paretic hand to qualify for enrollment into a CIMT protocol (Levy et al., 2002).

Post-Stroke Complications

Up to 75 percent of patients admitted to a rehabilitation unit may experience medical complications after a stroke (Moroz et al., 2004). Death within the first week of a stroke is attributed to the stroke itself in 90% of patients (Moroz et al., 2004). This may be from cerebral edema, mass effect, or herniation. The most common cause of death within the first 2 to 4 weeks post-stroke is pulmonary embolism. Pneumonia is the most common cause of death during the second and third months post stroke, with cardiac disease responsible thereafter. Patients remain at high risk for pulmonary embolism for up to 3 months after stroke (Moroz et al., 2004).

Secondary Prevention

Secondary prevention of stroke is an important aspect of rehabilitation management (O'Neill et al., 2004). The physiatrist must make recommendations to the patient and family members for prevention of subsequent strokes. Approximately 7% of all patients with a history of transient ischemic attack (TIA) or stroke will have a recurrent event each year. Risk factors for stroke include modifiable and unmodifiable factors. Modifiable risk factors include hypertension, diabetes, heart disease, TIA or prior stroke, hypercholesterolemia, obesity, sedentary lifestyle, cigarette smoking, alcohol abuse, and cocaine use. Nonmodifiable risk factors include age, gender, race, and family history. Furthermore, the use of antiplatelet agents, anticoagulation and carotid endarterectomy may be utilized for secondary stroke prevention in some patients. The careful identification and reduction of risk factors may significantly reduce the risk of recurrent stroke and patient/family education must be addressed as part of the rehabilitation program.

Conclusion

Many individuals are left with a combination of physical, cognitive, and psychosocial impairments following an acquired brain injury. The challenge for physiatrists specializing in neuro-rehabilitation is in applying the knowledge gathered from group studies to the management of each patient's unique pattern of deficits, which produce a broad array of disabilities and handicaps that may persist long after the initial injury (Whyte et al., 1998). The pattern of impairments varies greatly from patient to patient. Handicaps may be affected by differences in the social and physical environments to which the brain injury survivor returns providing further treatment challenges for the physiatrist specializing in neuro-rehabilitation (Whyte et al., 1998). Therefore, an interdisciplinary treatment approach that considers the complex and unique pattern of deficits seen in an individual patient is the best approach to treatment. Physiatrists must be able to communicate effectively with patients, families and staff and provide assessments of prognosis based on literature, prognostic parameters, and clinical experience. At the same time we must never take away hope (Zasler, 1999).

Much progress has been made in the area of brain-injury rehabilitation. Rehabilitation and community integration focus on helping the person achieve a new sense of "self." While we are often unable to "cure" those who have suffered a devastating acquired brain injury, we are capable of ameliorating the impact of physical and cognitive impairments on the individual's functional status. Physiatrists and the rest of the rehabilitation team provide individuals with the tools they require to adapt and adjust to their new circumstances.

Four weeks after beginning acute inpatient rehabilitation, Mr. Smith had made a considerable amount of gains in all the disciplines. He was on a regular diet. He was ambulating with a quad cane and he was able to transfer independently. He continued to have some cognitive deficits for which he required supervision during all his activities. However, his comprehension and awareness of his environment and people around him had improved drastically. He was able to recognize his wife and son, which was something he could not do initially. Mr. Smith was discharged home with a referral to comprehensive outpatient neuro-rehabilitation program for continued therapy, and he is continuing to make gains.

"Hospital discharge should be looked on as the beginning of a new life in which the patient faces the challenge of adopting different roles and relationships and search for new meaning in life" (Brandstater, 1998). Brain-injury survivors face many challenges to community living every day of their lives, which often include a combination of chronic physical, cognitive and psychosocial impairments. According to Gordon et al. (1999), these individuals experience the unique challenge of "walking the sometimes conflicting paths of who they were, who they are, and who they want to be." Helping to meet the complex, ongoing needs of this population is one of the key challenges for all involved in neuro-rehabilitation, including clinicians, survivors, as well as families and friends.

References

Association of Academic Physiatrists. (1999) *The History of Physiatry*. Available at: http://www.physiatry.org/about/history.html.

Bakay, R.A., Sweeney, K.M., Wood, J.H. (1986) Pathophysiology of cerebrospinal fluid in head injury. Part 1: Pathological changes in cerebrospinal fluid solute composition after traumatic injury. *Neurosurgery* 18:234–243.

Boake, C., Francisco, G.E., Ivanhoe, C.B., Kothari, S. (2000) Brain injury rehabilitation. In Braddom, R.L. (ed.): *Physical Medicine and Rehabilitation* Philadelphia: WB Saunders, pp. 1073–1116.

Bogey, R.A., Geis, C.C., Bryant, P.R., Moroz, A., O'Neill, B.J. (2004) Stroke and neurodegenerative disorders. 3. Stroke: Rehabilitation management. *Archives of Physical Medicine and Rehabilitation* 85(Suppl 1):S15–S20.

Brandstater, M.E. (1998) Stroke rehabilitation. In Delisa, J.A., Gans, B.M. (eds.): *Rehabilitation Medicine: Principles and Practice*. Philadelphia, PA: Lippincott Raven, pp. 1165–1189.

Brunnstrom S. (1970) *Movement Therapy in Hemiplegia: A Neurological Approach*. Harper & Row. New York, NY.

Choi, H., Sugar, R., Fish, D.E., Shatzer, M., Krabak, B. (eds.): (2003) In *Physical Medicine & Rehabilitation Pocketpedia*. Philadelphia, PA: Lippincott Williams & Wilkins, pp. 92–96.

Cotman, C.W., Berchtold, N.C. (2002) Exercise: A behavioral intervention to enhance brain health and plasticity. *Trends in Neurosciences* 25(6):295–301.

Cotman, C.W., Engesser-Cesar, C. (2002) Exercise enhances and protects brain function. *Exercise and Sport Sciences Reviews* 30(2):75–79.

Dobkin, B.H. (2004) Strategies for stroke rehabilitation. *The Lancet* 3:528–536.

Dromerick, A.W., Edwards, D.F., Hahn, M. (2000) Does the application of constraint-induced movement therapy during acute rehabilitation reduce arm impairment after ischemic stroke? *Stroke* 31:2984–2988.

Elovic, E., Baerga, E., Cuccurullo, S. (2004) Traumatic brain injury. In Cuccurullo, S. J. (ed.): *Physical Medicine and Rehabilitation Board Review* New York, NY: Demos Medical Publishing, pp. 47–80.

Flanagan, S.R., Kane, L., Rhoades, D. (2003) Pharmacological modification of recovery following brain injury. *Journal of Neurologic Physical Therapy* 27:129–136.

Gordon, W.A., Hibbard, M.R., Brown, M., Flanagan, S., Korves, M.C. (1999) Community integration and quality of life of individuals with traumatic brain injury. In Rosenthal, M., Griffith, E.R., Kreutzer, J.S., Pentland, B. (eds.): *Rehabilitation of the Adult and Child with Traumatic Brain Injury*. Philadelphia, PA: F.A. Davis Company, pp. 312–325.

Hesse, S., Bertelt, C., Schaffrin, A., Malezic, M., Mauritz, K. (1994) Restoration of gait in nonambulatory hemiparetic patients by treadmill training with partial body weight support. *Archives of Physical Medicine and Rehabilitation* 75:1087–1093.

Hovda, D.A., Feeney, D.M. (1984) Amphetamine with experience promotes recovery of locomotor function after unilateral frontal cortex injury in the cat. *Brain Research* 298:358–361.

Hovda, D.A., Sutton, R.L., Feeney, D.M. (1989) Amphetamine-induced recovery of visual cliff performance after bilateral visual cortex ablation in cats: Measurements of depth perception thresholds. *Behavioral Neuroscience* 103:574–585.

Johansson, B.B. (2000) Brain plasticity and stroke rehabilitation. *Stroke* 31:223–230.

Jorgensen, H.S., Nakayama, H., Raaschou, H.O., Olsen, T.S. (1995) Intracerebral hemorrhage versus infarction: stroke severity, risk factors, and prognosis. *Annals of Neurology* 38:45–50.

Katz, R.T., Dewald, J.P.A., Schmit, B.D. (2000) Spasticity. In Braddom, R.L. (ed.): *Physical Medicine and Rehabilitation*. Philadelphia, PA: WB Saunders, pp. 592–615.

Kikuchi, K., Nishino, K., Ohyu, H. (2000) Increasing CNS norepinephrine levels by the precursor L-DOPA facilitates beam-walking recovery after sensorimotor cortex ablation in rats. *Brain Research* 860:130–135.

Kline, A.E., Chen, M.J., Tso-Olivas, D.Y., Feeney, D.M. (1994) Methylphenidate treatment following ablation-induced hemiplegia in rat: Experience during drug action alters effects on recovery of function. *Pharmacology and Biochemistry of Behavior* 48:773–779.

Levy, C.E., Behrman, A., Rothi, L.G., Ring, H., Heilman, K. (2002) Fronteirs and fundamentals in neurorehabilitation. In O'Young, B.J., Young, M.A., Stiens, S.A. (eds.): *Physical Medicine and Rehabilitation Secrets*. Philadelphia, PA: Hanley & Belfus, pp. 220–233.

Malkmus, D., Booth, B.J., Kodimer, C. (1980) Rehabilitation of head injured adults: Comprehensive cognitive management. Downey, CA: Professional Staff Association of Rancho Los Amigos Hospital.

Malouin, F., Potvin, M., Prevost, J., Richards, C., Wood-Dauphinee, S. (1992) Use of an intensive task-oriented gait training program in a series of patients with acute cerebrovascular accidents. *Physical Therapy* 72:781–793.

McElligott, J.M., Greenwald, B.D., Watanabe, T.K. (2003) Congenital and acquired brain injury. 4. New frontiers: Neuroimaging, neuroprotective agents, cognitive-enhancing agents, new technology, and complementary medicine. *Archives of Physical Medicine and Rehabilitation.* 84(Suppl 1):S18–S22.

Meythaler, J.M., Brunner, R.C., Johnson, A., Novack, T.A. (2002) Amantadine to improve neurorecovery in traumatic brain injury-associated diffuse axonal injury: A pilot double-blind randomized trial. *Journal of Head Trauma Rehabilitation* 17(4):300–313.

Moroz, A., Bogey, R.A., Bryant, P.R., Geis, C.C., O'Neill, B.J. (2004) Stroke and neurodegenerative disorders. 2. Stroke: Comorbidities and complications. *Archives of Physical Medicine and Rehabilitation* 85(Suppl 1):S11–S14.

Mukand, J., Guilmette, T., Allen, D., Brown, L.K., Brown, S.L., Tober K.L., Van Dyck, N.R. (2001) Dopaminergic therapy with carbidopa L-DOPA for left neglect after stroke: a case series. *Archives of Physical Medicine and Rehabilitation* 82:1279–1282.

O'Neill, B.J., Geis, C.C., Bogey, R.A., Moroz, A., Bryant, P.R. (2004) Stroke and neurodegenerative disorders. 1. Acute stroke evaluation, management, risks, prevention, and prognosis. *Archives of Physical Medicine and Rehabilitation* 85(Suppl 1):S3–S10.

Roth, E.J. (1992) Medical rehabilitation of the stroke patient. *Be Stroke Smart* 8:8.

Roth, E.J. (2002) Stroke. In O'Young, B.J., Young, M.A., Stiens, S.A. (eds.): *Physical Medicine and Rehabilitation Secrets.* Philadelphia, PA: Hanley & Belfus, pp 167–177.

Roth, E.J., Harvey, R.L. (2000) Rehabilitation of stroke syndromes. In Braddom, R.L. (ed.): *Physical Medicine and Rehabilitation.* Philadelphia, PA: WB Saunders, pp. 1117–1160.

Russell, W.R. (1932) Cerebral involvement in head injury. *Brain* 35:549–603.

Stiens, S.A. (2002) The physiatric consultation: interdisciplinary intervention and functional restoration. In O'Young, B.J., Young, M.A., Stiens, S.A. (eds.): *Physical Medicine and Rehabilitation Secrets.* Philadelphia, PA: Hanley & Belfus, pp. 97–102.

Stiens, S.A., O'Young, B., Young, M.A. II. (2002) Person-centered rehabilitation: Interdisciplinary intervention to enhance patient enablement. In O'Young, B.J., Young, M.A., Stiens, S.A. (eds.): *Physical Medicine and Rehabilitation Secrets.* Philadelphia, PA: Hanley & Belfus, pp 4–9.

Schuanke, T., Barth, T.M. (1997) Amphetamine and task-specific practice augment recovery of vibrissae-evoked forelimb placing after unilateral sensorimotor cortical injury in the rat. *Journal of Neurotrauma* 14:459–468.

Twitchell, T.E. (1951) The restoration of motor function following hemiplegia in man. *Brain* 74:443–480.

Wade, D.T., Skilbeck, C.G., Hewer, R.L. (1983) Predicting Barthel ADL score at 6 months after an acute stroke. *Archives of Physical Medicine and Rehabilitation* 64:24–28.

Wagner, A.K., Fabio, T., Zafonte, R.D., Goldberg, G., Marion, D.W., Peitzman, A.B. (2003) Physical medicine and rehabilitation consultation: Relationships with acute functional outcome, length of stay, and discharge planning after traumatic brain injury. *American Journal of Physical Medicine and Rehabilitation* 82(7):526–536.

Watanabe, T.K., Millar, M.A., McElligott, J.M (2003) Congenital and acquired brain injury. 5. Outcomes after acquired brain injury. *Archives of Physical Medicine and Rehabilitaion* 84(Suppl 1):S23–S27.

Walker-Batson, D., Curtis, S., Natarajan, R., Ford, J., Dronkers, N., Salmeron, E., Lai, J., Unwin, D.H. (2001) A double-blind, placebo controlled study of the use of amphetamine in the treatment of aphasia. *Stroke* 32:2093–2098.

Wernig, A., Muller, S. (1992) Laufband locomotion with body weight support improved walking in persons with severe spinal cord injuries. *Paraplegia* 30:229–238.

Whyte, J., Hart, T., Laborde, A., Rosenthal, M. (1998) Rehabilitation of the patient with traumatic brain injury. In Delisa, J.A., Gans, B.M. (eds.): *Rehabilitation Medicine: Principles and Practice*. Philadelphia: Lippincott-Raven, pp. 1191–1239.

Zafonte, R.D., Lexell, J., Cullen, N. (2001) Possible applications for dopaminergic agents following traumatic brain injury: Part 2. *Journal of Head Trauma Rehabilitation* 16:112–116.

Zasler, N.D. (1999) Physiatric assessment in traumatic brain injury. In Rosenthal, M., Griffith, E.R., Kreutzer, J.S., Pentland, B. (eds.): *Rehabilitation of the Adult and Child with traumatic Brain Injury*. Philadelphia, PA: F.A. Davis Company, pp. 117–130.

Zorowitz, R., Baerga, E., Cuccurullo, S. (2004) Stroke. In Cuccurullo, S.J. (ed.): *Physical Medicine and Rehabilitation Board Review*. New York, NY: Demos Medical Publishing, pp. 47–80.

4

The Role of the Neurologist in Assessment and Management of Individuals with Acquired Brain Injury

ROBERT A. DUARTE AND OLGA FISHMAN

Introduction

The specialist in neurology is trained to make a targeted diagnosis of specific ailments involving the brain, spinal cord, and peripheral nerves by obtaining a thorough history and a detailed neurological examination. Additionally, neurologists work with other neuro-rehabilitation specialists in setting up a proper rehabilitation program designed to maximize the patient's physical and neuro-cognitive recovery, as well as provide the patient with tools to help cope with newfound deficits. Typical conditions that are evaluated and treated by a neurologist include traumatic brain injury (TBI), cerebrovascular accident (CVA), seizures, headaches, pain and sleep disorders.

Role of the Neurologist

Neurologists usually become involved with patients suffering from an ABI in the emergency room setting. Following a TBI, the patient's overall neurological status has been traditionally assessed by using the Glasgow Coma Scale (GCS) (See Chapter 2, Table 2.1). While GCS remains one of the most popular tools for assessment of patients with TBI, it is by no means the only one. Additionally, the usefulness of GCS in patients who are intubated is limited because their verbal responses may not be assessed properly. Wijdicks et al. (2005) recently proposed a Full Outline of UnResponsiveness (FOUR) score, which evaluates patients on the basis of eye response, motor response, brainstem reflexes (pupillary, corneal, and cough) and respiratory pattern, thus avoiding the limitations of the GCS score when evaluating patients with severe TBI who are intubated and therefore unable to communicate verbally (Table 4.1). GCS and FOUR scores are crucial to the initial assessment because they are well correlated with intracranial pathology and hence necessitate further investigation such as neuroimaging, looking for possible surgically correctable causes of depressed mental status. In addition to performing coma scales of choice, the neurologist must perform a detailed neurological

TABLE 4.1. FOUR score

Eye response	Motor response	Brainstem reflexes	Respiration
4 eyelids open or opened, tracking, or blinking to command	4 thumbs-up, fist or peace sign	4 pupil and corneal reflexes present	4 not intubated, regular breathing pattern
3 eyelids open, no tracking	3 localizing to pain	3 one pupil wide and fixed	3 not intubated, Cheyne-Stokes breathing
2 eyelids closed, but open to loud voice	2 flexion response to pain	2 pupil or corneal reflexes absent	2 not intubated, irregular breathing
1 eyelids closed, but open to pain	1 extension response to pain	1 pupil and corneal reflexes absent	1 breathes above ventilator rate
0 eyelids remain closed with pain	0 no response to pain or generalized myoclonus status	0 absent pupil, corneal and cough reflex	0 breathes at ventilator rate or apnea

Document each individual subsection score. For eye response (E), grade the best possible response after at least three trials in an attempt to elicit the best level of alertness. For motor response (M), grade the best possible response to pain. For brainstem reflexes (B), grade the best possible response. For respiration (R), observe patient's breathing pattern and grade appropriately.

Source: Adapted from Wijdicks, E.F., Bamlet, W.R., Maramattom, B.V., Manno, E.M., McClelland, R.L. (2005): New Coma Scale: The FOUR Score. *Annals of Neurology* 58:585–593.

examination, including but not limited to assessment of higher cortical function-ing, language, speech, spatial and temporal orientation, as well as signs of aphasia, apraxia, visual field cuts, and other signs of hemispheric dysfunction.

The neurological examination is the primary ancillary tool of every neurologist. Skilled examination combined with a thorough history provides clues to diagnosis in a majority of cases; therefore, proper examination techniques and ability to interpret findings become of paramount importance. Neurological evaluation is typically performed in a traditional sequence beginning with a mini-mental status examination, followed by cranial nerves, motor function, sensory testing, deep tendon reflexes, and lastly coordination and gait (Table 4.2).

The most common bedside test for assessing cognitive function is the Folstein Mini-Mental Status Examination (MMSE). MMSE (Table 4.3) is a brief screening tool that takes about 10 minutes to administer. It assesses several cognitive domains, namely orientation, memory, language, praxis, attention and concentration. The

TABLE 4.2. Components of the neurological examination

Mini-mental status (MMSE)
Cranial nerves I–XII
Motor (tone, bulk, strength, abnormal movements)
Sensory (touch, temperature, pain, vibration, proprioception)
DTRs (biceps, brachioradialis, triceps, patellar and Achilles; Babinski reflex)
Coordination and gait

TABLE 4.3. Folstein mini-mental state examination

Activity	Score
ORIENTATION—1 point for each answer	——
Ask: "What is the: (year)(season)(date)(day)(month)?"	
Ask: "Where are we: (state)(county)(town)(hospital)(floor)?"	
REGISTRATION—score 1–3 points according to how many are repeated	——
Name three objects: Give the patient 1 second to say each.	
Ask the patient to: repeat all three after you have said them.	
Repeat them until the patient learns all three.	
ATTENTION AND CALCULATION—1 point for each correct subtraction	——
Ask the patient to: begin from 100 and count backwards by 7.	
Stop after 5 answers. (93, 86, 79, 72, 65)	
RECALL—1 point for each correct answer	——
Ask the patient to: name the three objects from above.	
LANGUAGE	——
Ask the patient to: identify and name a pencil and a watch (2 points)	
Ask the patient to: repeat the phrase "No ifs, ands, or buts." (1 point)	
Ask the patient to: "Take a paper in your right hand, fold it in half, and put it on the floor" (1 point for each task completed properly)	
Ask the patient to: read and obey the following: "Close your eyes." (1 point)	
Ask the patient to: write a sentence. (1 point)	
Ask the patient to: copy a complex diagram of two interlocking pentagons. (1 point)	
TOTAL:	——

From: Folstein, M.F., Folstein, S.E., McHugh, P.R. (1975) "Mini-mental state," A practical method for grading the cognitive state of patients for the clinician. *Journal of Psychiatric Research* 12:189–198.

MMSE yields scores ranging from 0 to 30. Though MMSE score is dependent on a patient's level of education, a score below 24 points has been the traditional cut-off for patients with cognitive impairment. This test has often been criticized for poor sensitivity to subtle changes, as many brain injury patients may have a normal MMSE, but show significant cognitive impairments upon more detailed neuropsychological testing. Thus, good performance on the MMSE should be combined with testing (by a neuropsychologist) to ascertain a patient's ability to perform his or her pre-injury home, community, work or school roles.

Following the mental status examination, the nerves supplying the head and neck region must be evaluated. This portion of the examination is known as the cranial nerve (CN) examination. Cranial nerve I, commonly known as the olfactory nerve, is responsible for the sense of smell. Due to their location between the inferior frontal lobes and the base of the skull, olfactory nerves are often disrupted after a traumatic brain injury. A lesion within the olfactory pathway leads to alterations in sense of smell (parosmia) or total absence of smell (anosmia).

Cranial nerve II, optic nerve, carries visual information garnered in the retina by rods and cones to the lateral geniculate body, where neurons synapse and the optic pathway continues via temporal and parietal lobes to the occipital lobe. The function of the optic nerve is evaluated by testing visual acuity utilizing the

Snellen chart, pupillary reaction to light, color recognition and visual field testing. Lesions along the optic pathway may produce pupillary abnormalities, defects in visual fields and color desaturation. Fundoscopic examination is performed with the examiner using an opthalmoscope. Abnormalities in the fundus known as papilledema can reflect elevations in intracranial pressure, often seen in cerebral structural abnormalities such as brain tumors.

Cranial nerves III (ophthalmic), IV (trochlear), and VI (abducens) are usually tested together, as they work collectively to provide full range of eye movements. Testing begins by observing eyes in a position of primary gaze while observing for proper ocular alignment and presence of ptosis (droopy eyelid). Then, conjugate eye movement in six principal directions of gaze is observed by having the patient follow the target outlining the letter H. CN III palsy with unilateral eyelid drooping, dilated pupil and an externally deviated eye can be seen in a unilateral hemispheric lesion, such as a stroke or tumor.

CN VI (abducens) palsy frequently occurs in the setting of increased intracranial pressure, particularly due to its long intracranial course. Brain trauma frequently produces trochlear nerve palsy, wherein the patient may have trouble looking down and will frequently complain of trouble walking down the stairs.

Cranial nerve V (trigeminal) supplies sensation to the face and controls the muscles of mastication. Its function is usually evaluated by using a wisp of cotton for fine touch, pin to test for pain and cool tuning fork to test for temperature. Muscles of mastication are rarely affected in brain injury, unless facial injuries occur concomitantly.

Cranial nerve VII (facial) is responsible for the facial motor muscles and is evaluated by asking the patient to smile, show teeth, close the eyes tightly, and wrinkle the forehead. A lesion above the level of facial nerve nucleus located in the brainstem will spare the forehead, as it is bilaterally innervated. It is important to differentiate a lower motor nerve lesion from an upper motor nerve lesion of the facial nerve, with the latter implying hemispheric lesion, and the former a lesion within the brainstem or periphery.

Cranial nerve VIII (auditory) is necessary for hearing. Since hearing pathways project bilaterally early on, hearing is rarely affected in brain injury unless there is a fracture of the internal auditory canal, thus damaging the nerve itself. CN VIII is grossly tested by the examiner rubbing his/her fingers together next to the patient's ears, asking which stimulus the patient hears louder. The type of hearing disturbance can be further clarified using Weber and Rinne tests, which allow for distinction between sensorineural and conductive hearing loss.

CN IX (glossopharyngeal) and CN X (vagus) are usually tested together, as they provide coordination in the swallowing process. The patient will be typically asked to open his/her mouth wide, protrude the tongue and say "AAAAH," while the examiner observes for palatal movement. Gag reflex is tested by using a tongue depressor and touching the pharyngeal surface with a cotton swab, comparing side-to-side. While testing gag reflex is commonly taken to represent the function of IXth and Xth nerves, presence of gag does not provide any information about the patient's ability to swallow. Additionally, up to 20% of the normal healthy population may have a depressed or absent gag. The best known means of evaluation of swallowing is the modified barium swallow or cine-esophagram, which allows the observation of movement of the food bolus during deglutition and swallowing. These are usually performed in conjunction with the speech/swallow therapist and gastroenterologist. Voice hoarseness in the absence of laryngeal process may be an indication of bulbar dysfunction. Alternately, swallowing difficulties and hoarseness could be caused by diffuse bilateral hemispheric dysfunction.

Cranial nerve XI (spinal accessory nerve) innervates the trapezius and sternocleidomastoid muscles, and is usually tested by asking the patient to shrug his/her shoulders and to turn his/her head against resistance.

Cranial nerve XII (hypoglossal) is necessary for tongue movement, and is tested by asking the patient to protrude the tongue and move it side to side.

The motor examination usually consists of evaluating muscular bulk, tone, strength, and presence of involuntary movements. Presence of muscle atrophy usually indicates either primary muscle disorder or a peripheral denervating process. Atrophy may frequently coexist with muscle fasciculations. Muscle tone is the permanent state of partial contraction of a muscle and is assessed by passive movement. Increased tone can be divided into spasticity or rigidity both secondary to a brain or spinal cord injury known as an upper motor neuron lesion. Hypotonia is defined as decreased tone and may be seen in lower motor neuron lesions often seen in peripheral nerve injuries. Strength is typically graded on a scale from 0 to 5, where 0 signifies absence of voluntary muscle contraction, and 5 is full strength (Table 4.4). Patterns of muscle weakness can provide clues to lesion localization. For example, if weakness involves the face, arm and leg equally, then the lesion is likely affecting corticospinal tracts in a deep subcortical location; if weakness is more severe in the face and arm rather than leg, then the lesion is likely more cortical and superficial.

Sensory examination usually involves testing—touch, temperature, pain, vibration and proprioception. Touch is usually tested by touching the patient on the face, testing all 3 divisions of the trigeminal nerve separately, as well as touching the patient on the extremities and asking the patient to compare sensation from side to side. Pain is usually tested by a disposable pin in a similar manner. Vibration is tested by using a 256-Hz tuning fork. Temperature is tested by using a cool tuning fork or a reflex hammer, in a similar manner. Proprioception is tested by isolating the patient's joint of interest, such as the distal phalangeal joints, asking

TABLE 4.4. Grading of muscle strength in neurological examination

0	No muscle contraction is detected
1	A trace contraction is noted in the muscle by palpating the muscle while the patient attempts to contract it
2	The patient is able to actively move the muscle when gravity is eliminated
3	The patient may move the muscle against gravity but not against resistance from the examiner
4	The patient may move the muscle group against some resistance from the examiner
5	The patient moves the muscle group and overcomes the resistance of the examiner; this is normal muscle strength

the patient to close both eyes, and then, holding the patient's finger on the sides, move the finger up or down. The patient should be able to specify whether the finger is in the up or down position. If they have difficulty with small excursions, larger excursions should be attempted. If large excursions provide no clue to joint position, the examiner should move to a larger joint located more proximally, i.e., wrist or elbow. Lower extremities may be tested in a similar manner. Additionally, Romberg's sign, which was previously thought to be significant for cerebellar dysfunction, actually tests proprioception (knowing where one is in space) in lower extremities. The patient is asked to stand with his/her feet together and eyes closed; instability and falling over in this position is considered a positive Romberg's sign and is revealing of diminished lower extremity proprioception often seen in a patient with syphilis or vitamin B12 deficiency.

The portion of the deep tendon reflex examination (DTR) includes the biceps, brachioradialis and triceps involving the upper extremities and patellar and Achilles reflex in lower extremities. The presence of hyperactive DTRs in a weak extremity suggests corticospinal tract dysfunction, often seen in a stroke victim, whereas hypoactive DTRs are usually indicative of lower motor neuron dysfunction often seen in chronic diabetics with neuropathy. The Babinski reflex is tested by stroking the outer aspect of the sole from the heel toward the fifth digit on the foot; flexor response with downgoing toes is normal and extensor (upgoing) toe response is nonspecific, but indicative of corticospinal tract dysfunction. The presence of brisk reflexes with associated extensor plantar response and/or clonus is abnormal and should be further investigated.

Coordination is primarily a function of the cerebellum and its connection to the cortex. It is usually tested by asking the patient to alternately touch his/her nose and the examiner's finger that moves within the patient's visual field. The patient with cerebellar dysfunction will exhibit dysmetria; that is, he/she will point beyond the examiner's finger, or he/she will have marked oscillations on the way there. The lower extremity is usually tested by asking the patient to place the heel on the shin of the other leg and to slide the foot up and down the shin.

Stance is tested by asking the patient to stand with his/her eyes open and feet together. Then, the patient is asked to walk; with the examiner watching for circumduction of a lower extremity, which could be a sign of hemiparesis. Wide based gait is a sign of cerebellar dysfunction. The patient should also be asked, if possible, to walk on the tiptoes and heels; this allows for detection of subtle gastrocnemius and tibialis anterior weakness, respectively. Finally, the patient should be asked to walk one foot in front of another, known as tandem gait.

Neurological Work-Up

A typical work-up to evaluate for the presence of acquired brain injury involves an imaging study. Typically, computed tomography (CT) and magnetic resonance imaging (MRI) are utilized the most. CT scans are widely employed, and available in nearly every emergency room. CT scans are fast and reliable, and therefore remain a staple of the emergent neurological examination. Images in CT scans are acquired by means of thin X-ray beams rotating around examining part and detectors measuring the amount of radiation passing though. A computer analyzes these measurements, creating cross-sectional images of the area being scanned. By stacking these images—also known as "slices"—the computer can assemble three-dimensional models of the organs in a human body. Typically, a CT scan of brain without contrast material is the first neuro-imaging procedure utilized in the evaluation of a patient with a traumatic brain injury to rule out cerebral hemorrhage and identify possible skull fractures or bony lesions in the emergency setting. It is usually used to rule out cerebral hemorrhage and identify possible skull fractures in the setting of the Emergency Department. CT scan is superior to MRI in evaluation of bony lesions, and is just as good in evaluation for the presence of blood. For these purposes, CT scans are typically obtained without intravenous contrast.

While a CT scanner is composed of X-ray generator, detector array and process-ing unit, an MRI scanner consists of a large magnet, detector array, and processing unit. The MRI machine applies a radio frequency pulse that is specific only to hydrogen. The system directs the pulse toward the area of the body being exam-ined. Unlike CT scans, an MRI scanner does not expose the patient to ionizing radiation and has a greater resolution for soft tissues. Often enough MRI scans require contrast; it is typically Gadolinium-based and inert, and unlike CT contrast medium, which is usually iodinated, it is safe for kidneys and hypoallergenic.

However, MRI scanners have a few limitations. Namely, MRI scans are con-traindicated for someone with a pacemaker, old ferromagnetic aneurysm clips, or bullet fragments; the presence of extensive dental work, implants, or braces may introduce an artifact that will produce a poor quality image. Additionally, claus-trophobic patients and those who cannot lie supine may experience difficulties in a scanner, as the MRI examination will typically require the patient to stay still in a relatively closed space for 30–40 minutes at a time. Nonetheless, image quality obtained with an MRI is superior to that obtained with CT, and therefore justifies its preference by most physicians, and remains the gold standard in nonemergent evaluation of brain injury.

Additional testing modalities that are frequently employed by neurologists in-clude transcranial and carotid Doppler ultrasound, which will be discussed in the Stroke section of this chapter, and electroencephalography (EEG), which is dis-cussed in the Epilepsy section.

Seizures

Patient is a 49-year-old male who presented to the hospital after a motor vehicle accident at 40 miles/hour, in which the patient was unrestrained and his head struck the windshield. On initial examination, the patient's GCS is 8 (best eye score 2/4, best verbal score 2/5, best motor score 4/6) (Chapter 2, Table 2.1); there is marked bruising of the forehead with multiple facial lacerations. During evaluation in the emergency room, the patient is observed to have a single generalized tonic-clonic seizure lasting 45 seconds, associated with tongue biting. CT scan of the head revealed frontal and occipital hemorrhagic contusions. Patient was loaded with intravenous phenytoin (dilantin) and transferred to the intensive care unit for monitoring and neurological checks.

Seizures are a common complication of traumatic brain injury (TBI). A seizure is defined as a disturbance or disruption in the electrical activity of the brain, which results in uncontrollable changes to behavior, motor functions, or a change in sensory perception. The presence of intracranial pathology predisposes a patient to having seizures and consequently developing a seizure disorder. Epilepsy, as opposed to seizures, is usually defined as two or more unprovoked seizures. Early seizures are thereby defined as acute symptomatic, but they are not representative of epilepsy, as seizures are provoked by the presence of an acute lesion. Alcohol abuse, subdural hematoma, and presence of brain contusion are known independent risk factors for the development of early post-traumatic seizures (Wiedemayer et al., 2002).

As discussed earlier, TBI is a significant risk factor for developing early seizures, as well as late epilepsy. Studies have shown that the presence of severe TBI increases one's chances of developing epilepsy as much as 74 times over the baseline rate at 2-year post-injury mark, with maximal risk of seizures in the first 7 days post-injury, followed by slow decline over a 5-year period. Risk factors for the development of post-traumatic epilepsy in the brain-injured patient highly correlate with severity of injury and include: bilateral cortical contusions, especially in the parietal region, dural penetration with bone or metal fragments, multiple intracranial operations, intracerebral hematoma, subdural or epidural hematoma, midline shift >5 mm, depressed skull fracture, prolonged disturbance of consciousness, and early seizure (Temkin, 2003; Frey, 2003). In 2003, The American Academy of Neurology (AAN) published guidelines on antiepileptic drug prophylaxis in acute severe TBI (Chang & Lowenstein, 2003). It is recommended that patients with severe TBI be loaded with IV phenytoin (dilantin) as soon as possible after the injury in order to prevent post-traumatic seizures within the first 7 days. Continued prophylactic treatment should not extend beyond 7 days (level B recommendation).

In addition to TBI, any other ABI also substantially increases the risk of developing epilepsy. In various studies, incidence of epilepsy after stroke was estimated to be anywhere between 3% to 67% (Camilo & Goldstein, 2004). This accounts for the increased prevalence of epilepsy in older adults, as cumulative brain lesion load increases with age. There have been a few recent studies on the cellular mechanisms underlying acquired epilepsy, and it has been shown that injury-induced alterations in intracellular calcium concentration levels and calcium homeostatic mechanisms play a role in the development and maintenance of acquired epilepsy by producing long term neuroplasticity changes underlying epileptic phenotype (Delorenzo et al., 2004).

The patient has not had any further seizures after the first episode; his mental status improved over the next week, and CT of the brain has reflected initial stages of resolution. Phenytoin has been discontinued after 1 week and the patient has been successfully discharged to a rehabilitation facility. Seven months after the accident, the patient presented

to the emergency room with another seizure that started as a rhythmic twitch of the arm,
progressing into a generalized tonic-clonic seizure.

Epilepsy is classified according to the International League Against Epilepsy
(ILAE) classification as localization-related versus generalized (Engel, 2001).
Generalized epilepsy syndromes include primary generalized syndromes with typical childhood onset, and are beyond the scope of this discussion. Epilepsy caused
by acquired brain lesions is by definition localization related, i.e., originating from
an abnormal area of the brain, whether seizures themselves are focal or secondarily
generalized. Focal seizures, still often referred to as partial, may be motor, sensory,
visual, or autonomic in nature, and can be experienced as focal rhythmic activity or
tingling, or visual changes depending on the localization of a seizure focus. They
may also be isolated (i.e., simple partial) or complicated by impaired level of consciousness (i.e., complex partial seizures). Partial seizures may also secondarily
generalize into tonic-clonic seizures occurring in approximately one third of cases.
Obtaining a thorough history of seizures, evoking a history of *deja vu* or *jamais
vu*, olfactory sensations, intense fear or nausea preceding a seizure is essential, as
it would provide additional clues about localization of the epileptic lesion.

The workup for a patient who has suffered a seizure episode includes blood
tests, imaging studies, and electroencephalographic monitoring. Laboratory studies usually include a chemistry panel to evaluate for the presence of electrolyte and
glycemic abnormalities. Additionally, some epileptologists advocate obtaining a
serum prolactin level after a seizure. Recent AAN guidelines on use of prolactin
in diagnosing epileptic seizures (Chen et al., 2005) suggest that elevation of prolactin within 20 minutes of the event can be used as an adjunct in distinguishing
true seizures from a nonepileptic event. Elevations in prolactin levels can also
be seen in pregnancy, in cases of a prolactin-secreting tumor, and in patients on
dopamine-blocking agents. A complete blood count should be performed since an
elevation in the white blood cell count may point toward an underlying infection.
If infection is indeed considered, a lumbar puncture may need to be performed to
evaluate for the presence of encephalitis. Finally, both blood and urine toxicology
screens should also be performed in order to rule out possible environmental or
recreational drug use.

Routine electroencephalogram (EEG) is useful in the evaluation of a patient
with seizures. This test is painless, and usually takes a total of 60 minutes and is
usually administered by a technician. The treating physician may request the patient to be sleep-deprived prior to the procedure, as it may provoke the appearance
of epileptiform discharges. During an EEG, patients are typically asked to hyper-
ventilate for a short period of time, and they may also be requested to look at a
flashing strobe light. These maneuvers are known to elicit epileptiform discharges.
Approximately 50% of people with epilepsy will have normal results on their first
EEG, however the sensitivity goes up to 90% after the 3rd EEG (Binnie & Stefan,
1999). It is very rare that a seizure episode is captured during routine EEG, but
prolonged video EEG monitoring in a medically supervised environment allows
physicians to observe a patient's seizures directly. Observing seizure semiology

(i.e., appearance) coupled with EEG correlate makes it possible to characterize ictal events and differentiate bona fide seizures from nonepileptic events, and provides a longer time-sample for capture of epileptiform discharges. Nonetheless, electroencephalographic studies are not useful in predicting the likelihood of post-traumatic seizures in any given patient.

Treatment of epilepsy is essential in maintaining a patient's health and life style. Fortunately, the arsenal of a neurologist treating epilepsy has been significantly expanded over the last 15 years. In addition to standard drugs for epilepsy, i.e., phenytoin (Dilantin), valproic acid (Depakote), carbamazepine (Tegretol), and phenobarbital (Luminal), there have been a substantial number of new drugs developed and tested over the years. According to recent American Academy of Neurologists (AAN) guidelines on the efficacy and tolerability of newer drugs (French et al., 2004), several new generation medications are safe to start as a monotherapy for new onset epilepsy. Topiramate (Topamax) and oxcarbazepine (Trileptal) are FDA approved as monotherapy agents, and lamotrigine (Lamictal) can be used as an adjunct, followed by a switch to a single-agent regimen. Individual choice of Anti-Epileptic Drug (AED) therapy should indeed be guided by patient-specific co-morbidities, i.e., a patient with a prominent headache syndrome may benefit from topiramate, while patients with severe mood disturbances may benefit from mood-stabilizing properties of lamotrigine.

The patient was examined in the emergency room; routine laboratory studies as well as toxicology screen were negative. CT scan of the brain revealed the presence of encephalomalacia in regions of prior trauma. EEG was obtained and revealed frontal slowing with rare epileptiform discharges. Though the patient did not formally meet the criteria for epilepsy, the decision was made to start the patient on antiepileptic drugs, as this seizure most likely represented a remote symptomatic seizure originating from the focus of encephalomalacia. Since the patient has suffered from concomitant mood disturbances, the decision was made to start lamotrigine, which is noted for its mood-stabilizing properties. The patient was instructed not to drive. He was able to tolerate the medication well and did not develop a rash; he is currently maintained on 200 mg of lamotrigine twice a day and has not experienced any further seizures.

The question of whether a patient should be allowed the right to drive following a seizure remains an important issue. While the occurrence of a fatal motor vehicle accident due to a seizure is uncommon (Sheth et al., 2004), most authorities agree that a patient who suffered a seizure should not drive for a year after seizures have been stabilized. However, recently it has been shown that reduction of seizure-free period from 12 months to 3 months does not result in an increase in seizure-related motor vehicle crashes (Drazkowski et al., 2003). Legally, the rules regarding driving in seizure patients vary state by state. Therefore, each practitioner should check in with the state's motor vehicles authority regarding the proper procedure for reporting and counseling a patient. The neurologist should also gather input from the interdisciplinary team on the patient's attentional skills, processing abilities, and reaction time.

In New York State, patients who have had a seizure or have been unconscious following an ABI, must file an MV-80U.1 form with the Motor Vehicles Department in

Albany to be cleared to return to driving. Occupational therapists (see Chapter 12) will often refer patients for a specialized driving evaluation to assess safety awareness and driving skills post-ABI.

The patient suffering from epilepsy must be educated on the potential stressors that may precipitate a seizure. These include poor sleeping habits, alcohol or other recreational drug use, exposure to environmental, dietary, physical, or emotional stressors. Patients should be advised never to be alone when bathing, swimming or climbing heights. Family members need to be informed on how to manage their loved one who is having a seizure, with the emphasis on preventing a further brain injury. After a seizure, the patient should be turned to the side so as to allow any fluid in the oral cavity to drain, thus preventing aspiration. Most seizures are self-limited and last less than 5 minutes; however emergency services should be contacted for any prolonged seizure.

The risk of post-traumatic seizures decreases with time and reaches a normal value for the general population approximately 5 years after the brain injury. About half of the patients who develop late post-traumatic epilepsy have only 3 or fewer seizures and go into spontaneous remission thereafter. Nonetheless, a decision to stop anti-epileptic agents should be made after careful consideration of risks versus benefits.

Stroke

The patient is a 68-year-old female with a past medical history of hypertension and diabetes who was found by her family members lying on the floor next to her bed and unable to talk or get up. The patient was rushed to the emergency room, where she was found to have dense right hemiparesis, face and arm more than leg, and global aphasia. Since the time of onset was not known, the patient was excluded as a candidate for thrombolysis. Routine labs were within normal limits. CT of the head revealed the presence of a large hypodense area in the left fronto-temporal region. Since EKG revealed the new onset of atrial fibrillation, the patient was admitted to the telemetry service.

The impact of stroke on the health care system is staggering, costing an estimated 41 billion dollars annually in both direct health care cost and lost income. Stroke is the leading cause of disability in adults, with 30% of stroke survivors requiring assistance with activities of daily living, 20% requiring assistance with ambulation, and 16% needing institutionalized care (Biller & Love, 2004). With industrialized nations' ever-increasing life expectancy, it is obvious that stroke is becoming one of the most important and most expensive public health hazards. Cerebrovascular disease is a multifactorial disorder and the risk of a stroke could be greatly decreased by minimizing correctable factors, i.e., tightened glycemic control, blood pressure medication, smoking cessation, and aggressive cholesterol lowering treatments.

Most authorities agree upon stroke classification on the basis of vessel size ("small" vs. "large" vessel), mechanism of obstruction (thrombotic vs. embolic) or presence of bleeding (ischemic vs. hemorrhagic). Small vessel infarctions are representative of end-artery obstructions by microscopic cholesterol plaques within the lumen of the vessel. Large vessel strokes occur due to obstruction of a main territory-supplying vessel such as the middle cerebral artery. In large vessels, obstruction is typically caused by progressive accumulation of intra-arterial thrombus or by embolization from a remote source, i.e., carotid artery or heart. Recent research follows a logical conclusion by showing that the volume of infarcted tissue correlates with the degree of residual disability (Thijs et al., 2000). Common impairments caused by stroke include: motor weakness (77%), cognitive deficits (44%), dysphagia (45%), bladder/bowel dysfunction (48%) (Lawrence et al., 2001), visuo-spatial deficits (15%) (Linden et al., 2005) and dementia (28%) (Linden et al., 2004).

A typical diagnostic workup in a patient status post stroke involves CT or MRI of the brain in order to delineate the anatomy and observe the extent of the damage. If available, magnetic resonance angiography (MRA) of intracranial vessels is often advocated, as it allows determining the presence of intracranial vessel narrowing. While MRA is a static study of anatomical peculiarities, carotid doppler ultrasonography allows for evaluation of flow patterns within intracranial vessels and is considered useful in the evaluation of anterior circulation strokes. Transcranial Dopplers serve a similar purpose in posterior circulation strokes. A Holter monitor is useful in detection of atrial fibrillation, as the heart is the most common cause of embolism. Transesophageal echocardiogram (TEE) is the test of choice for detection of left atrial thrombus. Low ejection fraction and valvular disease predispose to cerebrovascular disease as well. Laboratory studies usually include lipid profile, as hyperlipidemia is a correctable risk factor and hemoglobin A1C as a screen for hyperglycemic state. Workup of a cerebrovascular event in a young person without risk factors deserves additional testing for the presence of hypercoagulable state, evaluation for presence of embolism from venous circulation to arterial circulation through patent foramen ovale, and possible search for venous outflow obstruction.

Until 1995, acute stroke therapy consisted of controlling modifiable risk factors and managing immediate and remote consequences of acute stroke. Based on randomized controlled trials, the Federal and Drug Administration (FDA)-approved the use of intravenous tissue plasminogen activator (tPA) for treatment of acute ischemic stroke in June of 1996, thereby giving neurologists a tool to potentially reverse the neurological deficits secondary to an ischemic stroke. Other novel therapies include combined use of intra-arterial and intravenous tPA, intra-arterial tPA alone, clot retrieval devices, glycoprotein IIb/IIIa inhibitors and neuroprotection through hypothermia.

While admitted, the patient had a complete neurological work-up. MRI of the brain revealed a large left fronto-temporal lesion on diffusion-weighted imaging sequence, corresponding to the CT finding. MRA of the brain showed drop-off of the signal in the left middle cerebral artery, likely due to a clot obstructing the lumen. Carotid Doppler ultrasonography revealed 60% reduction of flow in the area of the left internal carotid artery. Transesophageal echocardiogram showed large left atrium without clots present. Patient was anticoagulated with coumadin, and was discharged to the acute rehabilitation facility. Follow-up appointment with a vascular surgeon was made regarding carotid stenosis.

Secondary stroke prevention usually involves seeking out modifiable risk factors as well as placing a patient on an antiplatelet agent. According to AAN guidelines on anticoagulants and antiplatelet agents in acute ischemic stroke (Coull et al., 2002), a patient with acute ischemic stroke presenting within 48 hours of symptom onset should be given aspirin (160–325 mg/day) to reduce stroke mortalitiy and decrease morbidity. Further secondary prevention involves maintenance of the patient on an antiplatelet agent [aspirin, clopidogrel (Plavix)] or sustained release aspirin/dipyridamole (Aggrenox) combination) at the discretion of the treating neurologist. Hypertension, diabetes mellitus, heart disease, dyslipidemia, smoking, carotid stenosis, and oral contraceptive use are some of the modifiable risk factors that can be addressed in conjunction with the patient's primary care physician. The British Heart Study showed that 40 mg of simvastatin (Zocor) daily reduced stroke chance by 25% in patients with coronary artery disease and stroke and cholesterol levels above 140 mg/dL, making statin treatment an integral part of stroke prevention (Heart Protection Study Collaborative Group, 2002). Similarly, there was a significant stroke risk reduction in patients with hypertension that were treated with ramipril (Altace), although it is not clear whether the observed benefit was the result of a class effect (Yusuf et al., 2000). Most authorities agree that first line hypertension treatment for secondary stroke prevention is administration of angiotensin-converting enzyme (ACE) inhibitors, angiotensin receptor blockers, and thiazide diuretics.

In cases where carotid stenosis is identified, carotid endarterectomy may be indicated depending on the degree of obstruction. Based on North American Symptomatic Carotid Endarterectomy Trial (NASCET), carotid endarterectomy is recommended in symptomatic patients with greater than 70% stenosis. Ipsilateral stroke risk in 2 years was 9% with surgery and 26% with medical management only. Symptomatic patients with greater than 50–69% stenosis experience only marginal benefit, and therefore the decision is left to the discretion of the operating surgeon and the neurologist. In asymptomatic patients with greater than 60% stenosis the intervention is not indicated (Haynes et al., 1994).

It has been an accepted standard of care to anticoagulate patients with nonvalvular atrial fibrillation with warfarin (Coumadin). Cochrane review of available literature in 2001 showed that, assuming a baseline risk for 45 strokes per 1,000 patients, warfarin could prevent 30 incidences of stroke at the expense of 6 major bleeding episodes (Aguilar et al., 2005). Aspirin has been found to be efficacious as well, however less so, preventing only 17 incidences of stroke without an increase in bleeding complication. Additionally, it appears that younger patients with lone atrial fibrillation benefit less from warfarin, which supports the notion of using aspirin in this subset of patients. Treatment of atrial fibrillation in a stroke patient requires a multidisciplinary approach and should be done in conjunction with an internal medicine practitioner as well as a cardiologist.

Hyperbaric oxygen therapy (HBOT) has been evaluated as another potential avenue of treatment for patients with acute ischemic stroke. The primary purpose of HBOT is to increase the amount of salvageable tissue located within ischemic penumbra, as well as to provide neuroprotection through a decrease in edema. Recently, Cochrane (2000) cooperative has examined available data on utility of HBOT in acute ischemic stroke and in TBI (Bennett et al., 2004; McDonagh et al., 2004). It was shown that in application of HBOT in treatment of traumatic brain injury, the risk of death was substantially reduced without increase in functional recovery. However, HBOT provided no additional benefit in survival or functional recovery of patients with acute ischemic stroke, therefore this treatment is not currently recommended. Further research may define the role of HBOT in treatment of acute stroke and TBI.

Secondary complications following a stroke may include increased intracranial pressure, systemic hypertension, seizures, hemorrhagic transformation, and obstructive hydrocephalus. The issue of systemic hypertension in acute stroke has been a subject of frequent academic debates, as there are no official guidelines to that effect. Recent Cochrane Review done by Blood Pressure in Acute Stroke Collaboration (BASC, 2000) reported that there was not enough evidence to evaluate the effect of altering blood pressure on outcome during the acute phase of stroke. Additionally, there is not enough evidence to decide if antihypertensive drugs are helpful or harmful in the acute period after stroke. Most authorities do caution against decreasing blood pressure too rapidly and too aggressively as this might further compromise blood supply to ischemic penumbra and worsen the extent of the damage. Seizures in stroke can occur during both early and late stages. There is a wide discrepancy in reporting seizure incidence after stroke, much due to differences in time frames. Early seizures occur in 2–33% of patients suffering from acute stroke (Camilo & Goldstein, 2004); presence of subarachnoid hemorrhage and cortical location were common predictive factors for appearance of early seizures. It is obvious that seizures in stroke need to be addressed; however there is no clear answer regarding which medications are most effective for management of post-stroke epilepsy, how long a patient should be treated and whether prophylactic treatment of seizures is necessary. The Cochrane collaboration is expected to publish a review of antiepileptic drugs for the primary and secondary prevention of seizures after stroke, which hopefully will shed light on this issue and provide treating neurologists with statistical underpinnings for their clinical decisions.

Encephalopathies

Encephalopathy is a term that literally means "disease of brain," referring to an altered mental state. The differential diagnosis of encephalopathy is diverse and encompasses pathological conditions from every category of disease, and is one of the most common in-patient reasons for neurological consultation. Encephalopathy may be caused by an infectious agent, increased intracranial pressure, metabolic or mitochondrial dysfunction, exposure to toxins (including alcohol, drugs, radiation, industrial chemicals, and heavy metals), vitamin deficiencies, hormonal abnormalities, or hypoxia/hypoperfusion of the brain. Common neurological symptoms associated with encephalopathy are progressive loss of memory and cognitive ability, personality changes, difficulty with concentration, lethargy, and progressive loss of consciousness. The patient's neurological exam can be significant for presence of myoclonus, nystagmus, asterixis, tremor, dementia, seizures, or any other lateralizing signs. Routine blood tests, cerebrospinal fluid (CSF) examination by performing a lumbar puncture, imaging studies, and electroencephalograms are a few examples of diagnostic studies that may be useful in the differentiation of various causes of encephalopathy.

Herpetic encephalopathy is the most common, treatable cause of encephalopathy. Another example of encephalopathy is anoxic/hypoxic encephalopathy. Anoxic and hypoxic brain injuries are located on the same continuum; hypoxic injury is defined by relatively diminished oxygenation of the brain, and anoxic injury is defined by absent oxygenation of the brain. In contrast to focal hypoxemic injury, such as one sustained due to a stroke, anoxic/hypoxic injury usually happens due to systemic causes and therefore preferentially affects watershed areas of the brain. Specific lobes of the brain, the mesial temporal lobes, are particularly sensitive to hypoxia, thereby making short-term memory loss the most common complication of anoxic/hypoxic brain injury (Gibson et al., 1981). Degree of overall damage is highly dependent on the period of time that oxygenation was compromised.

While occasionally the cause of anoxic/hypoxic brain injury is apparent or is discovered during initial assessment, neurologists are usually called in to evaluate the patient. In this case the role of the neurologist is not to diagnose the condition, but to prognosticate meaningful recovery. Cardiopulmonary arrest is the single most common cause of anoxic brain injury with in-hospital mortality rates of up to 86% (McGrath, 1987). The duration of coma significantly correlates with mortality; individuals who are at least easily arousable within 12 hours of resuscitation will have the best prognosis among patients who sustained cardiopulmonary arrest. Nonetheless, there will still be 25% mortality even in this subselect group of patients, mostly related to their underlying cardiac disease. Coma or obtundation immediately post-resuscitation is generally a poor prognostic sign, with only 28% of patients surviving (Thomassen & Wernberg, 1979).

Pain and Headache

Pain is a complex multidimensional subjective experience mediated by emotion, attitude, and perception. Pain in ABI can appear early and resolve, or may linger, thereby becoming chronic. Early pain due to injury reflects underlying bodily injury as affecting discrete neuroanatomical pathways. It is thought to confer evolutionary advantage by alerting the organism to the need for recovery. Chronic pain is thought to be a result of maladaptation of the central nervous system to the injury, as no clear cause–effect relationships between severity of injury and severity of chronic pain exist, no particular survival benefits are conferred and muscular activity is avoided, thereby inhibiting successful recovery and restoration of function.

Central Pain Syndrome

The International Association for the Study of Pain has defined central pain caused by a lesion or dysfunction in the central nervous system. The lesion or disease process can occur anywhere along the neuraxis. Typical locations include cerebral hemispheres, brainstem and spinal cord. The clinician must have a certain degree of suspicion in order to make this diagnosis, especially if there is no identifiable lesion. In TBI, one may find an infarct or a hemorrhage in a patient with central pain syndrome. However, there appears to be no difference between hemorrhages and infarcts in regards to the tendency to induce central pain.

Typically, these patients describe a "neuropathic-type" pain—an unfamiliar, odd, dysesthetic (painful numbness), burning, lancinating sensation, with the skin often sensitive to simple touch; this phenomenon is known as allodynia. Central pain syndrome often begins shortly after the causative injury or damage, but may be delayed by months or even years, especially if it is related to post-stroke pain.

This condition is often refractory to standard analgesic medications and requires a combination of pharmacological agents including antiepileptics, antidepressants, and opioids in order to achieve adequate pain control. In addition to pharmacological therapies, patients should be seen in a comprehensive pain management center utilizing the services of a pain psychologist. If above measures are not effective, there has been some success with surgical interventions, such as deep brain stimulation and ablation procedures.

Headache

The patient is a 34-year-old female with a prior history of migraines who presents with worsening headache after she tripped and fell on the ground, sustaining a scalp laceration. Patient thinks she might have momentarily lost consciousness. Patient describes her headaches as unilateral and throbbing, typical of her usual migraines which were previously easily controlled with ibuprofen. However they have become increasingly more difficult to control, and patient reports that ibuprofen no longer relieves the headache. Since the incident happened 2 months ago, patient has missed 7 workdays due to headaches and she is anxious, as she is afraid to lose her job. Her neurological examination is significant for painful neck spasms.

The National Institute of Health consensus statement (1998) defines mild traumatic injury as a traumatically induced physiological disruption of brain function, as manifested by a least one of the following: (1) any period of loss of consciousness; (2) any loss of memory for events immediately before or after the accident; (3) any alteration in mental state at the time of the accident (e.g., feeling dazed, disoriented, or confused); and (4) focal neurological deficit(s) that may or may not be transient; but where the severity of the injury does not exceed the following: (a) post-traumatic amnesia (PTA) not greater than 24 hours; (b) after 30 minutes, an initial Glasgow Coma Scale (GCS) of 13–15; and (c) loss of consciousness of approximately 30 minutes or less.

Post-traumatic syndrome is common, and is characterized by headache and any of the following: personality change, impaired memory, impaired concentration, reduced attention span, easy distractibility, fatigue, apathy, insomnia, decreased sexual desire, dizziness or lightheadedness, and mood disturbances. These symptoms can range in severity from being quite subtle to very obvious.

Post-traumatic headache (PTHA) has been classified as a secondary headache disorder by the International Headache Society (Lipton et al., 2004). Examples of primary headache disorders, on the other hand, include migraine, tension-type, and cluster headaches. Most people who report having a headache following a TBI have a pre-existing primary headache disorder or an immediate relative with a primary headache. Post-concussive headache is the most common sequelum of brain trauma. In the acute stage of head and neck injury, headache prevalence is estimated to be 90%; this percentage point falls only to 44% at 6 months after the injury, and may persist in up to 20% of patients 4 years later (Ramadan & Keidel, 2000). Women have a 1.9-fold increased risk of developing post-traumatic headache compared to men. This may be secondary to the higher incidence of primary headache disorders among women.

Current studies, as summarized by Martelli et al. (1999), support the conclusion that the presence of post-concussive headache is generally negatively correlated with scores on neuropsychological testing. Decrements in information processing speed and complex attention are most frequently observed, while reductions in cognitive flexibility and verbal associative fluency, as well as learning and memory, appear to represent secondary findings that may be mediated by decreases in information processing and complex attention. Investigations of the effect of general, chronic pain on neuropsychological test results have produced similar results. Therefore, presence of chronic headache and pain are very likely to hinder recovery process from ABI. However, patients who sustain a severe brain injury with marked cognitive deficits may never truly complain of headaches until the cognitive deficits disappear. Hickling et al. (1992) found that 15 of 20 consecutive patients referred to a psychological practice for posttraumatic headache had post-traumatic stress disorder. Anxiety and depression further contribute to development of PTHA. The most frequently seen headache following traumatic brain injury resembles a tension-type headache, occurring in 85% of the patients. These headaches are characterized by a bilateral gripping, a nonthrobbing sensation not associated with nausea, vomiting, or marked light or sound sensitivity. A migraine with or without aura is the second-most-common type of headache following TBI. These headaches are often characterized by a unilateral throbbing sensation associated with nausea and/or vomiting usually interfering with an activity. The third most common headache presentation is that of occipital neuralgia. This frequently occurs following a whiplash injury where the occipital nerve is irritated. These headaches are characterized by a unilateral headache originating in the cervical region extending to the forehead often described as a shooting, lancinating sensation triggered by neck movement. In addition, these may be accompanied by paresthesias or dysesthesias. Less commonly, one may present with headaches triggered by marked position change known as low-pressure headaches or headaches secondary to intracranial hypotension. In these patients the headaches are characteristically triggered by sitting up or standing and dramatically relieved upon lying down. This could result from a cerebrospinal fluid leak through a dural sleeve tear or a cribriform plate fracture. Myofascial pain disorders are often underrecognized. These usually involve masseter, trapezius, or temporalis muscles and may occur following a traumatic brain injury.

Workup of headaches in clients with ABI should include an imaging study of the brain and cervical spine, especially in patients with a TBI, as presence of acute hemorrhage needs to be excluded. For this particular purpose, a CT scan is sufficient and is preferred over an MRI. Additionally, an X-ray or CT of the c-spine to rule out a cervical fracture should be performed. In the subacute or chronic stage, an MRI of the brain is the preferred test, as it provides a better, higher resolution image of intracranial structures without subjecting patients to radiation. If the headaches persist or there is an apparent cervicogenic component, an MRI of the cervical spine should be considered. An electroencephalogram (EEG) is generally not recommended in any patient presenting with headache unless there is a strong suspicion of a seizure disorder. Blood testing is generally not useful.

Patient has been referred for MRI of the brain, which was reportedly normal. As her headaches were now occurring more often than 4 times per month, a decision to start prophylactic treatment along with acute migraine management was made. Patient was started on nortriptyline (Pamelor) nightly, as well as sumatriptan (Imitrex) as needed for acute headaches, which she was able to tolerate well. She was additionally referred to physical therapy for management of neck spasm. Patient reported improvement in her headaches over the subsequent 2 months.

Treatment of acute headache following trauma depends upon the underlying pathogenesis, i.e., hemorrhage requiring immediate surgical intervention (see Chapter 2). Management of postconcussional headaches requires a multidimensional approach, combining pharmacotherapeutics with psychotherapy and relaxation techniques. The pharmacologic arsenal of headache treatment is very diverse, including multiple drugs in various categories including triptans, anti-inflammatory agents, selective serotonin reuptake inhibitors, tricyclic antidepressants, anticonvulsants, and beta-blockers. The choice of medication should be guided by the characteristics of a headache. If the headache appears to be migraine-like, then anti-migraine medications should be employed. If the frequency of a patient's episodic headaches is less than 4 times per month, a triptan should be considered, whereas if the headaches are more frequent, a preventive therapy should be employed. The choice of a preventive therapy is frequently influenced by associated co-morbidities, such as depression. For example, depressed patients who have insomnia may be a good candidate for antidepressant therapy for their chronic headaches. Tricyclic antidepressants such as amitriptyline (Elavil) and nortriptyline (Pamelor) are considered to be the drugs of choice. Their mode of action includes the inhibition of reuptake of the biogenic amines and through sodium channel blockade along the peripheral nerve. Unfortunately, these agents have many potential side effects which may interfere with recovery in a brain injured patient, such as orthostatic hypotension, sedation, and cognitive slowing. Therefore, judicial use of these agents is advocated.

The anticonvulsants are considered to be the class of choice in preventing migraine headaches. Sodium valproate (Depakote) and topiramate (Topamax) are FDA-approved for the prevention of migraines; gabapentin (Neurontin) is also widely used for this purpose. However, one must be aware of the potential side effects of topiramate, which include cognitive slowing and memory difficulties. Somnolence, tremor, and dizziness are the few well-known side effects of sodium valproate, therefore caution must be exercised when prescribing these drugs in patients with TBI. These agents may also prove to be helpful in post-traumatic headache patients with an associated mood disorder, due to their mood-stabilizing properties. Certain antihypertensive medications, such as the beta-blockers nadolol (Corgard) and propranolol (Inderal), can also be considered as a preventive agent for headache treatment. These agents are known to affect mood negatively, and are therefore contraindicated in patients susceptible to depression.

Headaches with a cervicogenic component may respond to a variety of physical therapy modalities, including myofascial techniques, relaxation strategies such as biofeedback and meditation. Electromyography (EMG) guided biofeedback has been shown to be beneficial in PTHA treatment when combined with cognitive behavioral therapy (CBT) and pharmacotherapeutics (Onorato & Tsushima, 1983). EMG biofeedback treatment of PTHA typically includes the forehead, trapezii, frontal-posterior neck, and neck; the goal of EMG reading is attainment of signal intensity of 2 μV or less, which usually indicates a relaxed muscle (Green & Shellenberger, 1991). In a small-scale study of 40 PTHA patients, a combination of various modalities of biofeedback has been shown to produce moderate pain improvement in at least half the patients. However, perhaps the greatest benefit of biofeedback is that it can facilitate a perception of self-control and reduce feelings of helplessness. In their retrospective biofeedback outcome study, Ham and Packard (1996) reported that the greatest treatment effects were obtained for general relaxation and for ability to cope with pain. Additionally, most patients continued to apply biofeedback skills learned in pain management to their daily lives. Guided imagery has also been shown to be beneficial in at least one small-scale study of PTHA patients (Daly & Wulff, 1987). While never tested for PTHA, cognitive-behavioral therapy, relaxation treatment, and hypnosis were all shown to be of use in treatment of chronic headaches (Holroyd & Andrasik, 1978; Tobin et al., 1998).

Acupuncture is an appealing alternative treatment for headache sufferers; however, its usefulness has not been measured until recently. Cochrane review recently suggested that existing evidence supports the use of acupuncture in idiopathic headache, although the quality of evidence is not fully convincing (Melchart et al., 2001). Most recently, the Journal of the American Medical Association (JAMA) published a randomized, controlled trial of acupuncture in migraine sufferers, which compared acupuncture versus sham acupuncture versus waiting list in migraine sufferers. Results have shown that while acupuncture was significantly better in reducing headaches as compared to no intervention, it was not better than sham acupuncture, i.e., placement of needles in nontherapeutic points (Linde et al., 2005). Similar results were observed in the study of acupuncture in tension-type headache, where the acupuncture group performed better than the no acupuncture group, but similar to the group that received minimal acupuncture (Melchart et al., 2005). Further studies are necessary in order to determine if indeed there is a role of acupuncture in chronic headache treatment, particularly in PTHA.

Additionally, dietary discretion, particularly avoidance of cheese, monosodium glutamate, caffeine, chocolate and wine, is also recommended in chronic headache sufferers, as tyramine heightens sympathetic arousal.

Sleep Disorder

Sleep disorders are a well-known complication of traumatic brain injury, as well as many other ABIs. Various studies found average prevalence of sleep disorders in post-TBI patients of about 50 % (Mahmood et al., 2004). Additionally, it is well known that excessive somnolence is a major cause of motor vehicle accidents, resulting in 36% of highway fatalities and up to 54% of collisions (Leger, 1994). In a recent small-scale study of ten patients with TBI and sleep complaints, all were found to have treatable sleep disorders. Seven patients were suffering from sleep disorders on the obstructive spectrum, two had narcolepsy and only one had post-traumatic hypersomnia (Castriotta & Lai, 2001). It has also been found that patients with obstructive sleep apnea may have significant impairment in daytime functioning, intellectual capacity, memory, and motor coordination, which could be exacerbating cognitive deficits sustained during ABI. Since presence of sleep disorder itself appears to be significantly correlated with ABI, and the majority of sleep disorders are treatable, it is imperative that patients suffering from sleep disorders are identified and treated as they potentially present a hazard to themselves and public health.

The Epworth Sleepiness Scale (Johns, 1991) is one of the most popular means of screening patients with daytime sleepiness for presence of potential sleep disorder, and can be performed by a general practitioner. Patients whose test results are suggestive of excessive daytime sleepiness should be evaluated by a neurologist or pulmonologist skilled in sleep evaluation. Further diagnostic workup usually involves polysomnography and multiple sleep latency tests. Patients diagnosed with obstructive sleep apnea should undergo titration of nasal airway pressure in the sleep laboratory, in order to determine the optimal pressure that prevents episodes of apnea, oxygen desaturation, and snoring.

While severe TBI tends to be associated with disorders of hypersomnia, mild to moderate TBI is frequently associated with insomnia, which is a perception that sleep quality is inadequate or nonrestorative despite the adequate opportunity to sleep. Additionally, as patients recover from TBI, hypersomnia pattern appears to change to insomnia pattern. Curiously, it appeared that patients with severe TBI had fewer sleep complaints than patients with mild to moderate TBI, which could be related to lack of awareness of limitation due to cognitive impairment. Additionally, patients with mild TBI are expected to resume their responsibilities much sooner than patients with moderate or severe TBI and are rarely afforded the time and resources necessary in order to fully reintegrate themselves into their daily routine. This appears to cause additional stress, which in turn triggers further insomnia.

Treatment of sleep disorders in ABI depends on the nature of the disorder. Hypersomnia during the acute stage of TBI can be successfully treated using modafinil (Provigil) and methylphenidate (Ritalin). Modafinil is a medication that is commonly used to treat excessive daytime somnolence associated with narcolepsy. The precise mechanism of action is not completely understood, since it appears to be nonreactive with any major class of receptors. However, modafinil has been found to inhibit GABA release in the basal ganglia (Smith, 2003). Given that hypersomnolence is a common complaint among TBI patients, and current experience with modafinil also suggests its usefulness for treatment of fatigue, this medication has become popular in the arsenal of pharmacological agents to augment functional recovery (See Chapter 6).

Methylphenidate is another medication that is used as a stimulant for excessive sleepiness and as a treatment of attention deficit hyperactivity disorder (ADHD). Frontal lobes are frequently damaged as a result of TBI; they are also implicated in ADHD. Both of those conditions have sleep disturbance as a common comorbidity, which suggests that sleep disorder is closely related to frontal lobe functioning. A study by Flanagan et al. (2003) demonstrated that the use of methylphenidate has a beneficial effect on processing speed, distractibility, vigilance, and sustained attention in patients with TBI. Walker-Batson et al. (2001) suggested that dextroamphetamine administration results in a significant improvement in language skills in a group of patients with stroke-induced aphasia when paired with speech-language therapy as compared to controls. Additionally, Cochrane review of amphetamines for improving recovery after stroke shows that there are trends toward benefit in language and motor recovery in stroke patients who were given amphetamines; however, further studies are required in order to statistically confirm its usefulness (Martinsson et al., 2003). Therefore, methylphenidate would be an acceptable choice of treating hypersomnolence in a patient with ABI and could potentially exert beneficial effects on other aspects of patient's functioning.

Treatment of insomnia in ABI is much more involved because of comorbidity of insomnia with other psychiatric conditions, particularly depression. Therefore, the approach to the patient with insomnia should be very similar to the approach to a patient with pain disorder. It requires pharmacotherapeutic intervention coupled with appropriate rehabilitation techniques, proper counseling, as well as maintenance of sleep hygiene. Keeping a sleep log for 2–4 weeks helps to establish a pattern of insomnia, further clarifying which approach would work best. The current arsenal of medications active against insomnia includes eszopiclone (Lunesta), zaleplon (Sonata), and zolpidem (Ambien). As nonbenzodiazepine receptor active medications, they offer an alternative to the use of short-acting benzodiazepine receptor agonists, which are commonly used in the treatment of insomnia, but contraindicated in clients with ABI. Recent meta-analyses showed that zaleplon and eszopiclone were safe choices in treatment of insomnia in the elderly, with improved profile of effect on psychomotor and cognitive performance (Glass et al., 2005). Cognitive-behavioral therapy, progressive relaxation, guided imagery, and biofeedback are useful as well (Smith et al., 2005).

Conclusion

In conclusion, the neurologist plays an integral role in the evaluation and management of patients with acquired brain injury. The primary role of the neurologist is to make an accurate diagnosis or, at least, confirm the diagnosis and assess the extent of injury by obtaining a comprehensive history and performing a detailed neurological examination. A neurological treatment plan is then formulated to help prevent further neurological sequelae and promote restoration of function. As an educator and advisor, the neurologist has a unique opportunity to discuss prognosis and recommend possible nonsurgical as well as surgical alternatives to patients and their families. Lastly, a key role of the neurologist is to interface with the multidisciplinary brain injury team focusing on the primary goal of facilitating maximum recovery.

References

Aguilar, M., Hart, R., Hart, R.M. (2005) Antiplatelet therapy for preventing stroke in patients with non-valvular atrial fibrillation and no previous history of stroke or transient ischemic attacks. *Cochrane Database of Systematic Reviews* (4), CD001925.

Bennett, M.H., Trytko, B., Jonker, B. (2004) Hyperbaric oxygen therapy for the adjunctive treatment of traumatic brain injury. *Cochrane Database of Systematic Reviews* (4), CD004609.

Bennett, M.H., Wasiak, J., Schnabel, A., Kranke, P., French, C. (2005) Hyperbaric oxygen therapy for acute ischaemic stroke. *Cochrane Database of Systematic Reviews* (3), CD004954.

Biller, J., Love, B.B. (2004) Vascular diseases of the nervous system: Ischemic cerebrovascular disease. In Bradley, W.G., Daroff, R.B., Fenichel, G.M., Marsden, C.D. (ed.): *Neurology in Clinical Practice*, 4th ed. Stoneham, MA: Butterworth Publishers, chap. 57A, p. 1197.

Binnie, C.D., Stefan, H. (1999) Modern electroencephalography: Its role in epilepsy management (Review). *Clinical Neurophysiology* 110(10):1671–1697.

Camilo, O., Goldstein, L.B. (2004) Seizures and epilepsy after ischemic stroke. *Stroke* 35(7):1769–1775.

Castriotta, R.J., Lai, J.M. (2001) Sleep disorders associated with traumatic brain injury. *Archives of Physical Medicine and Rehabilitation* 82(10):1403–1406.

Chang, B.S., Lowenstein, D.H., Quality Standards Subcommittee of the American Academy of Neurology. (2003) Practice parameter: Antiepileptic drug prophylaxis in severe traumatic brain injury: Report of the quality standards subcommittee of the american academy of neurology. *Neurology* 60(1):10–16.

Chen, D.K., So, Y.T., Fisher, R.S. (2005) Use of serum prolactin in diagnosing epileptic seizures: Report of the Therapeutics and Technology Assessment Subcommittee of the American Academy of Neurology (Review). *Neurology* 65(5):668–675.

Coull, B.M., Williams, L.S., Goldstein, L.B., Meschia, J.F., Heitzman, D., Chaturvedi, S., Johnston, K.C., Starkman, S., Morgenstern, L.B., Wilterdink, J.L., Levine, S.R., Saver, J.L., Joint Stroke Guideline Development Committee of the American Academy of Neurology; American Stroke Association. (2002) Anticoagulants and antiplatelet agents in acute ischemic stroke: report of the Joint Stroke Guideline Development Committee of the American Academy of Neurology and the American Stroke Association (a division of the American Heart Association). *Stroke* 33(7):1934–19420.

Daly, E., Wulff, J. (1987) Treatment of a post-traumatic headache. *The British Journal of Medical Psychology* 60(Pt 1):85–88.

Delorenzo, R.J., Sun, D.A., Deshpande, L.S. (2004) Cellular mechanisms underlying acquired epilepsy: The calcium hypothesis of the induction and maintenance of epilepsy. *Pharmacology and Therapeutics* 105(3):229 266.

Drazkowski, J.F., Fisher, R.S., Sirven, J.I., Demaerschalk, B.M., Uber-Zak, L., Hentz, J.G., Labiner, D. (2003) Seizure-related motor vehicle crashes in Arizona before and after reducing the driving restriction from 12 to 3 months. *Mayo Clinical Proceedings* 78(7):819–825.

Engel, J. Jr, International League Against Epilepsy (ILAE). (2001) A proposed diagnostic scheme for people with epileptic seizures and with epilepsy: Report of the ILAE Task Force on Classification and Terminology. *Epilepsia* 42(6):796–803.

Flanagan, S.R., Kane, L., Rhoades, D. (2003) Pharmacological modification of recovery following brain injury. *Journal of Neurologic Physical Therapy* 27:129–136.

French, J.A., Kanner, A.M., Bautista, J., Abou-Khalil, B., Browne, T., Harden, C.L., Theodore, W.H., Bazil, C., Stern, J., Schachter, S.C., Bergen, D., Hirtz, D., Montouris, G.D., Nespeca, M., Gidal, B., Marks, W.J. Jr, Turk, W.R., Fischer, J.H., Bourgeois, B., Wilner, A., Faught, R.E. Jr, Sachdeo, R.C., Beydoun, A., Glauser, T.A. Therapeutics and Technology Assessment Subcommittee of the American Academy of Neurology: Quality Standards Subcommittee of the American Academy of Neurology; American Epilepsy Society. (2004) Efficacy and tolerability of the new antiepileptic drugs I: Treatment of new onset epilepsy: Report of the Therapeutics and Technology Assessment Subcommittee and Quality Standards Subcommittee of the American Academy of Neurology and the American Epilepsy Society. *Neurology* 62(8):1252 1260.

Frey, L.C. (2003) Epidemiology of posttraumatic epilepsy: A critical review. *Epilepsia* 44(Suppl. 10):11–17.

Gibson, G.E., Pulsinelli, W., Blass, J.P., Duffy, T.E. (1981) Brain dysfunction in mild to moderate hypoxia. *American Journal of Medicine* 70(6):1247–1254.

Glass, J., Lanctot, K.L., Herrmann, N., Sproule, B.A., Busto, U.E. (2005) Sedative hypnotics in older people with insomnia: Meta-analysis of risks and benefits. *British Medical Journal* 331(7526):1162.

Green, R., Shellenberger, P. (1991) *Dynamics of Health and Wellness: A Biopsychosocial Approach.* Orlando,FL: Holt, Rinehart, & Winston, Inc.

Ham, L.P., Packard, R.C. (1996) A retrospective, follow-up study of biofeedback-assisted relaxation therapy in patients with post-traumatic headache. *Biofeedback and Self-Regulation*, 21:93–104.

Haynes, R.B., Taylor, D.W., Sackett, D.L., Thorpe, K., Ferguson, G.G., Barnett, H.J. (1994) Prevention of functional impairment by endarterectomy for symptomatic high-grade carotid stenosis. North American Symptomatic Carotid Endarterectomy Trial Collaborators. *JAMA* 271(16):1256–1259.

Heart Protection Study Collaborative Group. (2002) MRC/BHF Heart Protection Study of cholesterol lowering with simvastatin in 20,536 high-risk individuals: A randomized placebo-controlled trial. *Lancet* 360(9326):7–22.

Hickling, E.J., Blanchard, E.B., Silverman, D.J., Schwarz, S.P. (1992) Motor vehicle accidents, headaches and post-traumatic stress disorder: assessment findings in a consecutive series. *Headache* 32(3):147–151.

Holroyd, K.A., Andrasik, F. (1978) Coping and the self-control of chronic tension headache. *Journal of Consulting and Clinical Psychology* 5:1036–1045.

Interventions for deliberately altering blood pressure in acute stroke. (2000) Blood pressure in Acute Stroke Collaboration (BASC).*Cochrane Database of Systematic Reviews* (2), CD000039.

Johns, M.W. (1991) A new method for measuring daytime sleepiness: The Epworth sleepiness scale. *Sleep* 14(6):540–545.

Lawrence, E.S., Coshall, C., Dundas, R., Stewart, J., Rudd, A.G., Howard, R., Wolfe, C.D. (2001) Estimates of the prevalence of acute stroke impairments and disability in a multiethnic population. *Stroke* 32(6):1279–1284.

Leger, D. (1994) The cost of sleep-related accidents: a report for the National Commission on Sleep Disorders Research. *Sleep* 17:84–93.

Linden, T., Skoog, I., Fagerberg, B., Steen, B., Blomstrand, C. (2004) Cognitive impairment and dementia 20 months after stroke. *Neuroepidemiology* 23(1–2):45–52.

Linden, T., Samuelsson, H., Skoog, I., Blomstrand, C. (2005) Visual neglect and cognitive impairment in elderly patients late after stroke. *Acta Neurologica Scandinavica* 111(3):163–168.

Linde, K., Streng, A., Jurgens, S., Hoppe, A., Brinkhaus, B., Witt, C., Wagenpfeil, S., Pfaffenrath, V., Hammes, M.G., Weidenhammer, W., Willich, S.N., Melchart, D. (2005) Acupuncture for patients with migraine: A randomized controlled trial. *Journal of American Medical Association* 293(17):2118–2125.

Lipton, R.B., Bigal, M.E., Steiner, T.J., Silberstein, S.D., Olesen, J. (2004) Classification of primary headaches. *Neurology* 63(3):427–435.

Mahmood, O., Rapport, L.J., Hanks, R.A., Fichtenberg, N.L. (2004) Neuropsychological performance and sleep disturbance following traumatic brain injury. *Journal of Head Trauma Rehabilitation* 19(5):378–390.

Martelli, M.F., Grayson, R.L., Zasler, N.D. (1999) Posttraumatic headache: Neuropsychological and psychological effects and treatment implications. *Journal of Head Trauma Rehabilitation* 14(1):49–69.

Martinsson, L., Wahlgren, N.G., Hardemark, H.G. (2003) Amphetamines for improving recovery after stroke (Review). *Cochrane Database of Systematic Reviews* (3), CD002090.

McDonagh, M., Helfand, M., Carson, S., Russman, B.S. (2004) Hyperbaric oxygen therapy for traumatic brain injury: A systematic review of the evidence. *Archives of Physical Medicine and Rehabilitation* 85(7):1198–1204.

McGrath, R.B. (1987) In-house cardiopulmonary resuscitation—After a quarter of a century. *Annals of Emergency Medicine* 16:1365–1368.

Melchart, D., Linde, K., Fischer, P., Berman, B., White, A., Vickers, A., Allais, G. (2001) Acupuncture for idiopathic headache. *Cochrane Database of Systematic Reviews* (1), CD001218.

Melchart, D., Streng, A., Hoppe, A., Brinkhaus, B., Witt, C., Wagenpfeil, S., Pfaffenrath, V., Hammes, M., Hummelsberger, J., Irnich, D., Weidenhammer, W., Willich, S.N., Linde,

K. (2005) Acupuncture in patients with tension-type headache: Randomised controlled trial. *British Medical Journal* 331(7513):376–382.

Onorato, V.A., Tsushima, W.T. (1983) EMG, MMPI, and treatment outcome in the biofeed-back therapy of tension headache and posttraumatic pain. *American Journal of Clinical Biofeedback* 6:71–81.

Ramadan, N.H., Keidel, M. (2000) The Headaches. In J. Olesen, P. Tfelt-Hansen, P. Welch (eds): *The Headaches*, 2nd ed. Philadelphia: Lippincott Williams & Wilkins, pp. 771–780.

Sheth, S.G., Krauss, G., Krumholz, A., Li, G. (2004) Mortality in epilepsy: Driving fatalities vs other causes of death in patients with epilepsy. *Neurology* 63(6):1002–1007.

Smith, B.W. (2003) Modafinil for treatment of cognitive side effects of antiepileptic drugs in a patient with seizures and stroke. *Epilepsy and Behavior* 4:352–353.

Smith, M.T., Huang, M.I., Manber, R. (2005) Cognitive behavior therapy for chronic insomnia occurring within the context of medical and psychiatric disorders. *Clinical Psychology Review* 25(5):59–92.

Temkin, N.R. (2003) Risk factors for posttraumatic seizures in adults. *Epilepsia* 44(Suppl 10):18–20.

Thijs, V.N., Lansberg, M.G., Beaulieu, C., Marks, M.P., Moseley, M.E., Albers, G.W. (2000) Is early ischemic lesion volume on diffusion-weighted imaging an independent predictor of stroke outcome? A multivariable analysis. *Stroke* 31(11):2597–2602.

Thomassen, A., Wernberg, M. (1979) Prevalence and prognostic significance of coma after cardiac arrest outside intensive care and coronary units. *Acta Anaesthesiologica Scandinavica* 23(2):143–148.

Tobin, D.L., Holroyd, K.A., Baker, A., Reynolds, R.V.C., Holm, J.E. (1998) Development in clinical trial of a minimal contact, cognitive–behavioral treatment for tension headache. *Cognitive Therapy and Research* 12:325–339.

US National Institutes of Health. (1998) Rehabilitation of persons with traumatic brain injury. NIH Consensus Statement). http://consensus.nih.gov/cons/109/109_statement.htm, accessed March 1, 2006.

Walker-Batson, D., Curtis, S., Natarajan, R., Ford, J., Dronkers, N., Salmeron, E., Lai, J., Unwin, D.H. (2001) A double-blind, placebo controlled study of the use of amphetamine in the treatment of aphasia. *Stroke* 32:2093–2098.

Yusuf, S., Sleight, P., Pogue, J., Bosch, J., Davies, R., Dagenais, G. (2000) Effects of an angiotensin-converting-enzyme inhibitor, ramipril, on cardiovascular events in high-risk patients. The Heart Outcomes Prevention Evaluation Study Investigators. *New England Journal of Medicine* 342(3):145–153.

5
Voiding and Sexual Dysfunction after Acquired Brain Injury
The Role of the Neurourologist

MATTHEW E. KARLOVSKY AND GOPAL H. BADLANI

Introduction

In acquired brain injury (ABI), including both CVA (cerebrovascular accident) and TBI (traumatic brain injury) there can be profound effects on the genitourinary tract. A spectrum of voiding disorders may range from urinary retention to complex incontinence. Often, normal urinary or sexual changes are seen with aging, yet comorbid conditions are frequently present in the elderly that may complicate and predate CVA or TBI. These include diabetes mellitus, coronary artery and vascular disease, as well as other neurological conditions such as Alzheimer's and Parkinson's disease, all of which themselves have effects on urinary and sexual function. Sexual function, often overlooked in healthy elderly patients, is a neglected yet vital issue to full rehabilitation, especially in young patients. This chapter will cover pertinent anatomy, pathophysiology, workup, and treatment of individuals who suffer voiding and sexual dysfunction after CVA and TBI. The urologist is an integral part of patient care, and should be consulted early in the course of recovery. As will be addressed below, urologic management in the acute setting prior to stabilization may be simply handled by catheter drainage. Once the extent of injury is determined and rehabilitation begins, a urologic work up and treatment plan can help guide overall care and expedite social reintegration.

Review of Relevant Neuroanatomy of Micturition

The central nervous system (CNS) facilitates and inhibits the sacral voiding reflex, located at spinal levels S2–4. The main centers of control within the CNS are in the cortex and pons. Urinary storage and emptying is a complex coordination between these centers and peripheral sympathetic, parasympathetic and somatic innervation of the bladder and sphincter complexes. The primary function of the lower urinary tract is to store urine at low intravesical pressures until such time it is deemed socially appropriate to expel all in a coordinated fashion.

Afferent pathways (Table 5.1) from the bladder include: the parasympathetic pelvic nerve which conveys intravesical pressure and tension from detrusor muscle

TABLE 5.1. Afferent anatomy

Afferent Pathway	Nerve	Level	Signal	Fiber type
Parasympathetic	Pelvic	S2–4	Bladder distention	A-δ
Parasympathetic	Pelvic	S2–4	Pain	C
Sympathetic	Hypogastric	T10–L2	Sphincter tension	A-δ
Sympathetic	Hypogastric	T10–L2	Pain	C
Somatic	Pudendal	S2–4	Bladder/sphincter temp, distension, pain	A-δ

via myelinated Aδ fibers; the sympathetic hypogastric nerve, which conveys mechanoreceptor-mediated information; and somatic afferent signals via the pudendal nerve from the bladder and urethral sphincter carry sensations of temperature, pain, and distension. Both parasympathetic and sympathetic fibers carry pain signals mediated by small unmyelinated C-fibers. Efferent pathways (Table 5.2) are tripartite as well. Parasympathetic outflow is via sacral levels S2–4. Release of acetylcholine onto muscarinic receptors which are present throughout the detrusor results in bladder contraction. Sympathetic fibers arise from segments T10 to L2 and richly innervate the bladder base, neck and prostatic urethra, with sparse innervation of the detrusor. Baseline tonic sympathetic release of epinephrine mediates inhibition of parasympathetic signals, as well as maintains closure of the bladder neck. Efferent somatic signals via the pudendal nerve arise from Onuf's nucleus within S2–4 spinal segments and release acetylcholine onto nicotinic receptors on the striated muscle of the external sphincter.

The pons may be considered the coordinator of the micturition cycle. It coordinates detrusor contraction and sphincter relaxation. The medial pontine center (Barrington's nucleus) facilitates micturition, while the lateral and ventral centers maintain continence, and facilitate tonic contraction of the pelvic floor (guarding reflex).

The pre-optic nucleus of the hypothalamus, among other suprapontine structures, sends projections to Barrington's nucleus, and exerts control over micturition. When stimulated, the urethral sphincter is relaxed and bladder contractions

TABLE 5.2. Efferent anatomy

Efferent pathway	Nerve	Level	Function	Neurotransmitter	Receptor	Receptor Location
Parasympathetic	Pelvic	S2-4	Bladder contraction, erection	Acetylcholine	Muscarinic (M2, M3)	Detrusor
Sympathetic	Hypogastric	T10-L2	Bladder neck tone, emission	Epinephrine	Adrenergic (α, β)	α-bladder neck β-bladder body
Somatic	Pudendal	S2-4	External sphincter, ejaculation	Acetylcholine	Nicotinic	External sphincter

are elicited (Gjone, 1966). Barrington's nucleus (micturition) is under tonic cortical inhibition by gamma aminobutyric acid (GABA), and conversely is activated by the excitatory transmitter glutamate. In addition, central dopamine receptors can either be inhibitory (D1) or excitatory (D2) in regard to voiding (Seki et al., 2001).

Pathophysiology of Voiding Dysfunction

Lower urinary tract dysfunction can involve difficulties with emptying, storage, or both. Emptying dysfunction may result in difficulty initiating a stream, decreased force of stream, straining to void, incomplete emptying, hesitancy, or intermittency of flow. Storage dysfunction includes nocturia, urinary frequency, and urgency, with or without incontinence. Lower abdominal and pelvic pain may accompany these symptoms. Patients with a neurogenic bladder from CVA or TBI may also develop bladder decompensation in the form of urinary retention or incomplete bladder emptying, renal insufficiency, and recurrent urinary tract infections.

For practical purposes, control over storage and emptying is mediated and modified at three levels in the CNS. The sacral micturition center (S2–4) is influenced by the pontine micturition center, and both these centers are influenced by the suprapontine/cortical center. The effects of CVA and TBI result from insults to the suprapontine/cortical center or the pontine center. Cortical/suprapontine lesions result in detrusor overactivity from destruction of inhibitory influence. This leads to the urgent, frequent and often uncontrollable desire to void. However, detrusor overactivity after CVA and TBI is also associated with uninhibited striated sphincter relaxation, further impairing normal barriers to incontinence. Deficits in perception of stored urine or inability to process normal cues to void may exacerbate the incontinence. The bladder's detrusor muscle and the striated sphincter however maintain reflex coordination, whereas discoordination, or dyssynergia, typically develops from pontine or infrapontine spinal cord injury. Pontine lesions may effect the transmission of inhibitory control from higher centers, or may result in dyssynergia of the bladder and sphincter.

In animal models of cerebral infarction, detrusor overactivity and decreased bladder capacity were observed (Yokoyama et al., 1998). Cerebral infarction is believed to produce up-regulation of excitatory glutamate-mediated receptors. In addition, inhibitory D1 receptors are reduced, unmasking the excitatory D2 receptor signals (Yokoyama et al., 1999). In patients with detrusor overactivity, lesions are most often noted in the frontal cortex, internal capsule and basal ganglia (Burney et al., 1996). By contrast, cerebellar infarcts have resulted in detrusor areflexia (Burney et al., 1996). However, research has failed to prove that hemispheric dominance influences findings. Marinkovic and Badlani (2001) retrospectively evaluated 44 symptomatic patients admitted to a rehabilitation unit after a stroke. Mean age was 81.2 years and time from CVA to urodynamic evaluation was 1 to 12 months. No significant difference in bladder dysfunction was observed in dominant or nondominant hemispheric CVAs. However, the larger the infarct size, the more significant the risk of incontinence.

Clinical Findings

The symptoms of frequency, urgency, urge incontinence, and nocturia are present in up to 87% of stroke patients (Sakakibara et al., 2001). For the patient, the most striking and distressing finding is new-onset incontinence. Up to 70% have incontinence, yet only 35% will complain of incontinence (Brockelhurst et al., 1985). Importantly, baseline incontinence may pre-date a stroke or TBI and may be exacerbated after the neurological insult. In addition, if mentation is affected, incontinence may not be perceived. Incontinence may develop immediately or even months after the CVA or TBI. The presence of immediate onset incontinence after a stroke is known to be a poor overall prognostic sign. Increased risk of incontinence has been correlated with aphasia, cognitive impairment and infarct size (Nakayama et al., 1997). Early incontinence after stroke is associated with a 52% mortality rate at 6 months, versus 7% for those remaining continent (Nakayama et al., 1997), and early incontinence is the single best indicator of future disability (Taub et al., 1994).

Mrs. Jones, a 59-year-old woman with preexisting hypertension, suffered a stroke that left her with partial paralysis of her right arm and leg. She now complains of "being wet all the time" and refuses to socialize with friends and family due to embarrassing odor and the need to be close to the bathroom because of decreased mobility. She has become quite depressed by her situation. After evaluation it was discovered that Mrs. Jones takes many medications for her hypertension, including a diuretic, each with a glass of water. She reports that she cannot often sense the desire to void, and even so, does not arrive to the bathroom in time. A 24-hour voiding diary revealed that she drank too much fluid during the day. Fluid consumption was therefore restricted somewhat, and her diuretic was replaced by a different medication. In addition, she was placed on an anticholinergic once a day, and has noted a reduction in incontinence episodes, number of pads used, and an improvement in getting to the bathroom on time.

Urinary retention is known to occur immediately after any severe neurological insult, and is termed "shock bladder." Its cause is poorly understood, but it may result from a loss of consciousness, inability to communicate or ambulate from the injury, or simply originate from a purely neurological source.

Pathophysiology of Sexual Dysfunction

Sexual dysfunction after stroke is well described and is often multifactorial, including both organic and psychological/social factors. Although sexual activity is a vital part of normal life, society tends to ignore sexuality and/or sexual dysfunction in the elderly or physically disabled. However, regular coitus may continue into the seventh, eighth, and even ninth decades (Masters & Johnson, 1966). Erectile dysfunction from aging is most commonly vasculogenic, with neuropathic components. The pudendal arteries supply the corpora cavernosa via the cavernous arteries. These end-arteries are only 0.4 mm in diameter during penile flaccidity, and double in diameter during sexual excitement. Besides atherosclerosis and diabetes, medication for hypertension, depression, and neuroleptics often hinder erectile function.

Penile somatic sensory afferents deliver information to the sacral spinal cord, where sensory information is sent to suprasacral and cortical regions. Afferent signals complete the local erectogenic reflex arc by stimulating parasympathetic efferents that mediate cavernosal artery vasodilation leading to cavernosal smooth muscle engorgement and erection. Seminal emission and ejaculation are coordinated by sympathetic and somatic pudendal efferents in the prostatic urethra and bulbospongious muscles, respectively.

The pattern of genital neuromuscular activation is believed to be similar in women, where parasympathetic activity leads to clitoral and labial engorgement, and vaginal lubrication. Female orgasm is a result of sympathetic activity that leads to contraction of the uterus, fallopian tubes, paraurethral glands, and somatic nerve mediated contraction of pelvic floor musculature.

Both thalamus and cortical areas receive sensory input from the genitalia. Neurons from the paraventricular nucleus project to thoracolumbar and sacral nuclei involved with erection. Disruption of central centers may lead to decreased sexual perception and desire, while sparing the local sacral reflexes that mediate arousal from tactile input.

Psychosocial factors such as depression, fear of another stroke, loss of self-esteem and spousal relationship changes all influence sexuality after stroke. In a study (Korpelainen et al., 1999) of 192 stroke patients who had active sexual lives pre-stroke, 75% of men reported erectile dysfunction, 50% of women reported lack of vaginal lubrication, and 33% of men reported complete cessation of sex at 2 years after stroke. Orgasmic dysfunction is seen in 75% of women and 67% of men after stroke, and is more frequently seen in cases with aphasia (Lundberg et al., 2001). TBI affects sexual function in a similar fashion, with similar psychosocial changes, especially in young patients.

Evaluation of Voiding and Sexual Dysfunction

In the neurologically impaired patient a thorough patient history is required to identify previous neurological disease, cognitive deficits, associated medical problems, prior surgery, trauma, infection, baseline incontinence, and medications. Concomitant bowel and sexual function pre-and post-event should be elicited as well. The urological history must focus on the patient's initial voiding complaints in addition to those following CVA or TBI. History of prior urological surgeries such as transurethral resection of the prostate (TURP), prostate cancer, radiation treatment or incontinence surgeries must be elicited. Reversible causes of incontinence should be sought and treated (Table 5.3) (Resnick & Yalla, 1985). Symptoms may need to be elicited from caregivers if aphasia or impaired cognition is present. Patients may be unaware of urgency or incontinence episodes. Low or high volume

TABLE 5.3. "DIAPPERS": Reversible
Causes of Incontinence (Resnick &
Yalla, 1985)

D	Delerium/dementia
I	Infection
A	Atrophic vaginitis
P	Psychological (depression)
P	Pharmaceuticals
E	Endocrine (diabetes)
R	Restricted mobility
S	Stool impaction

incontinence and nocturia must be differentiated in order to distinguish between polyuria, and decreased bladder capacity.

The physical examination should include a neurological evaluation of sacral reflexes (S2–4) for motor and sensory deficits. Perineal sensation is tested with light touch and pinprick. Bulbocavernosus and anal reflexes test the integrity of pudendal nerve function. The bulbocavernosus reflex is present in 95% of men and 80% of women, and when absent in men suggests either spinal shock or peripheral neuropathy. Manual dexterity and visual acuity should be assessed if self-catheterization is being considered. A prostate exam in men, and evaluation of pelvic floor and possible introital changes from menopause should be noted in women. In addition, the following urologic evaluation must be included:

- Voiding diary—assesses oral fluid intake and voided volumes, frequency, and incontinence episodes. Provides objective documentation of symptoms and important in monitoring response to therapy. Especially useful in cognitively impaired patients.
- Urine analysis and culture.
- Renal function—BUN and creatinine levels and/or kidney imaging especially when hematuria or recurrent urinary tract infections are present.
- Cystoscopy and urodynamics—when appropriate.

Sexual health of patients and erectile history in male patients should be fully elicited in those who are ambulatory, with good mental status and manual dexterity, and who have been clinically stable for 6 months. Performance status regarding exercise tolerance is an important consideration before resumption of sexual activity. Voiding dysfunction, especially incontinence, must be addressed and treated prior to addressing sexual dysfunction. Individual counseling may prove valuable.

Urodynamics—What and When

Neurogenic bladder dysfunction is often nonspecific and often doesn't correlate well with reported voiding symptoms. Urodynamics can be used to help guide initial therapy, or if initial empiric therapy fails. One prospective study of 400 patients found that clinical assessment based on symptoms did not correlate with the objective urodynamic findings in 45% of patients thought to have storage problems and 54% thought to have emptying problems (Katz & Blaivas, 1983). Urodynamic results may then assume a greater role in treatment decisions. However, for objective data to be useful, it must reproduce the patient's symptoms during the study, which may be difficult in patients unable to easily follow commands or change positions.

Cystometry

The most useful urodynamic study is cystometry, which assesses intravesical pressure during a simulated filling phase. The test is performed while sitting or supine where sterile water is infused slowly through a thin small catheter. Bladder capacity, compliance, sensation and detrusor activity, whether over- or underactive, are detected by a pressure transducer at the tip of the catheter. Findings should be corroborated with subjective complaints. With suprapontine lesions (cortex/forebrain) detrusor overactivity (involuntary detrusor contractions) is the expected finding, which explains urge incontinence. Urgency and urge incontinence may or may not be sensed by the patient, but uniformly cannot be inhibited. They may be weak or strong contractions, but are usually sustained. Seventy percent of stroke survivors demonstrate detrusor overactivity (Nitti et al., 1996). Fifty to 70% of patients with detrusor overactivity will have uninhibited sphincteric relaxation on electromyography (see below) (Burney et al., 1996).

Post-Void Residual (PVR)

An important measurement, it is done in conjunction with cystometry to determine whether the bladder is emptying efficiently. An elevated PVR signifies a weak detrusor, an obstruction, or both. Elevated residual urine may lead to urgency, frequency, stress or urge incontinence, infection or hydronephrosis.

Uroflow and Pressure-Flow Studies

Uroflow will determine the voiding flow rate. It is dependent on a detrusor contraction and urethral resistance, to determine whether or not an obstruction is present. This is more important in men to rule out prostatic obstruction. The presence or absence of prostatic obstruction or detrusor function can appropriately guide potential drug and/or surgical therapy. Often, when detrusor areflexia is present abdominal straining will be noted.

Electromyography (EMG)

EMG is used to assess external or striated urethral function. After CVA or TBI, patients may demonstrate uninhibited relaxation of the urethral sphincter during a detrusor contraction. Uninhibited relaxation is reported to occur with lesions of the anterior cerebral cortex, internal capsule and basal ganglia (Siroky, 2003). The patient will typically be unable to voluntarily contract the pelvic floor (guarding reflex) during a detrusor contraction. If urgency is perceived, the patient may be unable to inhibit voiding through guarding, leading to incontinence. Typically, bladder–sphincter coordination is maintained after these lesions, as opposed to spinal cord injury where dyssynergia results with involuntary contraction of the striated urethral sphincter during a detrusor contraction. However, rare dyssynergia should be suspected in young TBI patients, where bladder outlet obstruction is demonstrated.

Abdominal Leak Point Pressure (LPP)

Abdominal or valsalva leak point pressure is the measure of urethral or outlet resistance. It is performed during cystometry with fluoroscopy, where the bladder is filled with contrast and coughing or valsalva are used to provoke high bladder pressures. Urine leakage during these maneuvers suggests incontinence to be stress related and not urge related.

Physician and Patient Expectations for Recovery

Several longitudinal studies have shown reasonable improvement of incontinence with time. Incontinence, and not gross motor deficits, is often the greatest impedence to recovery (Siroky et al., 2003). Incontinence is strongly associated with aphasia, increased disability, and depression, and acts as a psychosocial barrier to full recuperation. Of 151 stroke patients with an initial incontinence rate of 60%, rates decreased to 42% and 29% at 4 and 12 weeks, respectively (Borrie et al., 1986). In another study of 324 stroke patients, 61% of stroke survivors regained continence at 12 weeks (Patel et al., 2001). Improvement from post-stroke incontinence is more likely to occur in patients younger than 75 years and in those with smaller strokes (Patel et al., 2001). Premorbid conditions can determine the level and speed of recovery as well.

Treatment

When treating post-CVA or TBI voiding dysfunction, a perfect result may not be achievable or realistic, yet a flexible approach often is satisfactory to the patient, caregiver and physician. All patient factors should be carefully weighed including prognosis of underlying disease, age, limiting factors such as dexterity or cognition, desire and/or necessity of surgery, desire to regain sexual activity, psychosocial environment, motivation, and economic resources. Though incontinence may be the primary focus, sexual dysfunction should not be ignored, especially in young patients. Whether male or female, incontinence must be adequately treated prior to intervention for sexual dysfunction.

Polyuria

Careful attention to voided urine volumes and fluid consumption can help distinguish between polyuria and a diminished bladder capacity. A 24-hour urine diary is used to record these events at baseline, and at follow up to guide management. Nocturia is defined as awakening for frequent nighttime voiding, whereas nocturnal polyuria occurs when urine volume during an optimal 8-hour sleep period exceeds 33% of the total 24-hour urine volume. Noctural polyuria can occur despite normal 24-hour urine volumes. Nocturnal enuresis is defined as involuntary voiding in bed and often wakes the patient up. Incontinence during the day as well as night suggests an overactive/urge component, whereas a dry nighttime patient that is incontinent during the day may have a stress-predominant component. Fluid restriction, a voiding dairy, supervised timed voiding, leg elevation with or without compression stockings, and afternoon diuretic use can reduce nighttime urine production that occurs from third space shifting in patients with heart failure or leg edema.

Urinary Retention in Men

During the period of acute brain injury, urinary retention may occur, and during the initial phase, an indwelling catheter may be the simplest therapy. However, if retention persists for weeks to months, clean intermittent catheterization (CIC) every 4 to 6 hours is the best minimally invasive therapy. As spontaneous voiding returns and a PVR is less than 100 ml, it may be discontinued. When CIC is not feasible either by patient or caregiver, and indwelling catheter can be inserted and changed monthly. Similarly, a suprapubic catheter is often a good alternative if urethral meatal erosion or penile discomfort develops.

Clean intermittent catheterization works best when continence can be maintained between catheterizations, and when bladder compliance and capacity is sufficient, usually 300 mL. Fluid restriction should be limited to promote a reasonable catheterization schedule. Patients who do not recover full detrusor function, or who have borderline voiding that worsened after CVA or TBI, may benefit from post-void catheterizations to ensure complete bladder emptying. Moreover, if compliance and capacity are poor, the bladder can be chemically paralyzed with anticholinergic agents, so that all urine is removed with timed catheterization.

Problems that may arise with CIC include urethral trauma, urethral stricture and predisposition to bacteriuria and urinary tract infection. Urine cultured from patients who perform CIC will always show some degree of colonization, and should not be treated routinely with antibiotics. Antibiotics are indicated if infection is suspected by the presence of fever or other constitutional symptoms. To avoid development of a latex allergy, non-latex catheter use is recommended. Lubrication helps minimize pain and trauma. Condom catheters are not recommended for long-term use in patients with intact bladder neck or urethral sphincters. In addition, skin breakdown and excoriation can occur. Chronic indwelling urinary catheters are often employed in the severely debilitated, and are a risk factor for infection and bladder stone formation. In addition, they can lead to erosion of the urethral meatus if poorly cared for. A suprapubic tube is an adequate alternative for those who cannot perform self-catheterization. It is easier to maintain, avoids the groin, but needs to be changed like any urinary catheter on a monthly basis.

Urinary retention in men may be due to bladder outlet obstruction (BOO), most commonly from benign prostatic hyperplasia (BPH), or from detrusor areflexia from stroke or TBI. In young patients with TBI, BOO is uncommon, and urethral stricture may be present, or even rarely detrusor sphincter dyssynergia. Medical therapy for prostatic obstruction is with α1-receptor blockers, which can be started once medically stable. Older agents such as terazosin and doxazosin require slow titration to avoid hypotension. Tamsulosin is an α-1a receptor blocker that is more selective for the prostate and bladder neck and may be used in patients with borderline hypotension, yet can cause retrograde ejaculation in up to 30%. Alfuzosin, another α1-receptor blocker, achieves higher intraprostatic concentrations than the other agents, and causes minimal vasodilatory changes, (McKeage & Plosker, 2002) causes minimal retrograde ejaculation, and does not require dose titration. For these reasons, it is used as a first line medication.

Surgical intervention for men with retention secondary to prostatic obstruction is managed with transurethral resection of the prostate (TURP). It is indicated when medical therapy had failed or is not tolerated by the patient. Adequate detrusor contraction must be demonstrated on urodynamics for TURP to be successful. TURP carries a degree of morbidity including hematuria, urinary tract infection, hospitalization, and retrograde ejaculation. Laser-vaporization TURP minimizes many of the potential morbidities of standard TURP, including hematuria, absorption of irrigation fluids, and time to recovery. It may even be performed on patients taking aspirin or warfarin. For those patients where TURP is indicated yet are too frail for surgery, minimally invasive therapies are available. Microwave and radiofrequency thermoablation of the prostate are employed through specially designed catheters or cystoscopes, during a 1-hour office visit. Local anesthesia and a sedative are usually given, and post-procedure catheterization is usually required for less than a week to avoid retention that results from prostatic edema.

Mr. Smith is a 71-year-old man who suffered blunt head injury during a motor vehicle accident. He sustained an intracranial bleed that required emergent drainage. Upon eventual discharge from the hospital, Mr. Smith found it very difficult to void without straining. He had been taking an α-blocker for BPH prior to the accident and was only now restarted on it. Two months later he still complained of incomplete emptying and developed a urinary tract infection. Evaluation revealed a post-void residual of 500 mL. Cystometry revealed him to have an acontractile bladder and used abdominal straining to void. Prostatic surgery was not recommended and a self-catheterization regimen was commenced.

Prostatic stents are another minimally invasive alternative. They are placed via cystoscope on an outpatient basis. However, stents rely on active drainage, requiring adequate detrusor function. They are not useful for retention secondary to detrusor failure. Once in place, they are epithelialized within 6–8 weeks. They may be used in patients on antiplatelet therapy, but not warfarin. They are an attractive alternative for those with hope of recovery, or those who refuse surgery.

The urologist, however, should refrain from performing any prostatic procedures for 6 to 12 months after stroke or TBI because incontinence and morbidity may be increased. Several variables are associated with an unsatisfactory prostatectomy outcome (incontinence), such as patients 70 years and over, worsening neurological symptoms, and a CVA involving both hemispheres. These predict poor outcomes in greater than 50% of patients (Lum & Marshall 1982).

Urinary Retention in Women

Usually secondary to detrusor underactivity, urinary retention in women is best managed by CIC. It offers the best long-term management, either by the patient herself or a caregiver. Often, restricted mobility or poor dexterity limits this option. Indwelling or suprapubic catheters are secondary options, however they require monthly changes, and contribute to discomfort and infection. Proper groin skin care can avoid urethral or labial erosion and fungal infection.

Incontinence—Treatment

Patients with diminished sensation but who can still empty their bladders or patients with detrusor overactivity can be first treated with timed voiding. To this regimen can be added anticholinergic medication to increase voiding intervals. Injudicious use of these medications in men with concomitant bladder outlet obstruction or men and women with detrusor underactivity may result in urinary retention.

A variety of oral agents are available for urgency, frequency, and urge incontinence. The most widely prescribed include oxybutynin, tolterodine, dicyclomine and hyocyamine. Both oxybutynin and tolterodine have immediate release and delayed release preparations. The delayed release preparations were made available to simplify and improve patient compliance, and to decrease the side effects. Oxybutynin has been shown to decrease urinary urgency and the frequency of both incontinence episodes and voluntary urination (Dmochowski et al., 2002). Previous literature has supported the equivalent efficacy of oxybutynin and tolterodine (Giannitsas et al., 2004), however, with a lower side effect profile with tolterodine. Common side effects are dry mouth and constipation, but also include somnolence, nausea, dizziness, blurry vision, and palpitation. More recently, a transdermal preparation of oxybutynin has become available. The patch is applied every 72–96 hours, and erythema and pruritus rates occur 5.6% and 16.8%, respectively, at the application site (Dmochowski et al., 2002). Yet because the medication avoids the first pass effect through the gut and liver, the active metabolite concentration is significantly reduced, minimizing side effects. Transdermal oxybutynin has been shown to be pharmacologically and clinically equivalent to the immediate-release preparation of oxybutynin (Davila et al., 2001), the extended release preparation (Appell et al., 2003), and long-acting tolterodine (Dmochowski et al., 2003).

Trospium is a new oral antimuscarinic medication. It is a quaternary amine that is minimally metabolized, not highly protein-bound, and theoretically should not cross the blood brain barrier (Pak et al., 2003). Trospium significantly decreases average frequency of toilet voids and urge incontinent episodes compared to placebo. It significantly increases average volume per void, and decreases average urge severity and daytime frequency (Zinner et al., 2004). It is well tolerated in trials of patients with overactive bladders, however it has not been studied for efficacy and tolerability in neurologically impaired patients, nor has it been compared to the other oral agents. In addition two other newer agents, darifenacin and solifenacin are also antimuscarinic agents with greater selectivity for the bladder which theoretically reduces the side effect profile including dry mouth, constipation, confusion and blurry vision. Conversely, there is no effective pharmacotherapy for detrusor underactivity.

Surgical therapies for incontinence are usually directed at female patients with stress incontinence. They would include periurethral bulking agents or pubovaginal sling placement. Periurethral injection of collagen or carbon particles, result in short term subjective and objective improvements and is a first line minimally invasive treatment (Pichard et al., 2003). Results are short-lived prompting repeat injections often two to three times; however, it may represent a useful option in women too frail for more invasive surgery. Sling procedures are indicated for stress incontinence, with or without urge incontinence. Patient selection must be prudent to avoid exacerbating urgency and urge incontinence postoperatively. There are no FDA-approved medications available for stress incontinence.

Newer Therapies

Sacral neuromodulation using the InterStim Continence Control System (Medtronic, Minneapolis, MN) is a minimally invasive therapy that has become commercially available in the United States since 1997. Treatment is based on intercepting the bladder afferent sacral fibers that transmit the excitatory signal that ultimately results in bladder contraction. Electrical stimulation is transmitted via an implanted electrode that enters the S3 foramen and lies adjacent to, but not in contact with the S3 afferent nerve. The lead is attached to a pulse generator placed beneath the skin, once a 7-day test trial using a removable lead proves patient responsiveness. It is indicated for the treatment of urgency, frequency, and urge incontinence. These symptoms are often associated with pelvic floor muscle and external sphincter muscle dysfunction, and it is postulated that stimulation of these somatic muscle groups leads to feedback inhibition of the afferent stimuli responsible for bladder contraction, in effect, augmenting the guarding reflex, suppressing detrusor overactivity. About half of all patients with refractory symptoms respond to test stimulation and become candidates for the permanent implant (Bosch, et al., 1998). Patients become candidates for permanent lead placement if symptoms are reduced by more than 50%. Its applicability to the older urge-incontinent population was addressed in a small but recent study (Amundsen & Webster, 2002). Twelve of 25 patients responded to test stimulation, and at a mean of 7.8 months follow-up, there was a sustained reduction in greater than 50% of incontinent episodes, with over 80% reduction in heavy leakage, and 40% reduction in frequency episodes, with a low rate of revision of lead position and reprogramming. Though refinements in technique have reduced operative morbidity, and follow up on the earliest United States cases is still less than 10 years, the technology is promising with good short-term results.

Botulinum toxin (BTX) is a presynaptic neuromuscular blocking agent that causes reversible muscle weakness for several months when injected in small quantities intramuscularly. Its clinical application in recent years in treating spastic muscle disorders has grown.

Briefly, Botulinum toxin (types A, B, C1, D, E, F, G) is derived from the Gram-positive anaerobic bacterium *Clostridium botulinum*, and is the most powerful naturally occurring toxin (Rackley & Abdelmalak, 2004). Botulinum-A toxin, with the widest urologic application thus far, cleaves a motor nerve terminal protein, SNAP-25, which leads to chemical denervation by preventing exocytosis of acetylcholine, the neurotransmitter responsible for skeletal muscle contraction. This leads to muscle relaxation, an effect that generally lasts between 3 and 6 months before full strength returns, although clinical effects have been observed between 6 and 12 months.

Though not currently FDA-approved for urological application, intravesical injection of BTX into the detrusor muscle has been performed for the treatment of idiopathic overactive bladder, refractory to both medical and behavioral management. Numerous studies have shown an increase in functional capacity; decrease in urgency, frequency, and urge incontinence (Wyndaele, 2002); and decreases in daily pad usage and weight, incontinence episodes, and urinary quality of life, with no increase in urinary retention (Flynn et al., 2004). Formal studies in patients who are post-CVA and TBI have not been done. Reported adverse effects are rare but include systemic side effects such as hypostenia lasting 2–4 weeks, and generalized muscle weakness (Wyndaele, 2002). With continued development and dose standardization, it may fill an important treatment void for those failing all medical therapies including sacral neuromodulation.

Nursing Care

Sometimes, all that is necessary for successful incontinence therapy in the neurologically impaired patient is simple behavior modification, such as fluid restriction, a timed voiding schedule, and a voiding diary. Many patients with dementia, however, who no longer have socially appropriate behavior also benefit substantially from a prompted voiding schedule. Gelber et al. (1993) reported that 37% of severely disabled, incontinent patients had a normally functional bladder and even these debilitated patients benefited from prompted voiding and fluid restriction.

The drawback is the labor-intensive nature of this method of management which is most effective in a home environment with one-to-one patient attention.

There is a wide array of absorbent, containment and protective products available on the market. It is important to assess the patient's needs prior to discussing specific products. Consider the patient's size, mobility, self-care skills, finances, and motivations. Absorbent products, like pad and pant systems, have become popular and consist of disposable pads held in place by lightweight reusable briefs. Compression devices such as a penile clamp may be an alternative for keeping the patient dry. The clamp should be removed every 4 hours for bladder emptying and the penile shaft should be inspected for swelling or irritation. If possible, the clamp should be kept off at night.

External collection devices draining to a leg bag or a bedside bag are used by both men and women. Frequent inspection of the penile and vulvar skin should be made, and the uncircumcised foreskin should not be completely retracted in order to avoid para-phimosis. Excoriation, necrosis and gangrene can occur from an indwelling catheter or condom catheter. Condom catheters must be changed daily and the skin carefully inspected for irritation. Irritation and rashes must be dealt with promptly. A variety of water-soluble moisturizing creams and lotions are available, as well as barrier creams and salves.

Mr. Doe, a 47-year-old man, has been severely debilitated from a stroke for several years and currently lives in a care facility. His chronic urinary catheter is not well cared for and penile erosion has occurred so that the catheter has eroded the urethral meatus halfway down the shaft. After examination, it appeared the catheter was always on tension that leads to erosion of the penile skin. Mr. Doe failed several trials of void, and urodynamics were performed that demonstrated an atonic bladder. In order to prevent further penile injury, the decision was made to have a suprapubic tube placed.

Sexual Dysfunction

Though incontinence is the primary focus of treatment, sexual dysfunction should not be ignored in patients with CVA and TBI, especially in young patients. Sexual counseling with patients and their partners is an important part of rehabilitation.

In men surviving CVA or TBI, erectile dysfunction is no different than in any other patient group. Vascular insufficiency is the most common etiology. Hormone evaluation maybe indicated with decreased libido, although depression secondary to disability may be the cause of decreased desire. Therapeutic modalities of oral medication, injectables, and surgery must be individualized. Cardiac evaluation is recommended before beginning any therapy, as patients' exercise tolerance and medication profile vary. As a significant number of patients are on antiplatelet or anticoagulant medication, the use of vacuum devices or penile injections for erections is rare. We defer surgical implant till full potentials of rehabilitation are achieved and non-surgical therapies are exhausted. Due to potential mobility limitations, a semirigid prosthesis is the preferred implant when indicated.

Oral medications for erectile dysfunction such as sildenafil, vardenafil, and tadalafil are all phosphodiesterase-5 inhibitors, and thus are all contraindicated in patients taking nitroglycerin, whether scheduled or as needed for angina, for fear of hypotension. Common side effects include rhinitis, headache, dyspepsia, flushing, and ocular changes, although all are self-limited. All may be used with precaution in men with BPH taking α-blockers, as hypotension may potentially result. All medications require concomitant genital stimulation for erection, and patients must wait at least 30 minutes after ingestion prior to engaging in sexual intercourse.

All women with sexual dysfunction after CVA and TBI who show signs of estrogen deficiency should be given local hormone replacement therapy, if not contraindicated. Sexual counseling and vibratory stimulation may be helpful in general, or specifically in those with genital sensory disorder, paresis or mobility restrictions. Lubricating gels may be used to reduce pain if introital tissues show signs of atrophy. Androgen supplementation may be attempted with hypoactive arousal, in postmenopausal women or in those not seeking fertility, because of risk of masculinization.

Conclusion

Successful rehabilitation of bladder and sexual function requires long term commitments on the part of the physician, the patient, and his or her family as a high degree of motivation is necessary during frequently slow recovery periods. Early consultation and intervention by the urologist is recommended to help coordinate a treatment plan during all phases of the disease process. Stroke and TBI often result in similar voiding and sexual dysfunction. Urinary urgency, frequency, and urge incontinence difficulties can range in severity from mild to marked. It is important to allow adequate time for urinary symptom stabilization prior to instituting therapy, and to address urinary dysfunction prior to sexual dysfunction. It is also important to minimize reversible causes of incontinence when present. Overall debility and family involvement will direct care. Various behavioral, medical and surgical therapies are available and can be tailored as needed. A team approach between the patient, caregivers and physicians can set realistic goals for recovery of function. Sexual health should not be neglected regardless of age. Even severely debilitated patients can be managed successfully in order to minimize potential morbidity from the urinary tract. Regaining bladder and sexual function is very significant in maintaining mental health, avoiding isolation and promoting overall recovery.

References

Amundsen, C.L., Webster, G.D. (2002) Sacral neuromodulation in an older, urge incontinent population. *American Journal of Obstetrics and Gynecology* 187:1462–1465.

Appell, R.A., Chancellor, M.B., Zobrist, R.H., Thomas H., Sanders, S.W. (2003) Pharmacokinetics, metabolism and saliva output during transdermal and extended release oral oxybutynin administration in healthy subjects. *Mayo Clinical Proceedings* 78:696–702.

Borrie, M.J., Campbell A.J., Caradoc-Davies T.H., Spears, G.F. (1985) Urinary incontinence after stroke: A prospective study. *Age Ageing* 15:177–181.

Bosch, J.L.H.R. (1998) Sacral neuromodulation in the treatment of the unstable bladder. *Current Opinion in Urology.* 8:287–291.

Brockelhurst, J.C., Andrews, K., Richards, B., Laycock, P.J. (1985) Incidence and correlates of incontinence in stroke patients. *Journal of the American Geriatrics Society* 33:540–542.

Burney, T.L., Senapati, M., Desai, S., Choudhary, S.T., Badlani, G.H. (1996) Acute cerebrovascular accident and lower urinary tract dysfunction: A prospective correlation of the site of brain injury with urodynamic findings. *The Journal of Urology* 156:1748.

Davila, G.W., Daugherty, C.A., Sanders, S.W. (2001) A short term, multicenter, randomized double-blind dose titration study of the efficacy and anticholinergic side effects of transdermal oxybutynin compared to immediate release oral oxybutynin treatment of patients with urge urinary incontinence. *The Journal of Urology* 166:140–145.

Dmochowski, R.R., Davila, G.W., Zinner, N.R., Gittelman, M.C., Saltzstein, D.R., Lyttle, S., Sanders, S.W. (2002) Efficacy and safety of transdermal oxybutynin in patients with urge and mixed incontinence. *The Journal of Urology* 168:580–586.

Dmochowski, R.R., Sand, P.K., Zinner, N.R., Gittelman, M.C., Davila, G.W., Sanders, S.W. (2003) Comparative efficacy and safety of transdermal oxybutynin and oral tolterodine versus placebo in previously treated patients with urge and mixed urinary incontinence. *Urology* 62:237–242.

Flynn, M.K., Webster, G.D., Amundsen, C.L. (2004) The effect of botulinum-a toxin on patients with severe urge urinary incontinence. *The Journal of Urology* 172:2316–2320.

Gelber, D.A., Good, D.C., Laven, L.J., Verhulst, S.J. (1993) Cause of urinary incontinence after acute hemispheric stroke. *Stroke* 24:378–382.

Giannitsas, K., Perimenis, P., Athanasopoulos, A., Gyftopoulos, K., Nikiforidis, G., Barbalias, G. (2004) Comparison of efficacy of tolterodine and oxybutynin in different urodynamic severity grades of idiopathic detrusor overactivity. *European Urology* 46:776–782.

Gjone, R. (1966) Excitatory and inhibitory bladder response to stimulation of limbic, diencephalic and mesencephalic structures in the cat. *Acta physiologica Scandinavica* 66:91–102.

Katz, G.P., Blaivas, J. (1983) A diagnostic dilemma: When urodynamic findings differ from the clinical impression. *The Journal of Urology* 129:1170–4, 1983

Korpelainen, J.T., Neiminen, P., Myllyla, V.V. (1999) Sexual functioning among stroke patients and their spouses. *Stroke* 30:715–719.

Lum, S.K., Marshall, V.R. (1982) Results of prostatectomy in patients following a cerebrovascular accident. *British Journal of Urology* 54:186.

Lundberg, P.O., Ertekin, C., Ghezzi, A. (2001) Neurosexology: Guidelines for neurologists. *European Journal of Neurology* 8(Suppl 3):2–24.

Marincovic, S., Badlani, G. (2001) Voiding and sexual dysfunction after cerebrovascular accidents. *The Journal of Urology* 165:359–370.

Masters, W.H., Johnson, V.E. (1966) *Human Sexual Response.* Boston: Little Brown & Co.

McKeage, K., Plosker, G.L. (2002) Alfuzosin: A review of the therapeutic use of the prolonged-release formulation given once daily in the management of benign prostatic hyperplasia. *Drugs* 62:633–653.

Nakayama, H., Jorgensen, H.S., Pedersen, P.M., Raaschou, H.O., Olsen, T.S. (1997) Prevalence and risk factors of incontinence after stroke: The Copenhagen stroke study. *Stroke* 28:58–62.

Nitti, V.W., Adler, H., Combs, A.J. (2003) The role of urodynamics in the evaluation of voiding dysfunction in men after Cerebrovascular accident. *The Journal of Urology* 155:263–266.

Pak, R.W., Petrou, S.P., Staskin, D.R. (2003) Trospium chloride: A quarternary amine with unique pharmacologic properties. *Current Urology Reports* 4(6):436–440.

Patel, M., Coshall, C., Lawrence, E. (2001) Recovery from poststroke urinary incontinence: Associated factors and impact on outcome. *Journal of the American Geriatrics Society* 49:1229–1233.

Pickard, R., Reaper, J., Wyness, L., Cody, D.J., McClinton, S., N'Dow, J. (2003) Periurethral injection therapy for urinary incontinence in women. *Cochrane Database Systematic Reviews* (2):CD003881, 2003.

Rackley, R., Abdelmalak, J. (2004) Urologic applications of Botulinum toxin therapy for voiding dysfunction. *Current Urology Reports* 5:381–388.

Resnick, N.M., Yalla, S.V. (1985) Management of urinary incontinence in the elderly. *New England Journal of Medicine* 313(13):800–805.

Sakakibara, R., Shinotoh, H., Uchiyama, T., Sakuma, M., Kashiwado, M., Yoshiyama, M., Hattori, T. (2001) Questionnaire-based assessment of pelvic organ dysfunction in Parkinson's disease. *Autonomic Neuroscience: Basic & Clinical* 92:76–85.

Seki, S., Igawa, Y., Kaidoh, K. (2001) Role of dopamine D1 and D2 receptors in the micturition reflex in conscious rat. *Neurourology and Urodynamics* 20:105–113.

Siroky, M. (2003) Neurological disorders: Cerebrovascular disease and Parkinsonism. *The Urologic Clinics of North America* 30:27–47.

Taub, N.A., Wolfe, C.D., Richardson, E., Burney, P.G. (1994) Predicting the disability of first-time stroke sufferers at 1 year. 12 month follow up of a population-based cohort in southeast England. *Stroke* 25:352.

Yokoyama, O., Komatsu, K., Ishiura, Y. (1998) Change in bladder contractility associated with bladder overactivity in rats with cerebral infraction. *The Journal of Urology* 159:577–580.

Yokoyama, O., Yoshiyama, Y., Namiki, M., de Groat, W.C. (1999) Glutamatergic and dopaminergic contributions to rat bladder hyperactivity after cerebral artery occlusion. *The American Journal of Physiology* 276:R935-R942.

Wyndaele, J.J. (1993) Muscular weakness as side effect of Botulinum toxin injection for neurogenic detrusor overactivity. *Spinal Cord* 40:599–560.

Zinner, N., Gittelman, M., Harris, R., Susset, J., Kanelos, A., Auerbach, S. (2004) Trospium chloride improves overactive bladder symptoms: a multicenter phase III trial. *The Journal of Urology* 171(6 Pt 1):2311–2315.

6
Neuropsychiatry and Traumatic Brain Injury

Angela Scicutella

Introduction

Although the earliest descriptions of brain injuries date back to the ancient Egyptians (1700 B.C.) where 27 cases of head trauma are recorded in *The Edwin Smith Surgical Papyrus,* the neuropsychiatric concept that behavioral sequelae can result from brain injury was not understood, as this culture believed that the heart was the seat of emotion and thinking (Finger, 2000). Later on in the historical timeline, there appears to be some hint of recognition that the brain and human behavior may be linked when in 400 B.C., the Greek physician Hippocrates wrote *On Injuries of the Head* and described a patient with head trauma who subsequently experienced delirium and seizures (Hippocrates). More recently in 1848, the now well-known case of Phineas Gage, who suffered destruction of the left frontal lobe of his brain while at his job laying down track for a new railroad, was documented. Subsequent to his injury, he evidenced a change in personality marked by impulsivity and poor judgment. He was unable to resume his occupation where he had previously been highly regarded, as his colleagues noted, "He was no longer Gage." This landmark case in our modern era linked Gage's brain trauma as being etiologically responsible for his emotional changes (Barker, 1995). Subsequently, others such as Adolf Meyer in 1904, proposed that brain trauma from a variety of causes could lead to neuropsychiatric syndromes such as delirium, psychosis, memory problems, and mania, and he introduced the nosology "post-traumatic insanity" to try to define this phenomenon more precisely (Meyer, 1904). More recently, in 1972, the neuropsychologist Dr. Luria described the case of a Russian soldier, Leva Zasetsky, who had suffered a bullet wound to the left parieto-occipital area of his brain during combat in World War II. Dr. Luria worked with him for 25 years and recorded this patient's courageous struggle to recover some of his ability to function despite cognitive deficits and frightening hallucinations (Luria, 1972).

In the United States, about 2 million patients sustain head trauma each year due to vehicular accidents, falls, violence, or sports injuries (NIH Consensus Development Panel, 1999). Due to improved acute trauma care in hospitals, many patients survive the physical ravages of traumatic brain injury (TBI) but many subsequently experience neuropsychiatric disorders such as those described in the patients above. In this chapter, the modern neuropsychiatrist's role in the diagnosis and treatment of the psychiatric consequences of TBI such as mood and anxiety disorders, psychosis, agitation, arousal and attention, dementia, and sexual dysfunction will be reviewed.

Depression

Hopelessness and sadness are characteristic of the emotional state known as depression, which is a commonly observed neuropsychiatric condition after TBI. The psychiatrist's handbook, known as the *Diagnostic and Statistical Manual Text Revision* (DSM-IV-TR) (American Psychiatric Association, 2000), outlines the necessary symptoms which a patient must experience to be diagnosed with major depression. These include a depressed mood or loss of pleasure for 2 weeks, as well as the presence of four or more of the following symptoms: change in appetite or weight loss, insomnia or hypersomnia, fatigue or loss of energy, being restless or slowed down to a degree that is observable by others, feeling worthless, being unable to concentrate, or having suicidal thoughts, plan or attempt. However, patients suffering from various medical conditions such as TBI can have a prominent disturbance in their mood marked by many of the above characteristics and yet not fulfill the criteria for major depression. Such a patient would be categorized by DSM-IV-TR (American Psychiatric Association, 2000) criteria as having a mood disorder secondary to a general medical condition (TBI). In using this symptom profile, a study of 666 outpatients with TBI found that the three symptoms which most differentiated depressed from nondepressed patients were feeling hopeless, feeling worthless, and having difficulty enjoying activities (Seel et al., 2003).

The occurrence of depression after TBI has been estimated to be between 6% and 77% (Jorge & Robinson, 2003). Various methodological factors have been suggested to explain the wide range in statistics, including how the sample was chosen (i.e., referral to a specialty TBI clinic or a community population study); size of the sample (small or large); what subgroup of patients was assessed (i.e., mild, moderate, or severe TBI patients or some combination thereof); when studies were done in relation to injury (i.e., in the first few months after the incident or years or even decades later); what type of assessment tool was utilized (patient self-report questionnaire, family's report of the patient, or a clinician's structured diagnostic interview) (Newburn, 1998); and the medication status of patients at the time of the assessments (i.e., the effect narcotics, steroids, or benzodiazepines may have had on the rating of symptoms) (O'Donnell et al., 2003). Moreover, the diagnostic process is further complicated by the overlap between the two syndromes in that certain symptoms such as sleep and appetite changes as well as psychomotor agitation have been argued to be neurologic sequelae of the TBI itself, rather than the result of depression as a primary mood disturbance (Babin, 2003; Moldover et al., 2004).

Despite these issues in research protocols, what is significant in terms of clinical outcomes is that the risk of depression has been reported to remain elevated for decades following brain injury, as was highlighted in two recently published studies. In the first, the lifetime prevalence of major depression 50 years after closed-head injury for 520 veterans who had sustained TBI during World War II was noted to be 18.5%, while a current diagnosis of major depression was recorded in 11.2% of those same veterans (Holsinger et al., 2002). The second report of 60 patients who had been followed for 30 years post-TBI recorded a lifetime rate of major depression of 26.7%, with 10% having current illness at the time of the study (Koponen et al., 2002). However, a more recent report of TBI patients noted a decline in the frequency of psychiatric disorders over time, challenging the conclusion that the rate of psychiatric diagnoses, including depression, remains elevated years later. The researchers suggest that using cross-sectional, longitudinal, and cross-sequential assessments, where age and time post-injury are controlled for at enrollment to the study, may help to improve the accuracy of the epidemiological data in future studies with this population of patients (Ashman et al., 2004).

Several factors which have been suggested as being correlated with the development of depression after TBI include lesion location (left dorsal lateral frontal lesions and/or left basal ganglia lesions, as well as possibly parietal-occipital and right hemispheric lesions), poor social functioning (less than high school education, unstable employment, and relationship difficulties), and previous psychiatric history (depression and substance abuse) (Federoff et al., 1992; Gomez-Hernandez et al., 1997; Dikmen et al., 2004; Fann et al., 2004; Jorge et al., 2005). Since major depression among survivors of TBI is associated with diminished quality of life and poorer psychosocial functioning in studies which have examined patients in both the acute and chronic phases of TBI, the need for early recognition and treatment interventions in this patient population is a pressing one (Rapoport et al., 2003; Underhill et al., 2003; Hibbard et al., 2004).

Assessment

Assessing a patient begins with the taking of a thorough history to explore the details of the TBI incident and the subsequent treatment and hospital course which took place in the acute care setting. Past and present medical history other than TBI should be reviewed, as the clinician must consider the possibility that medical co-morbidity such as epilepsy, stroke, brain tumors, infections, endocrinologic disorders (thyroid, adrenal, and pituitary), systemic neoplasms, and cardiac or renal disease may be relevant and play a contributory role in the patient's presentation of depression. For example, a common co-morbid medical problem in TBI survivors which impacts on mood is hypopituitarism, especially growth hormone deficiency; with hormone replacement therapy, significant improvements in depression, anxiety, and fatigue have been observed (Popovic et al., 2005). A review of the patient's and his family's psychiatric history are key areas to explore, since other psychiatric disorders such as bipolar illness, anxiety syndromes, adjustment disorders, and substance abuse/dependence can either produce overlapping symptoms or be co-morbid with depression; this was observed in a recent study, where 76.7% of patients with TBI and depression also met criteria for a co-morbid anxiety disorder (Jorge et al., 2004). Pain and sleep problems are often present in TBI patients and can greatly affect mood, so a thorough assessment of these issues should also be explored when considering a possible diagnosis of depression (Branca & Lake, 2004; Oellet et al., 2004). The current medications taken by the patient must be reviewed, since many pharmacologic agents such as anticonvulsants, cardiac medications, steroids, hormones, and psychiatric medications can cause depression as a side effect. Of paramount importance to the history is an in-depth review of the patient's use of alcohol or illicit substances, as they too can play a role in the manifestation of depressive symptoms. Questions about psychosocial factors such as education, occupation, sexual history, current relationships, and avocations help the clinician to have a more complete portrait of the person as a human being, and not just a patient with TBI. To be thorough, the clinician should speak to the patient's family or friends to corroborate the history provided by the patient, so that the most accurate information guides the workup and treatment (Sadock & Sadock, 2005). Additionally, during the initial assessment process, the neuropsychiatrist should seek to communicate with other members of the treating team to discuss their observations of the patient as this may help the clinician to clarify diagnostic issues. Furthermore, this liaison approach is important in promoting a dialogue between the disciplines in order to enhance the patient's treatment as he or she progresses in the recovery process.

Pertinent to the differential diagnosis of depression in TBI patients is the syndrome of apathy (Andersson et al., 1999; Marin & Wilkosz, 2005). Symptoms such as lack of concern, emotional indifference, and reduced initiation and productivity can be assessed using the Apathy Evaluation Scale (AES) (Marin et al., 1991) in order to help differentiate mood disorder (depression) from motivational syndrome (apathy). In a recent study of 59 TBI patients, the prevalence of apathy without concomitant depression was reported to be 10.84% (Kant et al., 1998), whereas in two studies by Andersson and colleagues (Andersson et al., 1999; Andersson & Bergedalen, 2002), the prevalence of apathy in TBI patients using the AES was greater than 60%. Even across cultures, the concept of motivational deficits has been found to be a relevant construct, as was demonstrated in a later study of 80 TBI patients in a nonindustrialized country where the incidence of apathy as measured by the AES was reported to be 20% (Al-Adawi et al., 2004). Anatomically, apathy has been associated with dysfunctional activity in subcortical-frontal circuits which involve the basal ganglia, limbic structures, anterior cingulate, and prefrontal cortex (Masterman & Cummin, 1997).

In contrast to apathy, which is marked by emotional indifference, the clinician who is assessing for mood disorders should also be aware of patients with TBI who can exhibit uncontrollable outbursts of pathological laughing or crying (PLC), also known as emotional incontinence or pseudobulbar affect. These involuntary episodes are triggered by trivial stimuli which ordinarily would not result in such an extreme affective response (Zeilig et al., 1996). Since the patient's prevailing mood is neither one of depression nor euphoria, these incongruent responses can be a source of embarrassment. In a recent study, the prevalence of PLC was recorded as 10.9% during the first year after TBI (Tateno et al., 2004). Neuroanatomically, while brainstem nuclei mediate the acts of laughing and crying by integrating facial and respiratory functions, the motor cortex exerts control over the expression of these emotions. Therefore, a lesion along the pyramidal tracts between these brain regions can result in PLC (Wilson, 1924). An alternative hypothesis to account for PLC is that there is disruption of the cerebro-ponto-cerebellar pathways (Parvizi et al., 2001).

Subsequent to the history, the clinician performs a complete physical and neurologic exam, including a cognitive assessment which reviews orientation, attention, memory, language skills, visuospatial abilities, praxis, and frontal lobe tasks. During the psychiatric mental status exam, appearance, attitude, speech, motoric abnormalities (such as tremor), mood, psychotic symptoms (such as paranoia and hallucinations), homicidality (aggressive tendencies), and suicidality are assessed. This last entity must be emphasized, as a recent epidemiologic population study of TBI patients noted that the rates of death by suicide of these patients is between 2.7 and 4.1 times that of the general population (Teasdale & Engberg, 2001). Moreover, this same research indicated that the risk of suicide remained constant over the 15-year period that these patients were followed, highlighting the fact that suicide is not just an acute problem in the first few months subsequent to a devastating injury. When the three factors of hopelessness, suicidal ideation, and suicide attempts are present, the risk of suicide is increased, as was noted in another study of 172 TBI outpatients, whose post-injury suicide attempt rate over a 5-year follow-up period was 17.4% (Simpson & Tate, 2002). In more current research, patients who had a history of TBI, as well as a diagnosis of either major depression or bipolar disorder and suicidal behavior, were more likely to be males, to have a history of substance abuse, to be aggressive and hostile, and to have been diagnosed with narcissistic, borderline, antisocial, or histrionic personality disorders (Oquendo et al., 2004). After this thorough evaluation, the neuropsychiatrist may order appropriate lab tests based on his/her findings, such as a complete blood count (CBC), electrolytes, endocrine panel, electrocardiogram (EKG), electroencephalogram (EEG), and brain imaging to help clarify the diagnosis of depression.

Treatment

Drug treatment for depression in TBI patients is based on good clinical judgment, experience with psychotropic medications in other neurologic disorders, as well as limited studies and case reports on these agents in the TBI population. Pharmacotherapy should be administered at the lowest effective doses initially with gradual increases as clinically indicated, with the goal being to ameliorate target symptoms and to minimize troublesome side effects which can interfere with rehabilitation efforts and wreak havoc on the patient's quality of life. One option for treatment is the administration of tricyclic antidepressants (TCAs), which block the reuptake of norepinephrine and serotonin into the presynaptic neuron; examples of these drugs include amitriptyline (Elavil), nortriptyline (Pamelor), and desipramine (Norpramin). The latter drug was utilized in a small blinded, randomized, placebo-lead-in study and showed efficacy in improving symptoms of depression in ten patients with TBI (Wroblewski et al., 1996). Side effects of the TCAs include cardiac arrhythmias, sedation, and anticholinergic effects, such as dry mouth, confusion, and urinary retention. There is a potential for these medications to lower the seizure threshold, and therefore, in patients with TBI who are already at risk for this complication, vigilance in using the lowest doses possible should be the rule.

A newer class of antidepressant medications known as the SSRIs, which selectively inhibit serotonin reuptake by presynaptic neurons, includes fluoxetine (Prozac), sertraline (Zoloft), citalopram (Celexa), and paroxetine (Paxil); these provide another treatment choice. There are open-label studies and case reports of TBI patients whose depression improved when they were treated with the first three agents (Cassidy, 1989; Horsfield et al., 2002; Fann et al., 2000; Turner-Stokes et al., 2002; Perino et al., 2001), but there is a lack of rigorous double-blind, placebo-controlled studies using SSRIs. Recently, however, a 4-week double-blind parallel group trial with ten patients in each arm of the study was conducted involving sertraline, the stimulant methylphenidate (Ritalin) (see section below), and placebo which indicated that depressive symptoms in TBI patients improved significantly with either agent as compared to the placebo group (Lee et al., 2005). Of note, the SSRI class of medications has also been used successfully to treat PLC (Tateno et al., 2004; Muller et al., 1999). Side effects of SSRIs include diarrhea, nausea, vomiting, insomnia, sedation, tremors, and sexual dysfunction. The lack of cardiac side effects, a lower risk of inducing seizures, and fewer anticholinergic side effects makes this class a more attractive choice.

Venlafaxine (Effexor), which inhibits both serotonin and norepinephrine reuptake, has been reported anecdotally to be useful in treating depression in TBI patients. Nausea, constipation, dry mouth, and hypertension can be observed as side effects (Rao & Lyketsos, 2002). In one study there was limited evidence to recommend the treatment of TBI patients with phenelzine (Nardil), a member of the monoamine oxidase inhibitors (MAO-Is), a class of antidepressants which block the catabolism of norepinephrine and serotonin (Saran, 1985). However, with the risk of a hypertensive crisis if dietary sources of tyramine in foods such as cheese and wine are consumed, these agents are best avoided in TBI patients. Another agent, bupropion (Wellbutrin), which acts to increase the efficiency of the noradrenergic neurotransmitter systems, may be utilized in patients who have depression marked by apathy, but the risk of seizures at higher dosages of this medication makes it a less attractive choice in TBI patients (Shaughnessy, 1995).

If medications are not successful in treating depression, then electroconvulsive therapy (ECT), a nonpharmacologic option, is an alternative, as has been shown in a few case reports of TBI patients. A main concern with this therapy is that it can cause cognitive side effects which can be an issue for a TBI patient. However, the use of unilateral rather than bilateral electrodes may help to diminish this side effect (Ruedrich et al., 1983, Crow et al., 1996). Since TBI patients require support and education in order to help them cope with their injuries, psychotherapy as a treatment option for patients with depression and TBI cannot be overemphasized (Prigatano, 1991). Comprehensive neuropsychological rehabilitation programs which provide psychotherapy and cognitive remediation help to decrease symptoms of depression and anxiety in TBI patients, as has been recently demonstrated in a single-blind randomized controlled study (Tiersky et al., 2005). This topic is discussed in depth in the chapter on counseling patients with brain injury.

A related issue in the pharmacologic treatment of depression is that of sleep disturbance. The latter problem can be present as a symptom of depression or anxiety, but alternatively it can be due to a lesion in the neuronal pathways involved in regulating the sleep–wake cycle, a result of pain from the injury, or a medication side effect. If the sleep disturbance is due to depression, then sleep will likely improve when the patient is treated with one of the above-discussed antidepressant agents. However, if sleep problems persist because of other etiologies, it is recommended that adjustment of the patient's environment and sleep patterns be implemented and a trial of an agent such as trazodone (Desyrel), a relatively specific inhibitor of serotonin reuptake, be used. An important side effect to monitor with this medication is orthostatic hypotension. Hypnotics such as benzodiazepines (BZDs) (e.g., lorazepam [Ativan]) which broadly enhance gamma aminobutyric acid transmission, and non-benzodiazepines (e.g., zolpidem [Ambien]) which are selective BZD agonists, are best avoided due to side effects such as confusion, sedation, unsteady gait, and dependence issues (Oellet et al., 2004).

In patients with a predominant clinical picture of apathy rather than depression, medications which target the dopamine pathways in the brain should be utilized, since a disruption of dopamine transmission is implicated in the etiology of amotivation. Psychostimulants, which cause the release of catecholamines such as dopamine and norepinephrine from presynaptic neurons, have demonstrated benefits with regard to mood, cognition, and motivation in TBI patients, as has been noted in placebo-controlled studies of methylphenidate (Gualtieri & Evans, 1988; Plenger et al., 1996), as well as a chart review of dextroamphetamine (Cylert) (Hornstein et al., 1996). Side effects can include psychosis, anxiety, irritability, insomnia, and increases in heart rate and blood pressure. The potential for an increased rate of seizures, while present, has been uncommon clinically. Other agents which augment dopaminergic transmission and can be used in this population of patients, include amantadine (Symmetrel) (Nickels et al., 1994; van Reekum et al., 1995; Kraus & Maki, 1997), levodopa/carbidopa (Sinemet) (Lal et al., 1988), bromocriptine (Parlodel) (Muller & Von Cramon, 1994; Powell et al., 1996), and selegiline (Eldepryl) (Newburn & Newburn, 2005). Psychosis, gastrointestinal side effects and orthostatic hypotension can occur with these medications. Another option for patients with TBI and apathy is modafinil (Provigil), which promotes wakefulness and is approved for narcolepsy, but whose exact pharmacologic mechanism of action is unknown. It has shown the potential for increasing alertness and attention and improving cognition in an open-label trial of ten TBI patients (Teitelman, 2001). The most common side effect of modafinil is headache, but nausea, vomiting, and anxiety can also occur.

In addition to disruption of dopamine transmission in apathy, there is evidence to suggest that dysfunction of the cholinergic system can also lead to amotivation. This is based on the research done in Alzheimer's dementia (AD): patients with

AD are often apathetic, while biochemically they suffer from a deficiency of the neurotransmitter acetylcholine. Neuroanatomically, in both TBI and AD, cholinergic limbic–neocortical connections which are damaged can cause interference in the integration of cognitive and emotional processes (Cummings & Back, 1998). Therefore, cholinergic agents such as acetylcholinesterase-inhibitors (AchE-Is) which temporarily disrupt the hydrolysis of acetylcholine and thus increase its concentration in the synapse, have been shown to be beneficial in improving apathy in AD patients (Cummings, 2000). With this rationale, it was demonstrated that in one uncontrolled trial of four TBI patients in which the AchE-I donepezil (Aricept) was used, apathy scores on a structured rating scale improved (Griffin et al., 2003). Side effects of the AchE-Is include nausea, vomiting, and diarrhea. A patient example is provided to highlight some of these clinical issues.

A 53-year-old female was found unconscious at the bottom of a staircase in her home. In the emergency department, a head computerized tomography (CT) revealed an epidural hematoma of the right frontal-temporal region as well as bilateral frontal contusions. Several months later during her rehabilitation at a TBI unit, she was noted by the therapists working with her to have frequent crying spells and to be despondent over her cognitive deficits. During sessions she was often amotivated, displayed poor self-esteem, and complained of low energy and difficulty with concentration. After neuropsychiatric assessment, this patient was diagnosed with depression secondary to TBI, as the rest of the medical workup was negative. She was treated with an SSRI with improvement of her tearfulness, overall mood, and a notable increase in her participation in her rehabilitation classes.

Mania

After TBI, patients can experience an elevated mood state which is referred to as mania. In DSM-IV-TR (American Psychiatric Association, 2000) nosology this is defined as an elevated, expansive, or irritable mood which lasts at least 1 week. When the patient has an elevated mood, three of the following symptoms must also be present to make the diagnosis of mania, while when an irritable mood predominates, four additional symptoms are required. These include inflated self-esteem, decreased sleep, pressured speech, racing thoughts, poor attention, an increase in goal-related activity, and excessive involvement in pleasurable activities (e.g., spending sprees or sexual indiscretions) which could have painful repercussions. DSM-IV-TR (American Psychiatric Association, 2000) diagnostic categorization would classify such a patient as having bipolar I disorder. However, patients suffering from various medical conditions such as TBI can have an expansive or irritable mood and yet not meet full criteria for a manic episode or bipolar disorder. In such a case, mood disorder secondary to a general medical condition would be the diagnosis given. Secondary mania is a concept similar to the preceding one, and was first described by Klerman and Krauthammer (1978), who observed patients without previous psychiatric history who developed a psychotic disorder after a medical illness. Their definition of this syndrome included an elated or irritable mood in addition to only two of the above listed criteria.

The occurrence of mania after TBI has been estimated to be far less frequent than depression, in the range of 1.6–9% (Silver et al., 2001; Jorge et al., 1993). A recent study of 60 patients followed 30 years post-TBI revealed only one patient (1.7%) with a diagnosis of bipolar II disorder (Koponen et al., 2002), which by definition is an episode of depression and, at some time, an episode of hypomania (same symptoms as mania but the duration is at least 4 days but less than 1 week) (American Psychiatric Association, 2000). Although it is less likely to occur, some TBI patients have also been observed to experience rapid-cycling bipolar disorder in which at least four manic, hypomanic, or depressive episodes occur within 12 months (Monji et al., 1999; Murai & Fujimoto, 2003). Anatomically, an association has been made in TBI patients suffering from symptoms of mania and lesions which occur mainly in the right basotemporal or orbitofrontal regions (Jorge et al., 1993; Starkstein et al., 1988). However, several new case studies have noted TBI patients suffering manic episodes after left frontal or bilateral temporal lesions (Heinrich & Junig, 2004; Mustafa et al., 2005).

Assessment

When obtaining the history, the clinician should consider other medical conditions (In addition to TBI) which could present with symptoms of mania, such as epilepsy, brain tumors, central nervous system infections, thyroid disease, renal disease, and vitamin deficiencies. Other psychiatric illnesses to be screened for include substance abuse, since manic symptoms can be observed in patients who use opioids, hallucinogens, and cocaine. Diagnoses such as borderline or antisocial personality disorders also need to be considered since overlapping features of these syndromes such as irritability, aggressiveness, and impulsivity can mimic the manic state (Sadock & Sadock, 2005). Obtaining a list of medications, including over-the-counter preparations is essential, since agents such as antidepressants, steroids, and herbal preparations such as St. John's Wort and ginkgo biloba can precipitate manic symptoms as was reported in a recent case study of a TBI patient (Spinella & Eaton, 2002). The clinician's observations and findings after taking a careful history and neuropsychiatric evaluation (as outlined in the previous section on depression) will guide the ordering of appropriate tests such as brain imaging, lab tests, or EEG to further clarify the diagnosis.

Treatment

With the completion of this workup, the neuropsychiatrist is left with the decision of choosing an appropriate agent to treat the manic symptoms experienced by TBI patients. The literature in this area is sparse as there are no double-blind randomized placebo-controlled studies. Instead, clinical judgment is guided by the treatment of classical bipolar disorder and case reports of patients with TBI (Kennedy et al., 2001). Anticonvulsants such as valproic acid (Depakote) and car-bamazepine (Tegretol) have been used successfully in the treatment of the TBI manic patient and may be particularly good options if there is the presence of a seizure disorder as well (Monji et al., 1999; Pope et al., 1988; Stewart & Hemsath, 1988; Sayal et al., 2000; Kim & Humaran, 2002). Side effects of the former agent include weight gain, thrombocytopenia (low platelet count), and hepatic dysfunction while the latter can cause hyponatremia (low serum sodium) and hematologic dysfunction. Other anticonvulsants such as lamotrigine (Lamictal) and topiramate (Topamax) have also been shown to successfully treat bipolar disorder but there have been no studies which have used these agents in patients with TBI and mania (Calabrese et al., 1999; Marcotte, 1998). Side effects of lamotrigine include dizziness, sedation, ataxia, and most importantly, rash, which can then evolve into the potentially fatal condition known as Stevens–Johnson syndrome. Adverse effects of topiramate include sedation, decreased appetite, speech disorders, and cognitive impairment. Gabapentin (Neurontin) may also be a reasonable choice to treat manic symptoms based on its use in agitation with other types of neurologically impaired patients (Roane et al., 2000). However, as with the other pharmacologic agents already described, there are no controlled studies of its use with TBI patients. Common side effects of gabapentin include fatigue and dizziness. Although the mood stabilizer lithium (Eskalith) is used in classical bipolar disorder with much success and has been recommended for mania in relation to TBI, much caution must be utilized with this agent, as it can cause neurologic side effects such as tremor, ataxia, and confusion, which can worsen the condition of a TBI patient (Hale & Donaldson, 1982). In a placebo-controlled trial of one patient who suffered bilateral orbito-frontal and right temporo-parietal contusions, clonidine, an alpha-adrenergic receptor agonist which reduces the firing rate of noradrenergic neurons, successfully reversed the patient's manic symptoms (Bakchine et al., 1989). Side effects to monitor include dry mouth and eyes, sedation, hypotension, and constipation. The patient case below demonstrates some of these clinical features.

A 76-year-old male falls outside his internist's office and loses consciousness. The patient is rushed to the emergency room where a head CT reveals a right-frontal-temporal-parietal hemorrhage. A craniotomy is performed to evacuate the hemorrhage, and postoperatively, the patient does well. At home a few weeks later, he becomes agitated and accuses his wife of having affairs with several men in their apartment building. His wife noted that prior to this incident he had not been sleeping well for several nights. The patient is loud, irritable, and argumentative; and his speech is difficult to interrupt. His thoughts race from one topic to another and he grandiosely proclaims to anyone who will listen, that his doctor actually hit him over the head to cause the head injury in order to rob his money. After a neuropsychiatric evaluation, the patient was treated with valproic acid, which resulted in a decrease in his irritability and agitation.

Anxiety

Anxiety refers to a state of apprehension, uneasiness, or dread that occurs in anticipation of either internal or external threats which are perceived as unpredictable or uncontrollable. The four subcategories of anxiety in the DSM-IV-TR (American Psychiatric Association, 2000) include panic disorder (PD), obsessive-compulsive disorder (OCD), post-traumatic stress disorder (PTSD), and generalized anxiety disorder (GAD). When features of anxiety syndromes are present secondary to medical conditions such as in TBI, then anxiety secondary to medical illness is the DSM-IV-TR diagnosis to be used, as often the patient may have characteristics of several different types of anxiety syndromes present simultaneously (Hiott & Labbate, 2002). To understand the diagnostic issues involved better, each subcategory of anxiety will be described.

Panic attacks are defined as discrete periods of intense fear which develop abruptly and reach a peak within 10 minutes with the presence of at least 4 of the following 13 symptoms: palpitations, sweating, trembling, shortness of breath, the sensation of choking, chest pain, abdominal discomfort, dizziness, de-realization, chills, paresthesia, and fear of loss of control or death. To qualify for a diagnosis of PD, the patient must have recurrent panic attacks and be worried about having further episodes or be concerned about the consequences of an attack for at least one month after the initial panic attack. In some patients, the fear of having a panic attack in a situation or place from which they cannot escape creates marked discomfort and avoidant behavior known as agoraphobia (American Psychiatric Association, 2000). There are a limited number of studies where TBI and PD have been evaluated, and often this anxiety diagnosis is co-morbid with depression and alcohol dependence, as was observed by Deb and colleagues (Deb et al., 1999), who reported a 9% rate of PD in 120 patients aged 18–64 years 1 year after TBI. In several other epidemiologic studies which examined the frequency of anxiety diagnoses in patients with a TBI history, the rates of PD have been reported as 3.2%, 8.3%, and 11%, respectively, depending on whether lifetime prevalence (former) or post-TBI onset (latter two) was recorded (Silver et al., 2001; Koponen et al., 2002; Hibbard et al., 1998). Neuroanatomically the brain stem, limbic system, and prefrontal cortex have been implicated in the etiology of panic attacks (Scheutzow & Wiercisiewski, 1999).

In the DSM nomenclature (American Psychiatric Association, 2000), OCD is characterized by recurrent obsessions or compulsions that are excessive or unreasonable. Obsessions manifest as persistent impulses thoughts or images that are intrusive, inappropriate, and time-consuming, while compulsions are repetitive behaviors (checking, ordering) or mental acts (praying, counting) that the patient feels driven to perform in order to reduce the distress of the obsession. Two recent epidemiologic studies have reported rates of OCD from as low as 4.7% to as high as 14% in patients who had sustained TBI (Silver et al., 2001; Hibbard et al., 1998). Anatomically, the etiology of OCD has been linked to dysfunction of the orbital frontal cortex and subcortical circuits (Baxter et al., 1992; Grados, 2003). A study of ten patients with TBI and OCD observed that they exhibited a high frequency of obsessions which involved contamination and sexual themes as well as the need for symmetry and exactness. In addition to compulsive exercising, these patients also displayed cleaning/washing, checking and repeating compulsions. Co-morbid psychiatric diagnoses such as depression and other anxiety disorders were common, while on neuropsychological testing, these patients showed poor performance on general intelligence, attention, learning, memory, word-retrieval, and executive functions (Berthier et al., 2001).

PTSD in relation to TBI is an entity about which there has been much debate, since one of the essential criteria is that the patient who has been exposed to a threatening event must display re-experiencing symptoms, such as intrusive memories or distress when reminded about the particular trauma, recurrent dreams of the event, or the feeling that the trauma is recurring. Given that many TBI patients do not recall the event due to post-traumatic amnesia, which is a short interval after injury where the capacity to store and retrieve new information is lacking, one can argue that theoretically PTSD cannot occur in these patients. A study by Warden and colleagues reviewed 47 active-duty service members who had sustained moderate TBI with amnesia for the event. Using strict PTSD criteria, none of these patients qualified for the diagnosis, since no patient reported re-experiencing phenomena. However, when that part of the criteria was eliminated, then six patients (12.7%) received a diagnosis of PTSD (Warden et al., 1997). In a recent report of 100 patients involved in traffic accidents who sustained head injury with definite loss of consciousness, 48% reported PTSD at 3 months after the incident, and 33% suffered with this disorder one year later (Mayou et al., 2000). Some mechanisms to explain PTSD when there is a lack of recall of the traumatic event itself include: (1) recall of other distressing experiences associated with the event which occurred either before or after the period of amnesia that then serves as the "trauma"; (2) traumatic experiences may be processed by the limbic area of the brain at an implicit level outside awareness; and (3) learning of the traumatic event as told by others helps the patient to reconstruct the memory (Bryant, 2001; McNeil & Greenwood, 1996). Additional diagnostic criteria for PTSD include dissociative symptoms (de-realization, depersonalization, dissociative amnesia), marked avoidance of thoughts, feelings, or reminders of the trauma, as well as marked arousal, which can be observed as insomnia, irritability, poor concentration, hypervigilance, or a heightened startle response. To qualify for a diagnosis, these symptoms must cause impairment in functioning.

A more recently published epidemiologic study reported the rate of GAD in patients after TBI to be 1.7% (Koponen et al., 2002), but this is in contrast to other research which has noted rates in the range of 8–24% (Hibbard et al., 1998; Van Reekum et al., 1996; Fann et al., 1995). This syndrome is marked by excessive worry and anxiety about a number of issues that occur almost daily for at least 6 months. The patient is unable to control the worry and experiences at least three of six somatic symptoms which include restlessness, being easily fatigued, diminished concentration, irritability, muscle tension, or sleep disturbance. The symptoms of anxiety experienced by patients with TBI are usually attributed to the loss that patients feel in terms of their independence as well as the relation to their prior level of high functioning.

Assessment

During the evaluation of a patient with symptoms of anxiety, the neuropsychiatrist first obtains a thorough history from the patient and his family about the various situations in which apprehension is experienced, any pattern of avoidance behavior, and accompanying physical symptoms of anxiety such as those listed above in the descriptions of anxiety disorders. As there are many medical imposters of anxiety, such as cardiac, pulmonary, and endocrinologic disorders, the neuropsychiatrist must differentiate between these diagnostic challenges. In this population of patients with TBI, seizures are a particular concern for the clinician, since the presentation of seizures can mimic anxiety syndromes. For example, during the ictus, intense fear and dread can be the sole expression of a simple partial seizure or the aura of a complex partial seizure, while OCD symptoms such as perseverative thoughts (forced thinking) can also be experienced as the aura of a seizure (Scicutella, 2001). From the standpoint of the psychiatric differential diagnosis, the clinician must consider that the patient is suffering from more than one anxiety disorder or depression. In addition, certain personality disorders may overlap with a particular type of anxiety such as borderline in PTSD or obsessive-compulsive personality disorder with OCD. In GAD and PTSD, since there is the presence of autonomic hyperarousal, the clinician must consider the possibility of the abuse of stimulants or withdrawal from alcohol and sedatives. After a careful neuropsychiatric evaluation, the physician may also need to perform laboratory tests, including a CBC, metabolic studies, an endocrinologic screen, EKG, EEG, and brain imaging if warranted, to rule out medical etiologies of anxiety (Sadock & Sadock, 2005).

Treatment

Once the neuropsychiatrist has determined the type of anxiety that the patient is suffering from, the issue of treatment must be addressed. Because no randomized placebo-controlled studies of anxiety disorders in TBI patients have been done, the general pharmacologic principles for treating anxiety disorders in patients without neurologic compromise are used, with attention to dosing regimens, side effect profiles, and drug–drug interactions. The TCAs and SSRIs have been shown to be efficacious in the treatment of the four types of anxiety disorders (Janicak et al., 1993). In case reports of patients who have suffered TBI and anxiety, the successful use of SSRIs such as sertraline in the treatment of panic attacks (Scheutzow & Wiercisiewski et al., 1999) and fluoxetine to treat OCD (Stengler-Wenzke & Muller, 2002) has been demonstrated. Venlafaxine produced almost complete remission of compulsions in one patient with OCD after an epidural hematoma (Khouzam & Donnelly, 1998); this same agent has also been shown to be effective in the treatment of GAD (Derivan et al., 1998). Side effects of these medications have been reviewed previously. Additionally, TBI patients with GAD may respond to treatment with buspirone (Buspar), a partial serotonin (1A) agonist, whose side effects include nausea, dry mouth, dizziness, and nervousness (Gualtieri, 1991). Propranolol (Inderal), a beta-blocker, which reduces adrenergic receptor activation, can also be utilized in treating patients with GAD; its adverse reactions include weakness, hypotension, nausea, and depression (Emilien & Maloteaux, 1998). The BZD class of medications, of which lorazepam (Ativan) is an example, can be useful for treating PD and GAD, but the potential for tolerance, dependence, sedation, ataxia, memory disturbances, and occasional paradoxical disinhibition make this class less attractive for treating patients with TBI (Spier et al., 1986). MAO-I antidepressants have been of benefit in treating PTSD in patients without TBI. In addition to the potential for a hypertensive crisis as discussed earlier, more common side effects of these medications include orthostatic hypotension, edema, weight gain, insomnia, and sexual dysfunction (Sheehan et al., 1980). On occasion, antiepileptic drugs have been used to treat anxiety, but these are not first-line treatments and there are no studies using these agents in TBI patients specifically. For example, valproic acid has been used to treat PD (Woodman & Noyes, 1994), carbamazepine was successfully used to treat OCD (Koopowitz & Berk, 1997), and studies with lamotrigine (Hertzberg et al., 1999) and gabapentin (Hamner et al., 2001) have indicated some benefit in those patients suffering from PTSD. Side effects of these agents have been discussed previously. The neuropsychiatrist should also emphasize the beneficial role of psychotherapy, biofeedback, and support groups for TBI patients with anxiety in order to help them to better cope with their symptoms (Holland et al., 1999). The clinical case which follows describes some of these points.

A 70-year-old man fell off a 10-foot ladder while working at home and sustained a right temporal hemorrhagic contusion. A few months later, his family notes that he cannot stay in a closed room for any length of time. He becomes shaky, restless, and short of breath and needs to get out of the room urgently or he becomes agitated and will yell at his family. He also reports excessive worry about whether his grandchildren are safe, and he fears that they may hurt themselves. The patient is referred to the neuropsychiatrist for assessment and due to symptoms of both PD and GAD he was treated with a member of the SSRI class with marked improvement of his symptoms.

Psychosis

Psychosis is defined as the inability to distinguish reality from fantasy; or to put it another way, the psychotic patient demonstrates impaired reality testing. Clinically one can observe that patients have a thought disorder, or they may experience perceptual disturbances such as hallucinations, delusions, or paranoid ideation (Sadock & Sadock, 2005). In the DSM-IV-TR (American Psychiatric Association, 2000), psychosis is not a separate diagnostic category, but rather is a feature of a variety of other psychiatric disorders, including delirium and schizophrenia, which are particularly germane to a discussion of head trauma as will be discussed below.

Due to methodologic problems in the research of psychosis and TBI, including the type of population of patients used in studies (e.g., adults, children, open or closed head injuries) as well as the lack of standardized diagnostic criteria and variable periods of follow-up, it is difficult to assess the precise incidence and prevalence rates for psychosis and TBI (Arciniegas et al., 2003). An often-quoted study is that of Davison and Bagley, who in 1969 reviewed medical reports published between 1917 and 1960 and recorded that the rates of psychosis in these studies ranged from 0.07% to 9.8% (Davison & Bagley, 1969). Of interest are the disparate rates of psychosis recorded in two studies where follow-up had been lengthy; in a 10–15-year study, a rate of 20% was noted and in a longer 30-year study, 1.7% was recorded (Thomsen, 1984, Koponen et al., 2002). Risk factors predictive for the development of psychosis in TBI patients include premorbid neurologic or neurodevelopmental disorders as well as having sustained a head injury before adolescence (Fujii & Ahmed, 2001). A family history of psychosis in first-degree relatives and duration of loss of consciousness were also significantly associated with psychosis post-TBI (Sachdev et al., 2001). In a recent review of 69 published case studies of psychosis after TBI, certain features emerge which appear to be typical for this phenomenon: (1) it is more commonly observed in males; (2) persecutory or paranoid delusions are the most common type of psychotic symptoms, but auditory hallucinations are also frequently observed; (3) approximately 50% of patients demonstrate symptoms before the second year after TBI, while about 75% evidence psychosis within the first four years after TBI; and (4) abnormalities as recorded by EEG were most commonly temporal slowing, whereas brain imaging demonstrated frontal lobe lesions most often, but temporal lobe lesions were also observed (Fujii & Ahmed, 2002). Cognitively, patients with TBI and psychosis demonstrate impairments on neuropsychological testing in general intelligence, verbal memory, executive function, and vocabulary (Fujii et al., 2004).

Assessment

During the assessment of the patient with psychosis, the neuropsychiatrist once again explores the recent TBI incident and the course of events during the acute hospitalization, including episodes of delirium, the latter of which is a period of acute disturbance in consciousness marked by attentional and cognitive deficits, as well as perceptual disturbances such as delusions or hallucinations (American Psychiatric Association, 2000). The patient's medical history is reviewed for other potential etiologies of psychosis such as prior head injuries, infections, vitamin deficiencies, metabolic disease, strokes, or tumors. Particularly relevant in this differential diagnosis is post-traumatic epilepsy, which is often observed as a sequelae of TBI. Moreover, a frequent complication of temporal lobe epilepsy is psychosis, which can occur prior to (aura), during (ictally), or after the seizure (postictally, either periictally or interictally) (Trimble, 1991). Medications such as steroids and anticholinergic drugs (e.g., TCAs) can cause psychotic symptoms and should be reviewed.

Psychiatric diagnoses to consider in the psychotic patient with TBI include substance or alcohol abuse/dependence, mood disorders with psychotic features, dementia with hallucinations or delusions, and personality disorders such as paranoid type. Of particular importance in this category is schizophrenia, which is defined in DSM-IV-TR (American Psychiatric Association, 2000) by a period of at least 6 months of social or occupational dysfunction in which two or more of the following symptoms are present: (1) delusions; (2) hallucinations; (3) disorganized speech; (4) disorganized behavior; (5) lack of affect and avolition. In the context of TBI, there may be overlap with schizophrenia, since patients with the latter disorder may have sustained undocumented head injuries, or conversely, patients with schizophrenia may have cognitive deficits which make them more prone to sustain head injury. In these cases, it may be difficult to assess whether the head injury or schizophrenia is the etiology of the psychosis (Malaspina et al., 2001).

After a thorough history, the neuropsychiatrist proceeds with the physical, neurologic, cognitive, and mental status evaluation. Appropriate laboratory tests to perform include a CBC, metabolic panel, urine toxicology for substances, and when clinically indicated, EEG and brain imaging as well. If other etiologies cannot explain the patient's symptoms and it appears that the TBI is the cause of the psychosis, then the DSM-IV-TR diagnosis of psychotic disorder secondary to a general medical condition would be given.

Treatment

From a treatment standpoint, psychotic symptoms are treated with antipsychotic medications, also known as neuroleptics. As there are no randomized placebo-controlled studies of the treatment of psychotic syndromes occurring in the context of TBI, more general pharmacologic principles utilized in treating psychosis are employed. If the patient is judged to be in a state of delirium as when the patient is emerging from coma or due to another medical problem such as infection, then typical antipsychotics (dopamine receptor antagonists) such as haloperidol (Haldol) have traditionally been the drugs of choice. However, there is some controversy about using haloperidol in TBI patients due to a few reports that it negatively impacts on post-traumatic amnesia duration and cognition (Rao et al., 1985; Stanislav, 1997). Nevertheless, short-term use in delirium to improve confusion and psychosis, with appropriate tapering and discontinuation of the neuroleptic when the delirium clears, is acceptable. Side effects to be aware of include extra-pyramidal symptoms (EPS) (tremor, cogwheeling, and bradykinesia), dystonia (slow, sustained muscular contractions), akathisia (restlessness) (Sadock & Sadock, 2005), and the rarer but more serious outcome, neuroleptic malignant syndrome (NMS), which is marked by hyperthermia, rigidity, autonomic instability, and confusion (Kadyan et al., 2003). Tardive dyskinesia (TD) marked by involuntary movements of the head, limbs, and trunk can be observed as a delayed side effect of these medications usually only after years of treatment. Another concern is the fact that neuroleptics can lower the seizure threshold, making TBI patients potentially more prone to sustaining a seizure (Sadock & Sadock, 2005).

If psychosis develops at a point later in time and is unrelated to delirium, then it is advised to use atypical antipsychotics (serotonin-dopamine antagonists) which have less potential to cause EPS symptoms (Elovic et al., 2003). The common choices are risperidone (Risperdal), olanzapine (Zyprexa), quetiapine (Seroquel), and clozapine (Clozaril). Beneficial use of these agents, specifically in patients suffering from psychosis after TBI, has been recorded in a few case reports (Michals et al., 1993; Schreiber et al., 1998; Butler, 2000). Side effects to monitor with these medications include orthostatic hypotension, sedation, weight gain, hyperlipidemia, and impaired glucose tolerance. With clozapine, in particular, the increased risk of seizures and agranulocytosis make it a less attractive choice (Shaughnessy, 1995; Michals et al., 1993; Labbate & Warden, 2000). More recently there has been an association of an increased risk of stroke in patients who were treated with these medications for behavioral problems in dementia (Herrmann & Lanctot, 2005). Since patients with TBI may eventually go on to develop dementia over time, further research will be needed to guide the prescribing practice of these agents in this subset of patients. If low-potency typical antipsychotics such as chlorpromazine (Thorazine) or thioridazine (Mellaril) are utilized, EPS is less of an issue, but anticholinergic side effects are more problematic as they too can exacerbate cognitive deficits which may already be present in the traumatic brain injury population (Stanislav, 1997). A case study follows to illustrate some of these clinical points.

A 39-year-old male suffered traumatic brain injury as a result of a motor vehicle accident with brain damage in the right frontal-temporal brain regions. Subsequently, he developed delusions about being attacked by sharks and believed that he was no longer on earth but resided on Mars. These perceptions caused his attention to wander during therapy sessions and so a neuropsychiatry consult was sought. After a thorough evaluation, the patient was prescribed an atypical antipsychotic with a subsequent decrease in his delusional thinking and improvement in his ability to participate in his rehabilitation program.

Agitation

Agitation is a frequent behavioral problem associated with TBI patients and has been a source of debate in the field due to the lack of agreement about a standardized clinical definition. Since DSM-IV-TR (American Psychiatric Association, 2000) lacks a specific category for agitation, the closest approximation being personality change secondary to TBI (aggressive type), a proposal has been made to create a new diagnostic label, that of aggression, which could be subdivided into acute and chronic types. The former would be defined as lasting from a few weeks up to a few months and be essentially synonymous with delirium, while the latter would refer to the persistence of inappropriate verbal or physical behaviors beyond the two month time-frame (Silver et al., 2005). From the physiatry literature, an interdisciplinary definition has been suggested that would incorporate the elements of delirium, post-traumatic amnesia, and excesses of behavior that include some combination of aggression (verbal or physical), akathisia, disinhibition, and emotional lability (Sandel & Mysiw, 1996).

One way to help standardize the definition of agitation would be the utilization of valid and reliable scales, an example of which is the Agitated Behavior Scale (ABS) (Corrigan, 1989). This instrument includes 14 items which rate the patient's behavior in a variety of areas such as attention, impulsivity, irritability, violence, anger, wandering, pulling at tubes, and self-stimulating or self-abusing actions. Each observable behavior is rated from 1 to 4 (absent, slight, moderate, or extreme) with a cumulative score greater than 36 considered to be in the severe range of agitation. Another of these instruments is the Overt Agitation Scale (OAS), which measures verbal aggression as well as physical aggression to self, objects, and people. Each of these four areas is rated in a range from mild to severe (Brooke et al., 1992).

The incidence of agitation has been reported to be from 35% to 96% (Levin & Grossman, 1978; Rao et al., 1985) in the acute recovery period after TBI, and from 31% to 71% in patients who were followed 1–15 years after sustaining TBI (Oddy et al., 1985; McKinlay et al., 1981). A more current study of 158 subjects in an acute-care rehabilitation setting, most of whom had severe TBI, demonstrated that approximately 50% of these patients had post-traumatic agitation as measured by the ABS; this study noted that there were no statistically significant differences as regards to gender in terms of the frequency, duration, or presentation and extent of the post-TBI agitation (Kadyan et al., 2004). In another recent study by Tateno and colleagues (Tateno et al., 2003), it was found that 33.7% of 89 patients demonstrated significant aggressive behavior when measured with the OAS 6 months after their injury. Furthermore, the aggressive behavior was significantly associated with major depression, a history of alcohol or drug abuse, frontal lobe lesions, and poorer social functioning. The enormity of this problem is emphasized in a study by Bogner and colleagues, who reported that the presence of agitation in TBI patients receiving treatment in an acute rehabilitation center, was predictive of a longer length of stay and a decrease in functional independence from a cognitive standpoint at discharge (Bogner et al., 2001). Anatomically, agitation or aggression may be explained by damage to a number of different brain areas such as the hypothalamus, amygdala, medial temporal lobe, or orbito-frontal cortex as these regions and their connections are involved in the regulation of emotion (Arciniegas & Beresford, 2001).

Assessment

In acute agitation, the neuropsychiatrist must first assess if there are other underlying medical conditions (in addition to TBI) such as infections, metabolic imbalances, or medications such as narcotics, anticholinergic agents, or steroids which can be contributing to the patient's delirium. To treat the symptoms of acute agitation, neuroleptics such as haloperidol are used. Droperidol (Inapsine), an antipsychotic agent similar to halperidol, was recently reported to be effective in treating acute agitation in 27 patients with TBI (Stanislav & Childs, 2000). Other medications sometimes used in the acute setting include the BZDs such as lorazepam (Mysiw & Sandel, 1997). In a recent report of 11 TBI patients who were between 4 and 23 days post-injury, the treatment for acute agitation was the combined use of amantadine, methylphenidate, and trazodone. All the patients were noted to have resolution of their agitation as well as improvement in their cognitive function (Rosati, 2002). Additional randomized, controlled prospective studies are needed to determine the efficacy of this treatment approach.

The neuropsychiatrist who is asked to evaluate a patient with the chronic form of agitation in his/her office will need to take a thorough history and perform a complete neuropsychiatric examination as well as any necessary laboratory studies in order to be able to rule out other medical problems which may be the underlying etiology for the agitation. Included in the possible diagnoses would be a new episode of delirium, being post-ictal, pain syndromes, and the use of alcohol or illicit drugs. Psychiatric diagnoses in which aggression can be seen include major depression, bipolar disorder, anxiety disorders such as PTSD and GAD, and personality disorders such as antisocial type (Silver et al., 2005).

Treatment

There are few pharmacological agents with prospective studies of a randomized, placebo-controlled design which can definitively guide the treatment of agitation in TBI patients, but the beta-blocker propranolol and the stimulant methylphenidate have been exceptions in this regard. In separate studies of propranolol, it has been shown that there is either a statistically significant reduction in the maximum intensity of the episodes of agitation (Brooke et al., 1992) or in the actual number of aggressive episodes which occur (Greendyke et al., 1986). Stimulants such as methylphenidate have been used successfully to treat temper outbursts marked by belligerence and hostility in 38 male patients who had sustained TBI 2 years prior to the study (Mooney & Haas, 1993). Amantadine, a dopaminergic agent has been demonstrated to be of benefit in the treatment of aggressive behavior in TBI patients as noted in case reports (Chandler et al., 1988) as well as in a retrospective case analysis (Nickels et al., 1994). The anticonvulsants including carbamazepine (Kennedy et al., 2001; Azouvi et al., 1999; Chatham-Showalter, 1996), valproic acid (Wroblewski et al., 1997), gabapentin (Rybach & Rybach, 1995), and lamotrigine (Pachet et al., 2003) provide another option in the treatment of TBI patients with agitation, as has also been reported in case reports and open-label trials. Antidepressants, such as sertraline in the SSRI class (Kant et al., 1998), amitriptyline in the TCA group (Mysiw et al., 1988), trazodone (Rowland et al., 1992), and bupropion (Teng et al., 2001) have been noted to be useful in treating agitation and aggression in this population as well. Buspirone, in the anxiolytic class, has been observed to be effective in the treatment of angry outbursts and behavioral problems in TBI patients (Gualtieri, 1991; Holzer, 1998). The side effects of all these medications have been previously reviewed. Although other agents such as the mood stabilizer lithium (Glenn et al., 1989) or the benzodiazepines (Freinhar & Alvarez, 1986) have been used in the management of agitation, these medications are probably best avoided in the TBI population due to the potential neurotoxic effects (tremor, delirium, and seizures) of the former agent and possible cognitive disturbances (attention, alertness and memory) of the latter (Perna, 2004). The use of ECT as an alternative treatment to medication was found to help one patient with severe TBI and behavioral disturbance when he proved unresponsive to a variety of psychopharmacologic agents (Kant et al., 1995).

Finally, the neuropsychiatrist should also work in conjunction with the therapists on the rehabilitation team in order to be aware of the behavioral approaches which are being utilized to help the patient deal with agitation and aggression (Rothwell et al., 1999). These can include altering the environment to decrease provocative stressors, coping skills training, and behavior modification involving reinforcements for appropriate behavior (Watson et al., 2001). The family members should also be encouraged to seek supportive psychotherapy to help them cope with the injured loved one's behavioral disturbance and personality changes. A patient case can highlight some of these points.

A 70-year-old woman sustained head trauma when her car was broadsided by a truck. She sustained a left hemispheric subarachnoid hemorrhage with extension into the bilateral sylvian fissures as well as a left parietal/occipital subdural hematoma. Several months later when the patient was at the subacute rehabilitation facility, she became very angry when she felt that the staff did not appreciate that her abilities to perform tasks were much better than the rest of the patients there. She believed that she did not belong in the facility and was often packing her bags and threatening to leave the building. On one occasion, she ran out of the therapist's office into the parking lot with the staff in pursuit, and in another incident, while on a weekend pass to visit family, she refused to get in her daughter's car to be driven back to the rehabilitation center. She was physically aggressive towards family members, including biting, kicking, and hitting them. After evaluation with the neuropsychiatrist, valproic acid was used to treat the patient and she demonstrated a dramatic improvement in behavioral dyscontrol.

Arousal and Attention

When a patient sustains TBI, the physiologic state known as arousal, which is defined by the level of wakefulness and the intensity of stimulation needed to elicit a meaningful response by the individual, can be altered by varying degrees. Whereas in normal consciousness, the person is fully awake and able to respond cognitively and emotionally to both internal needs as well as to external stimuli, the drowsy patient sustains wakefulness only with the application of some form of external stimuli. These patients are often inattentive and confused. At the level of stupor, a patient can only be roused by vigorously repeated and often noxious stimuli; once the stimulus ceases the patient lapses back into unresponsiveness. The comatose patient appears to be asleep and incapable of being aroused by either external stimuli or their own internal needs, while the patient in a vegetative state undergoes alternate sleep–wake cycles, but doesn't regain awareness or purposeful behavior. When this condition extends beyond 1 month, the term *persistent vegetative state* is applied (Adams et al., 1997; Mesulam, 2000).

Overlapping with this concept is that of attention, since the ability to attend or concentrate on stimuli is predicated on one's degree of arousal. Impaired attention is a problem frequently observed in patients who have suffered TBI and its impact upon rehabilitation efforts is profound, since other cognitive processes such as encoding and storing items in memory, problem-solving, and language skills are dependent upon one's ability to focus on various stimuli (Stierwalt & Murray, 2002). The construct of attention is further divided into: (1) basic attention or the capacity to orient to simple stimuli; (2) selective attention, or the ability to prioritize some stimuli over others; (3) sustained attention, or vigilance, which represents the capacity to maintain attentional focus over time; and (4) divided attention, in which one must respond to or process multiple stimuli simultaneously (Niemann et al., 1996). Often after TBI, the basic attention abilities recover, but psychometric testing in a few recent studies reveal that TBI patients, several years post-injury, still struggle with cognitively challenging tasks when impairments in divided and sustained attention persisted (Stierwalt & Murray, 2002; Mangels et al., 2002; Dockree et al., 2004; Vanderploeg et al., 2005).

Anatomically, the arousal and attentional systems are complex and widely distributed through the brain and involve the ascending reticular formation of the brain stem, which extends from the medulla to the midbrain: the hypothalamus, thalamus, basal forebrain, limbic system, anterior cingulate, and parietal, temporal, and prefrontal cortical areas. Damage to any of these regions via mechanical injury or diffuse axonal impairment can disrupt the various neurotransmitter pathways (noradrenergic, dopaminergic, and cholinergic) which play key roles in the modulation of arousal and attention (Mesulam, 2000). Evidence for the latter neurotransmitter's role in this cognitive domain was highlighted in a recent study of TBI patients whose neuropsychological profile demonstrated decreases in sustained attention and reaction times while the morphometric analysis of their brain imaging revealed reduced gray matter density in the regions of all the major cholinergic pathways (Salmond et al., 2005).

Assessment

The neuropsychiatrist who evaluates the patient with arousal and attention deficits needs to conduct a thorough history with regard to factors which can induce a decreased level of awareness, such as infections, metabolic abnormalities, seizures, strokes, drug intoxication, and medications (Adams et al., 1997). A careful neurologic examination will include testing cranial nerves for pupillary reactivity, ocular motor movements, and oculovestibular reflexes to gauge brain stem function. Additionally, the level of arousal is assessed via the patient's ability to respond verbally, motorically, or via eye opening to various stimuli. Then, depending upon the patient's degree of alertness and ability to participate, a bedside cognitive evaluation which highlights tests of attention should be performed. Some examples of these tests include the digit-span (repetition of a list of numbers in which 7 ± 2 digits forward and 5 ± 1 digit in reverse is normal); a continuous performance test (the patient lifts his/her arm whenever the letter "A" is read aloud amongst a group of letters); trail-making tests (the patient connects in proper sequence an array of numbers or alternating numbers and letters which are arranged haphazardly on a paper); and an alternating sequences task (the patient must imitate a series of three hand gestures—palm, fist, edge of hand—repetitively without error). These tests help to determine if there are attentional deficits as manifested by distractibility, perseveration, or response inhibition (Mesulam, 2000). For more extensive cognitive evaluation, a neuropsychological battery should be ordered which can further assess the subsets of attention with more sophisticated measures, sometimes using computerized auditory or visual stimuli (Stierwalt & Murray, 2002; Cicerone,

2002). An alternative approach to assessing attention that can be helpful in an acute rehabilitation setting, is the use of a rating scale based on the staff's observations of patients in everyday activities. As has been discussed, a patient may have deficits in various subtypes of attention and thus performance on different tasks may help to categorize what these impairments might be. Examples of these include the neurobehavioral rating scale (NRS) (Levin et al., 1987), which documents alertness, attention, and fatigability, while the Moss Attention Rating Scale includes items for arousal, alertness, sustained attention, distractibility, and divided attention (Whyte et al., 2003). Laboratory workup to elucidate the etiology of a diminished level of arousal should include routine blood tests, urinalysis, toxicology, brain imaging, lumbar puncture if warranted, and an EEG, as an alteration in brain waves occurs in virtually all disturbances of consciousness (Adams et al., 1997).

Treatment

Increasing a patient's level of arousal and attention after TBI has been attempted with medications as well as through nonpharmacologic means. An example of the latter is the study by Wilson and colleagues (Wilson et al., 1996), who provided environmental sensory enhancement to 24 patients in a vegetative state. A more robust response, as measured by frequency of eye-opening and body movements, was noted when each of the five senses was stimulated at each treatment session, as compared to when just a single sense was stimulated. In addition, an increased level of arousal was also observed when the individual was exposed to personal favorite stimuli such as foods, songs, or photos as contrasted with the use of neutral stimuli. To improve attention, nonpharmacologic approaches that have been utilized include teaching compensatory strategies, such as reducing distracting elements in the environment and taking breaks to maximize one's performance (Mateer et al., 1999), as well as learning to anticipate task demands, to repeat information, and to get clarification when having to manage tasks in the setting of time constraints (Cicerone, 2002).

In the pharmacologic treatment of patients with deficits in arousal and attention, one approach that has been used is based on the idea of enhancing neurotransmitter systems which have been disrupted secondary to TBI. As discussed previously, psychostimulants such as methylphenidate and dextroamphetamine serve to augment the concentration of dopamine and norepinephrine by increasing their release and blocking their reuptake in the synapse. Controlled studies have been conducted with both of these agents (Plenger et al., 1996; Evans et al., 1987), but the most frequently documented positive effect in neuropsychologic tests of attention was in processing speed (Whyte et al., 1997), while the benefit of these medications to increase attention or reduce distractibility has been less certain (Whyte et al., 2002, 2004). Case studies of TBI patients, including individuals in the persistent vegetative state or minimally conscious state, have indicated that amantadine, another dopaminergic agent, improves attention, concentration, and arousal (Nickels et al., 1994; Kraus & Maki, 1997; Zafonte et al., 1998). Other dopaminergic agents which have been shown to be useful in enhancing alertness include levodopa and bromocriptine (Lal et al., 1988; Powell et al., 1996). Modafinil, which appears to activate limbic areas and is approved for narcoplepsy, is an obvious potential choice for treating underarousal in TBI (Teitelman, 2001; Elovic, 2000). Antidepressants with noradrenergic effects such as amitriptyline and desipramine have also been demonstrated to improve arousal and responsiveness in three patients with severe TBI (Reinhard et al., 1996). The side effects of these medications have been reviewed in previous sections.

Since TBI often results in the dysfunction of the cholinergic system in the hippocampus and frontal cortical areas, regions which play a pivotal role in the cognitive function of attention (Salmond et al., 2005; Arciniegas et al., 1999), the use of AchE-Is may also be useful pharmacologic agents in treating these deficits, as several studies have indicated (Griffin et al., 2003; Kaye, 2003; Zhang et al., 2004). Side effects of these medications have already been reviewed. It is noteworthy that there is an overlap in both the neuroanatomic structures and the neurotransmitter systems which play key roles in the biology of arousal and attention, as well as motivation, since the latter provides an individual with the drive to respond to stimuli once he is alert and able to concentrate. Therefore the use of similar pharmacologic agents to treat disorders of these functions appears to be a sound clinical approach. A case vignette highlights the issues involved in patients with problems of arousal and amotivation.

A 34-year-old male with a history of cardiomyopathy suffered a cardiac arrest with a pro longed period of unresponsiveness of unknown duration. He was resuscitated and placed on life support and subsequently underwent successful cardiac transplantation. After recovery from his surgery, he was noted to be fatigued and sleepy a lot of the time. He would close his eyes during rehabilitation sessions and say, "I want to sleep," in a monotone voice. Left to his own devices, he would immediately return to his room to sleep. He needed a great deal of repeated external stimulation by his therapists to enable him to remain alert and concentrate on a task for even brief periods. In addition, due to the anoxic encephalopathy which he suffered as a result of the cardiac arrest, his short-term memory was poor, and he lacked drive to do things spontaneously. The patient was treated with a variety of stimulants, including methylphenidate, with only slight improvement. Subsequently, the patient was placed on high-dose venlafaxine, as his clinicians thought his symptoms were consistent with depression, and on this medication, he did show some improvement. Later in his course of treatment, donepezil and modafinil were added sequentially to help increase his level of attention. Therapists in the rehabilitation center who work with him have noted an improved level of alertness and ability to concentrate as well as increased spontaneity in answering questions with this combination of pharmacologic medications.

Dementia

The cardinal feature of dementia as defined by DSM-IV-TR (American Psychiatric Association, 2000) is a deficit in memory. In addition, there must be a decline in at least one other cognitive sphere such as aphasia (disorder of language), apraxia (inability to perform a previously learned motor activity such as teeth brushing, despite having intact motor and sensory abilities), agnosia (impaired recognition of visual, auditory, or tactile stimuli which cannot be attributed to sensory loss, language disturbance or global cognitive deficits), or finally executive function (organizing, planning, sequencing skills). Furthermore, these deficits impact on social or occupational functioning and represent a significant decline from the person's baseline. In the acute period just after TBI, cognitive deficits can be present secondary to delirium or post-traumatic amnesia. Dementia is a more insidious process and refers to residual deficits which persist for months or years post-TBI. The prevalence of dementia after TBI is not precisely known but has been reported to occur at a rate of between 5% and 17.5% (Koponen et al., 2002; Gualtieri & Cox, 1991), whereas the prevalence of memory disturbances alone, the most common cognitive problem after TBI, ranges from 23–79% (Levin, 1990). Dementia in TBI patients may be due to damage of the frontal anterior and medial- temporal cortices as well as the underlying white matter which connects cortical to subcortical areas (Arciniegas & Beresford, 2001). In addition, since acetylcholine-rich hippocampal regions which are responsible for short-term memory function are frequently damaged in TBI, cholinergic dysfunction is believed to be etiologically related to the memory impairment seen in these patients (Arciniegas et al., 1999). Whether TBI is a definite risk factor for Alzheimer's disease (AD) remains controversial, as some research has shown an increased risk for AD in patients with head injury and other studies have not (Plassman et al., 2000; Williams et al., 1991; Mehta et al., 1999). One possible mechanism to explain the neuropathological overlap in these two entities suggests that the presence of the apo-lipoprotein E (epsilon) 4 allele which retards neural repair after trauma, serves in turn as a risk factor for the deposition of beta-amyloid protein and the subsequent formation of neurodegenerative plaques in AD (Koponen et al., 2004; Jellinger, 2004; Luukinen et al., 2005). In an epidemiologic study of TBI patients, it was found that the observed time from the brain injury incident to the development of AD was less than expected (Nemetz et al., 1999), implying that TBI may hasten the yet undetermined cascade of events necessary to precipitate AD in those patients who are ultimately predisposed to its development. This study gives support to the Satz model of cognitive reserve, which hypothesizes that the brain capacity which is available to carry on the basic ability to function as a human being differs for each person. Therefore dementia would occur at the point where there is a critical reduction in those neurons necessary to carry on these basic functions; this decrease in neurons could be due to normal aging, disease, or external factors such as toxins or TBI (Satz, 1993).

Assessment

The evaluation of a patient with cognitive decline begins with a thorough history about the current TBI incident and its subsequent treatment as well as a review of medical and surgical problems including whether there have been prior TBIs, falls, seizures, or strokes. Additionally, the patient's psychiatric history, family history of neurologic and psychiatric problems, medications, and social history, including level of education, alcohol and drug use, and driving issues should also be assessed. Questions about the impact of the cognitive deficits on the patient's ability to function safely and independently at home, socially, or in the workplace if applicable are key points to address. A comprehensive physical and neurologic examination, as well as a cognitive assessment which tests for attention, memory, and frontal lobe functions, is vital, as is a thorough mental status exam which assesses for psychiatric symptoms. Laboratory tests include a CBC, electrolytes, liver function tests, B12 and folate, as well as brain imaging such as an MRI (magnetic resonance imaging). Neuropsychological testing can help to establish the patient's baseline in terms of current cognitive strengths and weaknesses. The neuropsychiatrist must perform a thorough evaluation to rule out other possible etiologies in the differential diagnosis of cognitive decline, such as hydrocephalus, strokes, neoplasm, subdural hematoma, vitamin deficiencies, delirium, depression, and endocrine abnormalities such as hypothyroidism (Small et al., 1997; Frederiks et al., 2002) as well as hypopituitism, which has been reported in TBI patients with cognitive impairment (Popovic et al., 2005; Springer & Chollet, 2001).

Treatment

An important issue to address in treating TBI patients who have cognitive deficits is whether a concomitant diagnosis of depression is present. In a recent study, 28.4% of 74 patients with mild or moderate TBI who also suffered from major depression were found to have significantly lowered scores on measures of working and verbal memory, processing speed, and executive function as compared to patients without this diagnosis (Rapoport et al., 2005). In another study of 15 patients with mild TBI and depression, neuropsychological tests were noted to improve when their mood symptoms had been successfully treated with the antidepressant sertraline (Fann et al., 2001). Since TBI may produce cognitive impairment neurochemically via the disruption of cholinergic function, it has been suggested that using cholinergic-enhancing medications such as choline precursors or AchE-Is may be an appropriate pharmacologic approach. Cytidine 5'diphosphocholi is a choline precursor which has been reported to be effective in improving cognition after TBI in both case studies (Spiers & Hochanadel, 1999; Leon-Carrion et al., 2000) as well as in a randomized double-blind placebo-controlled study of fourteen patients (Levin, 1991). Although physostigmine, an AchE-I, has not been shown to be consistently effective in the treatment of memory deficits of TBI patients in several different studies (Goldberg et al., 1982; Levin et al., 1986), donepezil, another member of the AchE-I class, has been reported to improve memory in TBI patients in open-label and case study reports (Taverni et al., 1998; Whitlock, 1999; Whelan et al., 2000; Masanic et al., 2001; Morey et al., 2003). More recently in a 24-week randomized, placebo-controlled, double-blind, cross-over trial with 18 patients who had sustained TBI less than 6 months prior to the study, Zhang and colleagues documented that donepezil significantly increased neuropsychological testing scores in short-term memory and sustained attention (Zhang et al., 2004). In a non-randomized, open-label study of 111 outpatients with TBI who either received donepezil or one of the two newer AchE-Is, namely, rivastigmine

(Exelon) or galantamine (Reminyl), the areas of vigilance, concentration, initiation and general function were noted to be subjectively markedly improved in 61% and modestly improved in 39% of this population (Tenovuo, 2005). Furthermore, AchE-Is have also been shown to benefit mood, affect, and social interaction in brain-injured patients (Kaye, 2003; Whelan et al., 2000). Large-scale randomized, double-blind placebo controlled studies are needed to clarify the benefits of these agents in TBI patients. A patient case provides an example of this clinical problem.

A 50-year-old male sustained a left frontal temporal brain injury 3 years ago. Despite cognitive remediation and the use of compensatory strategies such as a memory book in which he writes his daily activities, his memory is still poor. He has trouble organizing what tasks he must complete and requires a lot of supervision from his wife. Due to his cognitive deficits, he was unable to return to his occupation as a clerk in an insurance company. After neuropsychiatric assessment, the patient decided to be started on donepezil with modest improvement in his memory.

Sexual Dysfunction

After TBI, a patient's sexuality can be altered in a variety of ways and he or she can experience difficulties not only with libido and the physical sexual act, but also develop problems with self-esteem and relationship skills. The clinical categorization of the various subtypes of sexual dysfunction as per DSM-IV-TR (American Psychiatric Association, 2000) nosology is beyond the scope of this chapter. For the purposes of this discussion, the focus of the sexual problems reviewed will be those commonly observed in relation to TBI; hence the appropriate diagnostic label would be sexual dysfunction secondary to TBI. In TBI patients, the rate of sexual dysfunction has been reported to be in the range of 4–71% (Sandel et al., 1996). While most often patients suffer from hyposexuality as a result of the brain injury, hypersexuality can also occur as was noted in 14% of subjects in one study (Kreutzer & Zasler, 1989). Of note, in a small minority of men with TBI, sexually aberrant behaviors such as inappropriate touching, exhibitionism, or overt sexual aggression has also been reported (Simpson et al., 1999). Neuroanatomically, hyposexuality has been related to lesions of the medial orbital gyrus of the frontal lobe, hippocampus, anterior thalamus, and hypothalamus (Elliott & Biever, 1996), while hypersexuality can occur with damage to the frontal lobe and bilateral temporal lobes (Zencius et al., 1990, Wesolowski et al., 1993). A clinical example of a sexual problem in this population of patients can serve to illustrate some key issues.

A 40-year-old male suffered traumatic brain injury after a motor vehicle accident which caused injury to the right frontal-temporal brain regions. Subsequent to this he was observed exposing himself and making inappropriate sexual overtures to female staff as well as family members. He began to masturbate in public places while using pornographic materials. His behavior is disruptive to his rehabilitation efforts and he is referred to the neuropsychiatrist for evaluation.

Assessment

As with other neuropsychiatric conditions, obtaining a history to try to narrow down the diagnostic possibilities is key, as sexual dysfunction after neurologic insults can be due to either genital and/or nongenital causes. The patient and his/her sexual partner should be asked about the patient's premorbid and post-TBI sexual history, including marital status, sexual preference, sexual activities, sexual abuse, quality of relationships, libido, arousal, and physiologic function (erection, ejaculation, vaginal lubrication, orgasm). Any sexually intrusive behaviors—which can range from inappropriate remarks to aggressive behavior, including rape—should also be explored in the TBI patient (Bezeau et al., 2004). Since many medications have sexual side effects and because diseases such as diabetes or sexually transmitted diseases can cause sexual dysfunction, inquiry into these topics is pertinent. Endocrinologic function is also particularly relevant since brain injuries which affect the pituitary gland, and hence hormonal levels, could be responsible for a patient's sexual problems. Decreased sensation or hypersensitivity, decreased mobility secondary to paralysis or orthopedic injuries, as well as tremor or balance problems, are all obvious impediments to sexually pleasurable activity and must be addressed as well. Prior psychiatric illness is relevant, as decreased or increased libido can be observed within the constellation of mood and anxiety disorders (Zasler & Martelli, 2005). A history of seizures is important to inquire about as epilepsy is a common sequelae of TBI (about 12% in severe TBI) (Annegers et al., 1980), and those with temporal lobe epilepsy often suffer with hyposexuality. Since cognitive-behavioral and emotional problems can limit one's ability to effectively maintain an intimate relationship, it is important in the examination of the TBI patient to explore the impact of relevant issues such as poor concentration, memory deficits, motivation, lack of confidence, excessive dependency and loss of equality in the relationship, disinhibition, and insensitivity to a partner's needs. As part of the neuropsychiatrist's role, he/she can order lab tests such as hormone levels (follicle-stimulating hormone [FSH], leutinizing hormone [LH], estrogen, testosterone) and then target appropriate ancillary consultations to the physiatrist, endocrinologist, gynecologist, or urologist (see the chapter on neurourology) to address those sexual issues which do not appear to be under his/her purview (Zasler & Martelli, 2005; Oddy, 2001).

Treatment

If the nature of the problem is ultimately determined to lie in the neuropsychiatric domain, the professional in this field can utilize different approaches to help the patient and his/her partner. In the above clinical case where hypersexuality is the clinical problem, one form of treatment would be to take advantage of the sexual side effects of antidepressants such as the SSRIs, which are known to decrease libido and cause problems in achieving ejaculation, orgasm, and erections (Krueger & Kaplan, 2002). Sometimes, mood stabilizers, especially anticonvulsants, are used to treat hypersexuality if this symptom is viewed as part of a manic or hypomanic state. If these fail, then sexual desire can be diminished with anti-androgens such as medroxyprogesterone (Britton, 1998) or depot-leuprolide acetate (Lupron) (Krueger & Kaplan, 2002) as was successfully done in the above-described clinical scenario. These medications are gonadotropin-releasing hormone analogs which cause a reduction in the pituitary production of LH and FSH, which in turn leads to a decrease in testosterone. Prior to starting this treatment, the patient requires baseline hormonal levels and a bone density evaluation, as bone loss can be a side effect of these agents (Krueger & Kaplan, 2002). A behavioral plan focused on modification of these inappropriate actions should also be undertaken as part of the treatment.

Hyposexuality is a more common sexual dysfunction problem. Antidepressants, antipsychotics, anticonvulsants, but also antihypertensives, stimulant medications, and anticholinergics can be the source of decreased libido; therefore, dosage modification or elimination of the medication entirely may help to improve a patient's sexual interest and performance (Aloni & Katz, 1999). Conversely, the neuropsychiatrist must also assess whether depression is the underlying cause of the sexual dysfunction, in which case appropriate treatment may improve the patient's desire. Utilizing medications which do not have sexual side effects, such as bupropion or nefazadone (Serzone), an inhibitor of serotonin and norepinephrine reuptake in the synapse whose primary adverse effect is sedation, may be more beneficial in this scenario (Hirschfeld, 1999). Psychotherapy, which can include both individual and couple's counseling to help the patient and his partner deal with the practical issues of sexual relations as well as emotional issues, should be part of the treatment paradigm. Since the reported rates of marital breakup after TBI are high, the role of psychotherapy in this area must be underscored. With a TBI group therapy format, patients can practice social skills with peers and have the opportunity to discuss common sexual problems and how to cope with them (Katz & Aloni, 1999), while the availability of sexuality handbooks which address these topics can also be valuable resources for TBI patients who have sufficient cognitive abilities to benefit from this approach (Simpson & Long, 2004). Finally, in those cases of TBI patients with sexually intrusive behaviors, behavioral programs which focus on establishing clear boundaries in relationships, encourage adaptive and appropriate behaviors, and provide a relapse prevention plan have been demonstrated to be successful (Bezeau et al., 2004).

Conclusion

As has been observed from the patient vignettes in this chapter, the neuropsychiatric complications of TBI are numerous and complex. In reviewing our progress along the neuropsychiatric historical timeline, it is observed that we have advanced from the point where there was merely a glimmer of understanding about the possible existence of a relationship between brain and behavior, to our more sophisticated, modern ideas about the brain and its definitive roles in emotion and cognition. Yet despite learning about brain–behavior connections through the deficits suffered by

TBI patients, much research still needs to be done to understand the intricate nature of these neuronal ties, as well as to improve the outcomes of our patients who have suffered these injuries. There is debate in the literature about whether cognitive and psychiatric sequelae of TBI are the result of specific brain lesions, psychologic reactions to trauma, pre-morbid psychiatric illness [as was proposed in a study which noted an increased relative risk of 1.6 for subsequent TBI in patients who had had any indicator of psychiatric illness in the year prior to TBI (Fann et al., 2002)], or a combination thereof. For this reason, future studies of patients should be prospective in design using standardized diagnostic criteria which will more accurately categorize both the degrees of TBI (mild, moderate, severe) as well as the specific psychiatric syndrome. This will help to better predict outcomes of psychiatric co-morbidity, cognitive impairment and functional status, as well as to allocate resources appropriately to assist these patients in repairing their lives In addition, randomized, blinded, placebo-control studies of psychopharmacologic agents are crucial to providing a rational, consistent approach to treating the various neuropsychiatric consequences of TBI. With these improvements as a start, patients who have had the misfortune of sustaining TBI can have the hope of enjoying an improved quality of life.

References

Adams, R.D., Victor, M., Ropper, A.M. (1997) *Principles of Neurology*, 6th ed. NY: McGraw-Hill Company chapter 17, pp. 344–366.

Al-Adawi, Dorvlo A., Burke, D.T., Huynh, C.C., Jacob, L., Knight, R., Shah, M.K., Al-Hussaini, A. (2004) Apathy and depression in cross-cultural survivors of traumatic brain injury. *Journal of Neuropsychiatry & Clinical Neurosciences* 16:435–442.

Aloni, R., Katz, S. (1999) A review of the effect of traumatic brain injury on the human sexual response. *Brain Injury* 13:269–280.

American Psychiatric Association (2000). *Diagnostic and Statistical Manual of Mental Disorders*, 4th ed.(Text Review) Washington, DC: American Psychiatric Press.

Andersson, S., Bergedalen, A.M. (2002) Cognitive correlates of apathy in traumatic brain injury. *Neuropsychiatry Neuropsychology and Behavioral Neurology* 15:184–191.

Andersson, S., Krogstad, I M., Finset, A. (1999a) Apathy and depressed mood in acquired brain damage: Relationship to lesion localization and psychophysiological reactivity. *Psychological Medicine* 29:447–456.

Andersson, S., Gundersen, P.M., Finset, A. (1999b) Emotional activation during therapeutic interaction in traumatic brain injury: Effect of apathy, self-awareness and implications for rehabilitation. *Brain Injury* 13:393–404.

Annegers, J.F., Grabow, J.D., Groover, R.V., Laws, E.R. (1980) Seizures after head trauma: A population study. *Neurology* 30:683–689.

Arciniegas, D.B., Beresford, T.P. (2001) *Neuropsychiatry–An Introductory Approach*. New York: Cambridge University Press, p. 376.

Arciniegas, D., Adler, L., Topkoff, J., Cawthra, E., Filley, C.M., Reite, M. (1999) Attention and memory dysfunction after traumatic brain injury: Cholinergic mechanisms, sensory gating and a hypothesis for further investigation. *Brain Injury* 13:1–13.

Arciniegas, D.B., Harris, S.N., Brousseau, K.M. (2003) Psychosis following traumatic brain injury. *International Review of Psychiatry* 15:328–340.

Ashman, T.A., Spielman, L.A., Hibbard, M.R., Silver, J.M., Chandna, T., Gordon, W.A. (2004) Psychiatric challenges in the first six years after traumatic brain injury: Cross sequential analyses of axis I disorders. *Archives of Physical Medicine and Rehabilitation* 85:S36–S42.

Azouvi, P., Jokic, C., Attal, N., Denys, P., Markabi, S., Bussel, B. (1999) Carbamazepine in agitation and aggressive behavior following severe closed-head injury: Results of an open trial. *Brain Injury* 13:797–804.

Babin, P.R. (2003) Diagnosing depression in persons with brain injuries: A look at theories, the DSM-IV and depression measures. *Brain Injury* 17:889–900.

Bakchine, S., Lacomblez, L., Benoit, N., Parisot, D., Chain, F., Lhermitte, F. (1989) Manic-like state after bilateral orbitofrontal and right temporoparietal injury: Efficacy of clonidine. *Neurology* 39:777–781.

Barker, F.G. (1995) Phineas among the phrenologists: The American crowbar case and nineteenth century theories of cerebral localization. *Journal of Neurosurgery* 82:672–682.

Baxter, L.R., Schwartz, J.M., Bergman, K.S., Szuba, M.P., Guze, B.H., Mazziotta, J.C., Alazraki, A., Selin, C.E., Ferng, H.K., Munford, P., Phelps, M.E. (1992) Caudate glucose metabolic rate changes with both drug and behavior therapy for obsessive-compulsive disorder. *Archives of General Psychiatry* 49:681–689.

Berthier, M.L., Kulisevsky, J., Gironell, A., Lopez, O.L. (2001) Obsessive-compulsive disorder and traumatic brain injury: Behavioral, cognitive and neuroimaging findings. *Neuropsychiatry, Neuropsychology, and Behavioral Neurology* 14:23–31.

Bezeau, S.C., Bogod, N.M., Mateer, C.A. (2004) Sexually intrusive behavior following brain injury: Approaches to assessment and rehabilitation. *Brain Injury* 18:299–313.

Bogner, J.A., Corrigan, J.D., Fugate, L., Mysiw, W.J., Clinchot, D. (2001) Role of agitation in prediction of outcomes after traumatic brain injury. *American Journal of Physical Medicine & Rehabilitation* 80:636–644.

Branca, B., Lake, A.E. (2004) Psychological and neuropsychological integration in multidisciplinary pain management after TBI. *The Journal of Head Trauma Rehabilitation* 19:40–57.

Britton, K.R. (1998) Medroxyprogesterone in the treatment of aggressive hypersexual behavior in traumatic brain injury. *Brain Injury* 12:703–707.

Brooke, M.M., Questad, K.A., Patterson, D.R., Questad, K.A., Bashak, K.J. (1992a) Agitation and restlessness after closed head injury: A prospective study of 100 consecutive admissions. *Archives of Physical Medicine & Rehabilitation* 73:320–323.

Brooke, M.M., Patterson, D.R., Questad, K.A., Cardenas, D., Farrel-Roberts, L. (1992b) The treatment of agitation during initial hospitalization after traumatic brain injury. *Archives of Physical Medicine & Rehabilitation* 73:917–921.

Bryant, R.A. (2001) Post-traumatic stress disorder and mild brain injury: Controversies, causes and consequences. *Journal of Clinical and Experimental Neuropsychology* 23:718–728.

Butler, P.V. (2000) Diurnal variation in Cotard's syndrome (copresent with Capgras delusion) following traumatic brain injury. *Aust NZ J Psychiatry* 34:684.

Calabrese, J.R., Bowden, C.L., McElroy, S.L., Cookson, J. (1999) Spectrum of activity of lamotrigine in treatment-refractory bipolar disorder. *American Journal of Psychiatry* 156:1019–1023.

Cassidy, J.W. (1989) Fluoxetine: A new serotonergically active antidepressant. *The Journal of Head Trauma Rehabilitation* 4:67–69.

Chandler, M.C., Barnhill, J.L., Gualtieri, C.T. (1988) Amantadine for the agitated head-injury patient. *Brain Injury* 2:309–311.

Chatham-Showalter, P.E. (1996) Carbamazepine for combativeness in acute traumatic brain injury. *Journal of Neuropsychiatry & Clinical Neurosciences* 8:96–99.

Cicerone, K.D. (2002) Remediation of 'working attention' in mild traumatic brain injury. *Brain Injury* 16:185–195.

Corrigan, J.D. (1989) Development of a scale for assessment of agitation following traumatic brain injury. *J Clinical Experiment Neuropsychology* 11:261–277.

Crow, S., Meller, W., Christenson, G., Mackenzie, T. (1996) Use of ECT after brain injury. *Convulsive Therapy* 12:113–116.

Cummings, J.L. (2000) Cholinesterase inhibitors: A new class of psychotropic compounds. *American Journal of Psychiatry* 157:4–15.

Cummings, J.L., Back, C. (1998) The cholinergic hypothesis of neuropsychiatric symptoms in Alzheimer's disease. *American Jounal of Geriatrics Psychiatry* 6:S64–S78.

Davison, K., Bagley, C.R. (1969) Schizophrenia-like psychoses associated with organic disorders of the central nervous system: A review of the literature. In Herrington, R.N. (ed.): *Current Problems in Neuropsychiatry. Schizophrenia, Epilepsy, the Temporal Lobe.* London: Headley, pp. 113–184.

Deb, S., Lyons, S.I., Koutzoukis, C., Ali, I., McCarthy, G. (1999) Rate of psychiatric illness one year after traumatic brain injury. *American Journal of Psychiatry* 156:374–378.

Derivan, A., Haskins, T., Rudolph, R. Pallay, A., Aguiar, L. (June 1998) Double-blind placebo-controlled study of once daily venlafaxine XR in outpatients with generalized anxiety disorder. *Abstract presented at the American Psychiatric Association Annual Meeting*, Toronto, Canada.

Dikmen, S.S., Bombardier, C.H., Machamer, J.E. Fann, J.R., Temkin, N.R. (2004) Natural history of depression in traumatic brain injury. *Archives of Physical Medicine and Rehabilitation* 85:1457–1464.

Dockree, P.M., Kelly, S.P., Roche, R.A.P., Hogan, M.J., Reilly, R.B., Robertson, I.H. (2004) Behavioral and physiological impairments of sustained attention after traumatic brain injury. *Cognitive Brain Research* 20:403–414.

Elliott, M.L., Biever, L.S. (1996) Head injury and sexual dysfunction. *Brain Injury* 10:703–717.

Elovic, E. (2000) Use of provigil for underarousal following TBI. *The Journal of Head Trauma Rehabilation* 15:1068–1071.

Elovic, E.P., Lansang, R., Li, Y., Ricker, J.H. (2003) The use of atypical antipsychotics in traumatic brain injury. *The Journal of Head Trauma Rehabilation* 18:177–195.

Emilien, G., Maloteaux, J.M. (1998) Current therapeutic uses and potential of beta-adrenoceptor agonists and antagonists. *European Journal of Clinical Pharmacology* 53:389–404.

Evans, R.W., Gualtieri, C.T., Patterson, D. (1987) Treatment of chronic closed head injury with psychostimulant drugs: A controlled case study and an appropriate evaluation procedure. *The Journal of Nervous and Mental Disease* 175:106–110.

Fann, J.R., Katon, W.J., Uomoto, J.M., Esselman, P.C. (1995) Psychiatric disorders and functional disability in outpatients with traumatic brain injuries. *American Journal of Psychiatry* 152:1493–1499.

Fann, J.R., Uomoto, J.M., Katon, W.J. (2001) Cognitive improvement with treatment of depression following mild traumatic brain injury. *Psychosomatics* 42:48–54.

Fann, J.R., Leonetti, A., Jaffe, K., Katon, W.J., Cummings, P., Thompson, R.S. (2002) Psychiatric illness and subsequent traumatic brain injury: A case control study. *Journal of Neurology, Neurosurgery, and Psychiatry* 72:615–620.

Fann, J.R., Uomoto, J.M., Katon, W.J. (2000) Sertraline in the treatment of major depression following mild traumatic brain injury. *Journal of Neuropsychiatry & Clinical Neurosciences* 12:226–232.

Fann, J.R., Burington, B., Leonetti, A., Jaffe, K., Katon, W.J., Thompson, R.S. (2004) Psychiatric illness following traumatic brain injury in an adult health maintenance organization population. *Archives of General Psychiatry* 61:53–61.

Federoff, J.P., Starkstein, S.E., Forrester, A.W., Geisler, F.H., Jorge, R.E., Arndt, S.V., Robinson, R.G. (1992) Depression in patients with acute traumatic brain injury. *Americal Journal of Psychiatry* 149:918–923.

Finger, S. (2000) *Minds Behind the Brain—A History of the Pioneers and their Discoveries.* New York: Oxford University Press, 9:13–15.

Frederiks, C., Hofmann, M.T., Reichard, R. (2002) Advances in diagnosis and treatment of Alzheimer's disease. *Hosp Physician* 38:47–54.

Freinhar, J.P., Alvarez, W.A. (1986) Clonazepam treatment of organic brain syndromes in three elderly patients. *Journal of Clinical Psychiatry* 47:525–526.

Fujii, D.E., Ahmed, I. (2001) Risk factors in psychosis secondary to traumatic brain injury. *Journal of Neuropsychiatry & Clinical Neurosciences* 13:61–69.

Fujii, D., Ahmed, I. (2002) Characteristics of psychotic disorder due to traumatic brain injury: An analysis of case studies in the literature. *Journal of Neuropsychiatry & Clinical Neurosciences* 14:130–140.

Fujii, D., Ahmed, I., Hishinuma, E. (2004) A neuropsychological comparison of psychotic disorder following traumatic brain injury, traumatic brain injury without psychotic disorder and schizophrenia. *Journal of Neuropsychiatry & Clinical Neurosciences* 16:306–314.

Glenn, M.B., Wroblewski, B., Parziale, J., Levine, L., Whyte, J., Rosenthal, M. (1989) Lithium carbonate for aggressive behavior or affective instability in ten brain-injured patients. *American Journal of Physical Medicine and Rehabilitation* 68:221–226.

Goldberg, E., Gertsman, L.J., Mattis, S., Hughes, J.E., Sirio, C.A., Bilder, R.M. (1982) Selective effects of cholinergic treatment on verbal memory in post-traumatic amnesia. *J Clin Neuropsychol* 4:219–234.

Gomez-Hernandez, R., Max, J.E., Kosier, T., Paradiso, S., Robinson, R.G. (1997) Social impairment and depression after traumatic brain injury. *Archives of Physical Medicine and Rehabilitation* 78:1321–1326.

Grados, M.A. (2003) Obsessive-compulsive disorder after traumatic brain injury. *International Review of Psychiatry* 15:350–358.

Greendyke, R.M., Kanter, D.R., Schuster, D.B., Verstreate, S., Wootton, J. (1986) Propranolol treatment of assaultive patients with organic brain disease. A double-blind crossover, placebo-controlled study. *The Journal of Nervous and Mental Disease* 174:290–294.

Griffin, S.L., van Reekum, R., Masanic, C. (2003) A review of cholinergic agents in the treatment of neurobehavioral deficits following traumatic brain injury. *Journal of Neuropsychiatry & Clinical Neurosciences* 15:17–26.

Gualtieri, C.T. (1991a) Buspirone for the behavior problems of patients with organic brain disorders. *J Clin Psychopharmacol* 11:280–281.

Gualtieri, C.T. (1991b) Buspirone: Neuropsychiatric effects. *The Journal of Head Trauma Rehabilitation* 6:90–92.

Gualtieri, T.C., Evans, R.W. (1988) Stimulant treatment for the neurobehavioral sequelae of traumatic brain injury. *Brain Injury* 2:273–290.

Gualtieri, T., Cox, D.R. (1991) The delayed neurobehavioral sequelae of traumatic brain injury. *Brain Injury* 5:219–232.

Hale, M.S., Donaldson, J.O. (1982) Lithium carbonate in the treatment of organic brain syndrome. *The Journal of Nervous and Mental Disease* 170:362–365.

Hamner, M.B., Brodrick, P.S., Labbate, L.A. (2001) Gabapentin in PTSD: A retrospective, clinical series of adjunctive therapy. *Annals of Clinical Psychiatry* 13:141–146.

Herrmann, N., Lanctot, K.L. (2005) Do atypical antipsychotics cause stroke? *CNS Drugs* 19:91–103.

Heinrich, T.W., Junig, J.T. (2004) Recurrent mania associated with repeated brain injury. *General Hospital Psychiatry* 26:490–492.

Hertzberg, M.A., Butterfield, M.I., Feldman, M.E., Beckham, J.C., Sutherland, S.M., Connor, K.M., Davidson, R.T. (1999) A preliminary study of lamotrigine for the treatment of posttraumatic stress disorder. *Biological Psychiatry* 45:1226–1229.

Hibbard, M.R., Uysal, S., Kepler, K., Bogdany, J., Silver, J. (1998) Axis I Psychopathology in individuals with traumatic brain injury. *The Journal of Head Trauma Rehabilitation* 13:24–39.

Hibbard, M.R., Ashman, T.A., Spielman, L.A., Chun, D., Charatz, H.J., Melvin, S. (2004) Relationship between depression and psychosocial functioning after traumatic brain injury. *Archives of Physical Medicine and Rehabilitation* 85:S43–S53.

Hiott, D.W., Labbate, L. (2002) Anxiety disorders associated with traumatic brain injuries. *Neuro Rehabilitation* 17:345–355.

Hippocrates. *On Injuries of the Head*. 400 BCE, parts 13 and 19.

Hirschfeld, R.M. (1999) Care of the sexually active depressed patient. *Journal of Clinical Psychiatry* 60(Suppl 17):32–35.

Holland, D., Witty, T., Lawler, J., Lanzisera, D. (1999) Biofeedback-assisted relaxation training with brain-injured patients in acute stages of recovery. *Brain Injury* 13:53–57.

Holsinger, T., Steffens, D.C., Phillips, C., Helms, M.J., Havlik, R.J., Breitner, J.C.S., Guralnik, J.M., Plassman, B.L. (2002) Head injury in early adulthood and the lifetime risk of depression. *Archives of General Psychiatry* 59:17–22.

Holzer, J.C. (1998) Buspirone and brain injury. *Journal of Neuropsychiatry & Clinical Neurosciences* 10:113.

Hornstein, A., Lennihan, L., Seliger, G., Lichtman, S., Schroeder, K. (1996) Amphetamine in recovery from brain injury. *Brain Injury* 10:145–148.

Horsfield, S.A., Rosse, R.B., Tomasino, V., Schwartz, B.L., Mastropaolo, J., Deutsch, S.I. (2002) Fluoxetine's effects on cognitive performance in patients with traumatic brain injury. *Int J Psych Med* 32:337–344.

Janicak, P.G., Davis, J.M., Preskorn, S.H., Ayd, F.J. (eds.): (1993) *Principles and Practice of Psychopharmacotherapy* Baltimore: Williams and Wilkins.

Jellinger, K.A. (2004) Head injury and dementia. *Current Opinion in Neurology* 17:719–723.

Jorge, R.E., Robinson, R.G. (2003) Mood disorders following traumatic brain injury. *International Review of Psychiatry,* 15:317–327.

Jorge, R.E., Robinson, R.G., Starkstein, S.E., Arndt, S.V., Forrester, A.W., Geisler, F.H. (1993) Secondary mania following traumatic brain injury. *American Journal of Psychiatry* 150:916–921.

Jorge, R.E., Robinson, R.G., Moser, D., Tateno, A., Crespo-Facorro, B., Arndt, S. (2004) Major depression following traumatic brain injury. *Archives of General Psychiatry* 61:42–50.

Jorge, R.E., Starkstein, S.E., Arndt, S., Moser, D., Crespo-Facorro, B., Robinson, R.G. (2005) Alcohol misuse and mood disorders following traumatic brain injury. *Archives of General Psychiatry* 62:742–749.

Kadyan, V., Colachis, S.C., Depalma, M.J., Sanderson, J.D., Mysiw, W.J. (2003) Early recognition of neuroleptic malignant syndrome during traumatic brain rehabilitation. *Brain Injury* 17:631–637.

Kadyan, V., Mysiw, W.J., Bogner, J.A., Corrigan, J.D., Fugate, L.P., Clinchot, D.M. (2004) Gender differences in agitation after traumatic brain injury. *American Journal of Physical Medicine & Rehabilitation* 83:747–752.

Kant, R., Bogyi, A.M., Carosella, N.W., Fishman, E., Kane, V., Coffey, C.E. (1995) ECT as a therapeutic option in severe brain injury. *Convulsive Therapy* 11:45–50.

Kant, R., Duffy, J.D., Pivovarnik, A. (1998a) Prevalence of apathy following head injury. *Brain Injury* 12:87–92.

Kant, R., Smith-Seemiller, L., Zeiler, D. (1998b) Treatment of aggression and irritability after head injury. *Brain Injury* 12:661–666.

Katz, S., Aloni, R. (1999) Sexual dysfunction of persons after traumatic brain injury: Perceptions of professionals. *International Journal of Rehabilitation Research* 22: 45–53.

Kaye, N.S. (2003) An open-label trial of donepezil (Aricept) in the treatment of persons with mild traumatic brain injury. *Journal of Neuropsychiatry & Clinical Neurosciences* 15:383–384.

Kennedy, R., Burnett, D.M., Greenwald, B.D. (2001) Use of antiepileptics in traumatic brain injury: A review for psychiatrists. *Annals of Clinical Psychiatry* 13:163–171.

Kim, E., Humaran, T.J. (2002) Divalproex in the management of neuropsychiatric complications of remote acquired brain injury. *Journal of Neuropsychiatry & Clinical Neurosciences* 14:202–205.

Khouzam, H.R., Donnelly, N.J. (1998) Remission of traumatic brain injury-induced compulsions during venlafaxine treatment. *General Hospital Psychiatry* 20:62–63.

Koopowitz, L.F., Berk, M. (1997) Response of obsessive compulsive disorder to carbamazepine in two patients with comorbid epilepsy. *Annals of Clinical Psychiatry* 9:171–173.

Koponen, S., Taiminen, T., Portin, R., Himanen, L., Isoniemi, H., Heinonen, H., Hinkka, S., Tenovuo, O. (2002) Axis I and II psychiatric disorders after traumatic brain injury: A 30 year follow-up study. *American Journal of Psychiatry* 159:1315–1321.

Koponen, S., Taiminen, T., Kairisto, V., Portin, R., Isoniemi, H., Hinkka, S., Tenovuo, O. (2004) APOE-e4 predicts dementia but not other psychiatric disorders after traumatic brain injury. *Neurology* 63:749–750.

Kraus, M.F., Maki, P.M. (1997) Effect of amantadine hydrochloride on symptoms of frontal lobe dysfunction in brain injury: Case studies and review. *Journal of Neuropsychiatry & Clinical Neurosciences* 9:222–230.

Krauthammer, C., Klerman, G.L. (1978) Secondary mania: Manic syndromes associated with antecedent physical illnesses or drugs. *Archives of General Psychiatry* 35:1333–1339.

Kreutzer, J., Zasler, N. (1989) Psychosexual consequences of traumatic brain injury: Methodology and preliminary findings. *Brain Injury* 3:177–186.

Krueger, R.B., Kaplan, M.S. (2002) Behavioral and psychopharmacological treatment of the paraphilic and hypersexual disorders. *Journal of Psychiatric Practice* 8:21–32.

Labbate, L.A., Warden, D.L. (2000) Common psychiatric syndromes and pharmacologic treatments of traumatic brain injury. *Current Psychiatry Reports* 2:268–273.

Lal, S., Merbtiz, C.P., Grip, J.C. (1988) Modification of function in head-injured patients with sinemet. *Brain Injury* 2:225–233.

Lee, H., Kim, S.W., Kim, J.M., Shin, I.S., Yang, S.J., Yoon, J.S. (2005) Comparing effects of methylphenidate, sertraline and placebo on neuropsychiatric sequelae in patients with traumatic brain injury. *Human Psychopharmacology Clinical and Experimental* 20:97–104.

Leon-Carrion, J., Dominguez-Roldan, J.M., Murill-Cabezas, F., Dominguez-Morales, M.R., Munoz-Sanchez, M.A. (2000) The role of citicholine in neuropsychological training after traumatic brain injury. *Neurorehabilitation* 14:33–40.

Levin, H.S. (1990) Memory deficit after closed head injury. *Journal of Clinical and Experimental Neuropsychiatry* 12:129–153.

Levin, H.S. (1991) Treatment of postconcussional symptoms with CDP-choline. *Journal of Neurological Sciences* 103:S39–S42.

Levin, H.S., Grossman, R.G. (1978) Behavioral sequelae of closed head injury: A quantitative study. *Archives in Neurology* 35:720–727.

Levin, H.S., Peters, B.H., Kalisky, Z., High, W.M., von Laufen, A., Eisenberg, H.M., Morrison, D.P., Gary, H.E. (1986) Effects of oral physostigmine and lecithin on memory and attention in the closed head injured patient. *Central Nervous System Trauma* 3:333–342.

Levin, H.S., High, W., Goethe, K.E., Sisson, R.A. (1987) The Neurobehavioral Rating Scale: Assessment of the behavioral sequelae of head injury by the clinician. *Journal of Neurology, Neurosurgery, and Psychiatry* 50:183–193.

Luria, A.R. (1972) *The Man With a Shattered World. The History of a Brain Wound.* New York: Basic Books, p. 38.

Luukinen, H., Viramo, P., Herala, M., Kervinen, K., Kesaniemi, Y.A., Savola, O., Winqvist, S., Jokelainen, J., Hillborn, M. (2005) Fall-related brain injuries and the risk of dementia in elderly people: A population based study. *European Journal of Neurology* 12:86–92.

Malaspina, D., Goetz, R.R., Friedman, J.H., Kaufmann, C., Faraone, S.V., Tsuang, M., Cloninger, C.R., Nurnberger, J.I., Blehar, M.C. (2001) Traumatic brain injury and schizophrenia in members of schizophrenia and bipolar disorder pedigrees. *American Journal of Psychiatry* 158:440–446.

Mangels, J.A., Craik, F.I.M., Levine, B., Schwartz, M.L., Sluss, D.T. (2002) Effects of divided attention on episodic memory in chronic traumatic brain injury: A function of severity and strategy. *Neuropsychologia* 40:2369–2385.

Marcotte, D. (1998) Use of topiramate, a new anti-epileptic as a mood stabilizer. *Journal of Affective Disorders* 50:245–251.

Marin, R.S., Wilkosz, P.A. (2005) Disorders of diminished motivation. *The Journal of Head Trauma Rehabilitation* 20:377–388.

Marin, R.S., Biedrzycki, R.C., Firinciogullaari, S. (1991) Reliability and validity of the apathy evaluation scale. *Psychiatry Research* 38:143–162.

Masanic, C.A., Bayley, M.T., van Reekum, R., Simard, M. (2001) Open-label study of donepezil in traumatic brain injury. *Archives of Physical Medicine & Rehabilitation* 82:896–901.

Masterman, D.L., Cummings, J.L. (1997) Frontal-subcortical circuits: The anatomic basis of executive, social and motivated behaviors. *Journal of Psychopharmacology* 11:107–114.

Mateer, C.A., Kerns, K.A., Eso, K.L. (1999) Management of attention and memory disorders following traumatic brain injury. *Journal of Learning Disabilities* 29:618–632.

Mayou, R.A., Black, J., Bryant, B. (2000) Unconsciousness, amnesia and psychiatric symptoms following road traffic accident injury. *British Journal of Psychiatry* 177:540–545.

McKinlay, W.W., Brooks, D.N., Bond, M.R., Martinage, D.P., Marshall, M.M. (1981) The short-term outcome of severe blunt head injury as reported by the relatives of the injured person. *Journal of Neurology, Neurosurgery, and Psychiatry* 44:527–533.

McNeil, J.E., Greenwood, R. (1996) Can PTSD occur with amnesia for the precipitating event? *Cognitive Neuropsychiatry* 1:239–246.

Mehta, K.M., Ott, A., Kalmijn, S., Slooter, A.J.C., van Duijn, C.M., Hofman, A., Breteler, M.M.B. (1999) Head trauma and risk of dementia and Alzheimer's disease—the Rotterdam study. *Neurology* 53:1959–1962.

Mesulam, M.M. (2000) Principles of Behavioral and Cognitive Neurology, 2nd ed. NY: Oxford University Press, chapter 2–3, pp. 121–256.

Meyer, A. (1904) The anatomical facts and clinical varieties of traumatic insanity. *American Journal of Insanity* 60:373–441.

Michals, M.L., Crismon, M.L., Roberts, S., Childs, A. (1993) Clozapine response and adverse effects in nine brain-injured patients. *Journal of Clinical Psychopharmacology* 13:198–203.

Mooney, G.F., Haas, L.J. (1993) Effect of methylphenidate on brain injury-related anger. *Archives of Physical Medicine & Rehabilation* 74:153–160.

Morey, C.E., Cilo, M., Berry, J., Cusick, C. (2003) The effect of Aricept in persons with persistent memory disorder following traumatic brain injury: A pilot study. *Brain Injury* 17:809–815.

Moldover, J.E., Goldberg, K.B., Prout, M.F. (2004) Depression after traumatic brain injury: A review of evidence for clinical heterogeneity. *Neuropsychology Review* 14:143–154.

Monji, A., Yoshida, I., Koga, H., Tashiro, K., Tashiro, N. (1999) Brain injury-induced rapid-cycling affective disorder successfully treated with valproate. *Psychosomatics* 40:448–449.

Muller, U., Von Cramon, Y. (1994) The therapeutic potential of bromocriptine in neuropsychological rehabilitation of patients with acquired brain damage. *Progress in Neuro-Psychopharmacology & Biological Psychiatry* 18:1103–1120.

Muller, U., Murai, T., Bauer-Wittmund, T., Von Cramon, D.Y. (1999) Paroxetine versus citalopram treatment of pathological crying after brain injury. *Brain Injury* 13:805–811.

Murai, T., Fujimoto, S. (2003) Rapid cycling bipolar disorder after left temporal polar damage. *Brain Injury* 17:355–358.

Mustafa, B., Evrim, O., Sari, A. (2005) Secondary mania following traumatic brain injury. *Journal of Neuropsychiatry & Clinical Neurosciences* 17:122–124.

Mysiw, W.J., Sandel, M.E. (1997) The agitated brain injured patient: Part 2: Pathophysiology and treatment. *Archives of Physical Medicine and Rehabilitation* 78:213–20.

Mysiw, W.J., Jackson, R.D., Corrigan, J.D. (1988) Amitryptyline for post-traumatic agitation. *American Journal of Physical Medicine & Rehabilitation* 67:29–33.

Nemetz, P.N., Leibson, C., Naessens, J.M., Beard, M., Kokmen, E., Annegers, J.F., Kurland, L.T. (1999) Traumatic brain injury and time to onset of Alzheimer's disease: A population-based study. *American Journal of Epidemiology* 149:32–40.

Newburn, G. (1998) Psychiatric disorders associated with traumatic brain injury: Optimal treatment. *CNS Drugs* 6:441–456.

Newburn, G., Newburn, D. (2005) Selegiline in the management of apathy following traumatic brain injury. *Brain Injury* 19:149–154.

Nickels, J.L., Schneider, W.N., Dombovy, M.L., Wong, T.M. (1994) Clinical use of amantadine in brain injury rehabilitation. *Brain Injury* 8:709–718.

Niemann, H., Ruff, R.M., Kramer, J.H. (1996) An attempt towards differentiating attentional deficits in traumatic brain injury. *Neuropsychological Review* 1:11–46.

NIH Consensus Development Panel on Rehabilitation of Persons with Traumatic Brain Injury. (1999) *Journal of the American Medical Association* 282:974–983.

Oddy, M. (2001) Sexual relationships following brain injury. *Sexual and Relationship Therapy* 16:247–259.

Oddy, M., Coughlan, T., Tyerman, A., Jenkins, D. (1985) Social adjustment after closed head injury: A further follow-up seven years after injury. *Journal of Neurology, Neurosurgery, and Psychiatry* 48:564–568.

O'Donnell, M.L., Creamer, M., Bryant, R.A., Schnyder, U., Shalev, A. (2003) Posttraumatic disorders following injury: An empirical and methodological review. *Clinical Psychology Review* 23:587–603.

Oellet, M.C., Savard, J., Morin, C.M. (2004) Insomnia following traumatic brain injury: A review. *Neurorehabilitation and Neural Repair* 18:187 198.

Oquendo, M.A., Friedman, J.H., Grunebaum, M.F., Burke, A., Silver, J.M., Mann, J.J. (2004) Suicidal behavior and mild traumatic brain injury in major depression. *The Journal of Nervous and Mental Disease* 192:430–434.

Pachet, A., Friesen, S., Wenkelaar, D., Gray, B. (2003) Beneficial behavioral effects of lamotrigine in traumatic brain injury. *Brain Injury* 17:715–722.

Parvizi, J., Anderson, S.W., Martin, C.O., Damasio, H., Damasio, A.R. (2001) Pathological laughter and crying. A link to the cerebellum. *Brain* 124:1708–1719.

Perna, R. (2004) Benzodiazepines and antipsychotics: Cognitive side-effects. *The Journal of Head Trauma Rehabilitation* 19:516–518.

Perino, C., Rago, R., Cicolin, A., Torta, R., Monaco, F. (2001) Mood and behavioral disorders following traumatic brain injury: Clinical evaluation and pharmacological management. *Brain Injury* 15:139–148.

Plassman, B.L., Havlik, R.J., Steffens, D.C., Helms, M.J., Newman, T.N., Drosdick, D., Phillips, C., Gau, B.A., Welsh-Bohmer, K.A., Burke, J.R., Guralnik, J.M., Breitner, J.C.S. (2000) Documented head injury in early adulthood and risk of Alzheimer's disease and other dementias. *Neurology* 55:1158–1166.

Plenger, P.M., Dixon, C.E., Castillo, R.M., Frankowski, R.F., Yablon, S.A., Levin, H.S. (1996) Subacute methylphenidate treatment for moderate to moderately severe traumatic brain injury: A preliminary double-blind placebo-controlled study. *Archives of Physical Medicine & Rehabilitation* 77:536–540.

Pope, H.G., McElroy, S.L., Satlin, A., Hudson, J.I., Keck, P.E., Kalish, R. (1988) Head injury, bipolar disorder and response to valproate. *Comprehensive Psychiatry* 29:34–38.

Popovic, V., Aimaretti, G., Casanueva, F.F., Ghigo, E. (2005) Hypopituitarism following traumatic brain injury. *Growth Hormone & IGF Research* 15:177–184.

Powell, J.H., Al-Adawi, S., Morgan, J., Greenwood, R.J. (1996) Motivational deficits after brain injury: Effects of bromocriptine in 11 patients. *Journal of Neurology, Neurosurgery, and Psychiatry* 60:416–421.

Prigatano, G.P. (1991) Disordered mind, wounded soul. The emerging role of psychotherapy in rehabilitation after brain injury. *The Journal of Head Trauma Rehabilitation* 64:1–10.

Rapoport, M.J., McCullagh, S., Streiner, D., Feinstein, A. (2003) The clinical significance of major depression following mild traumatic brain injury. *Psychosomatics* 44:31–37.

Rapoport, M.J., McCullagh, S., Shamni, P., Feinstein, A. (2005) Cognitive impairment associated with major depression following mild and moderate traumatic brain injury. *Journal of Neuropsychiatry & Clinical Neurosciences* 17:61–65.

Rao, V., Lyketsos, C.G. (2002) Psychiatric aspects of traumatic brain injury. *Psychiatric Clinics of North America* 25:43–69.

Rao, N., Jellinek, H.M., Woolston, D.C. (1985) Agitation in closed head injury: Haloperidol effects on rehabilitation outcome. *Archives of Physical Medicine & Rehabilitation* 66:30–34.

Reinhard, D.L., Whyte, J., Sandel, M.E. (1996) Improved arousal and initiation following tricyclic antidepressant use in severe brain injury. *Archives of Physical Medicine Rehabilitation* 77:80–83.

Roane, D.M., Feinberg, T.E., Meckler, L., Miner, C.R., Scicutella, A., Rosenthal, R.N. (2000) Treatment of dementia-associated agitation with gabapentin. *Journal of Neuropsychiatry & Clinical Neurosciences* 12(1):40–43.

Rosati, D.L. (2002) Early polyneuropharmacologic intervention in brain injury agitation. *American Journal of Physical Medicine & Rehabilitation* 81:90–93.

Rothwell, N.A., LaVigna, G.W., Willis, T.J. (1999) A non-aversive rehabilitation approach for people with severe behavioral problems resulting from brain injury. *Brain Injury* 13:521–533.

Rowland, R.T., Mysiw, W.J., Bogner, J.A. (1992) Trazodone for post-traumatic agitation [abstract]. *Archives of Physical Medicine & Rehabilitation* 73:963.

Ruedrich, S.L., Chu, C.C., Moore, S.L. (1983) ECT for major depression in a patient with acute brain trauma. *American Journal of Psychiatry* 140:928–929.

Rybach, R., Rybach, L. (1995) Gabapentin for behavioral dyscontrol. *American Journal of Psychiatry* 152:1399–1401.

Sachdev, P., Smith, J.S., Cathcart, S. (2001) Schizophrenia-like psychosis following traumatic brain injury: A chart-based descriptive and case–control study. *Psychological Medicine* 31:231–239.

Sadock, B.J., Sadock, V.A. (eds.). (2005) *Kaplan & Sadock's Comprehensive Textbook of Psychiatry*, 8th ed. New York: Lippincott Williams & Wilkins.

Sandel, M.E., Mysiw, W.J. (1996) The agitated brain injured patient. Part I. Definitions, differential diagnosis and assessment. *Archives of Physical Medicine & Rehabilitation* 77:617–623.

Saran, A.S. (1985) Depression after minor closed head injury: Role of dexamethasone suppression test and antidepressants. *Journal of Clinical Psychiatry* 46:335–338.

Salmond, C.H., Chatfield, D.A., Manon, D.K., Pickard, J.D., Sahakian, B.J. (2005) Cognitive sequelae of head injury: Involvement of basal forebrain and associated structures. *Brain* 128:189–200.

Sandel, M.E., Williams, K.S., Dellapietra, L., Derogatis, L.R. (1996) Sexual functioning following traumatic brain injury. *Brain Injury* 10:719–728.

Satz, P. (1993) Brain reserve capacity on symptom onset after brain injury: A formulation and review of evidence for threshold theory. *Neuropsychology* 7:273–295.

Sayal, K., Ford, T., Pipe, R. (2000) Case study: Bipolar disorder after head injury. *Journal of the American Academy of Child and Adolescent Psychiatry* 39:525–528.

Scheutzow, M.H., Wiercisiewski, D.R. (1999) Panic disorder in a patient with traumatic brain injury: A case report and discussion. *Brain Injury* 13:705–714.

Schreiber, S., Klag, E., Gross, Y., Segman, R.H., Pick, C.G. (1998) Beneficial effect of risperidone on sleep disturbance and psychosis following traumatic brain injury. *International Clinical Psychopharmacology* 13:273–275.

Scicutella, A. (2001) Anxiety Disorders in Epilepsy. In Ettinger, A.B. & Kanner, A.M. (eds.): *Psychiatric Issues in Epilepsy A Practical Guide to Diagnosis and Treatment.* Philadelphia: Lippincott Williams and Wilkins, pp. 95–109.

Seel, R.T., Kreutzer, J.S., Rosenthal, M., Hammond, F.M., Corrigan, J.D., Black, K. (2003) Depression after traumatic brain injury: A national institute on disability and rehabilitation research model systems multicenter investigation. *Archives Physical Medical Rehabilation* 84:177–184.

Shaughnessy, R. (1995) Psychopharmacotherapy of neuropsychiatric disorders. *Psychiatr Annals* 25:634–640.

Sheehan, D.V., Ballenger, J., Jacobsen, G. (1980) Treatment of endogenous anxiety with phobic, hysterical, and hypochondriacal symptoms. *Archives of General Psychiatry* 37:51–59.

Simpson, G., Tate, R. (2002) Suicidality after traumatic brain injury: Demographic, injury and clinical correlates. *Psychological Medicine* 32:687–697.

Simpson, G., Long, E. (2004) An evaluation of sex education and information resources and their provision to adults with traumatic brain injury. *The Journal of Head Trauma Rehabilitation* 19:413–428.

Simpson, G., Blaszczynski, A., Hodgkinson, A. (1999) Sex offending as a psychosocial sequelae of traumatic brain injury. *The Journal of Head Trauma Rehabilitation* 14:567–580.

Silver, J.M., Kramer, R., Greenwald, S., Weissman, M. (2001) The association between head injuries and psychiatric disorders: Findings from the New Haven NIMH epidemiologic catchment area study. *Brain Injury* 15:935–945.

Silver, J.M., Yudofsky, S.C., Anderson, K.E. (2005) Aggressive disorders. In Silver, J.M., McAllister, T.W., Yudofsky, S.C. (eds.). *Textbook of Traumatic Brain Injury.* Washington DC: American Psychiatric Press, pp. 259–277.

Small, G.W., Rabins, P.V., Barry, P.P., Burkholtz, N.S., DeKosky, S.T., Ferris, S.H., Finkel, S.I., Gwyther, L.P., Khachaturian, Z.S., Lebowitz, B.D., McRae, T.D., Morris, J.C., Oakley, F., Schneider, L.S., Streim, J.E., Sunderland, T., Teri, L.A., Tune, L.E. (1997) Diagnosis and treatment of Alzheimer's disease and related disorders: Consensus statement of the American Association for Geriatric Psychiatry, The Alzheimer's Association and the American Geriatrics Society. *Journal of American Medical Association* 278:1363–1371.

Spier, S.A., Tesar, G.E., Rosenbaum, J.F., Woods, S.W. (1986) Treatment of panic disorder and agoraphobia with clonazepam. *Journal of Clinical Psychiatry* 47:238–242.

Spiers, P.A., Hochanadel, G. (1999) Citicholine for traumatic brain injury: Report of two cases, including my own. *Journal of International Neuropsychological Society* 5:260–264.

Spinella, M., Eaton, L.A. (2002) Hypomania induced by herbal and pharmaceutical psychotropic medicines following mild traumatic brain injury. *Brain Injury* 16:359–367.

Springer, J., Chollet, A. (2001) A traumatic car crash. *Lancet* 357:1848.

Stanislav, S.W. (1997) Cognitive effects of antipsychotic agents in persons with traumatic brain injury. *Brain Injury* 11:335–341.

Stanislav, S.W., Childs, A. (2000) Evaluating the usage of droperidol in acutely agitated persons with brain injury. *Brain Injury* 14:261–265.

Starkstein, S.E., Boston, J.D., Robinson, R.G. (1988) Mechanisms of mania after brain injury: 12 case reports and review of the literature. *The Journal of Nervous and Mental Disease* 176:87–100.

Stengler-Wenzke, K., Muller, U. (2002) Fluoxetine for OCD after brain injury. *American Journal of Psychiatry* 159:872.

Stewart, J.T., Hemsath, R.H. (1988) Bipolar illness following traumatic brain injury: Treatment with lithium and carbamazepine. *Journal of ClinicalPsychiatry* 49:74–75.

Stierwalt, J.A.G., Murray, L.L. (2002) Attention impairment following traumatic brain injury. *Seminars in Speech and Language* 23:129–138.

Tateno, A., Jorge, R.E., Robinson, R.G. (2003) Clinical correlates of aggressive behavior after traumatic brain injury. *Journal of Neuropsychiatry & Clinical Neurosciences* 15:155–160.

Tateno, A., Jorge, R.E., Robinson, R.G. (2004) Pathological laughing and crying following traumatic brain injury. *The Journal of Neuropsychiatry & Clinical Neurosciences* 16:426–434.

Taverni, J.P., Seliger, G., Lichtman, S.W. (1998) Donepezil-mediated memory improvement in traumatic brain injury during post acute rehabilitation. *Brain Injury* 12:77–80.

Teasdale, T.W., Engberg, A.W. (2001) Suicide after traumatic brain injury: A population study. *Journal of Neurology, Neurosurgery and Psychiatry* 71:436–440.

Teitelman, E. (2001) Off-label uses of modafinil. *Am J Psychiatry* 158:1341.

Teng, C.J., Bhalerao, S., Lee, Z., Farber, H.M., Foran, T., Tucker, W. (2001) The use of bupropion in the treatment of restlessness after a traumatic brain injury. *Brain Injury* 15:463–467.

Tenovuo, O. (2005) Central acetylcholinesterase inhibitors in the treatment of chronic traumatic brain injury—clinical experience in 111 patients. *Progress in Neuro-Psychopharmacology & Biological Psychiatry* 29:61–67.

Tiersky, L.A., Anselmi, V., Johnston, M.V., Kurtyka, J., Roosen, E., Schwartz, T., DeLuca, J. (2005) A trial of neuropsychologic rehabilitation in mild-spectrum traumatic brain injury. *Archives in Physical Medicine & Rehabilitation* 86:1565–1574.

Thomsen, I.V. (1984) Late outcome of very severe blunt head trauma: A 10–15 year second-follow-up. *Journal of Neurology, Neurosurgery, and Psychiatry* 47:260–268.

Trimble, M.R. (1991) Interictal psychoses of epilepsy. *Advances in Neurology* 55:143–152.

Turner-Stokes, L., Nibras, H., Pierce, K., Clegg, F. (2002) Managing depression in brain injury rehabilitation: The use of an integrated care pathway and preliminary report of response to sertraline. *Clinical Rehabilation* 16:261–268.

Underhill, A.T., Lobello, S.G., Stroud, T.P. Terry, K.S., Devivos, M.J., Fine, P.R. (2003) Depression and life satisfaction in patients with traumatic brain injury: A longitudinal study. *Brain Injury* 17:973–982.

Van Reekum, R., Bayley, M., Garner, S. Burke, I.M., Fawcett, S., Hart, A., Thompson, W. (1995) N of 1 study: Amantadine for the amotivational syndrome in a patient with traumatic brain injury. *Brain Injury* 9:49–53.

Van Reekum, R., Bolago, I., Finlayson, M.A.J., Garner, S., Links, P.S. (1996) Psychiatric disorders after traumatic brain injury. *Brain Injury* 10:319–327.

Vanderploeg, R.D., Curtiss, G., Belanger, H.G. (2005) Long-term neuropsychological outcomes following mild traumatic brain injury. *Journal of International Neuropsychological Society* 11:228–236.

Warden, D.L., Labbate, L.A., Salazar, A.M., Nelson, R., Sheley, E., Staudenmeier, J., Martin, E. (1997) Posttraumatic stress disorder in patients with traumatic brain injury and amnesia for the event? *Journal of Neuropsychiatry & Clinical Neurosciences* 9:18–22.

Watson, C., Rutterford, N.A., Shortland, D., Williamson, N., Alderman, N. (2001) Reduction of chronic aggressive behavior 10 years after brain injury. *Brain Injury* 15:1003–1005.

Wesolowski, M.D., Zencius, A., Burke, W.H. (1993) Effects of feedback and behavior contracting on head trauma person's inappropriate sexual behavior. *Behavourial Residential Treatment* 8:89–96.

Whelan, F.J., Walker, M.S., Schultz, S.K. (2000) Donepezil in the treatment of cognitive dysfunction associated with traumatic brain injury. *Annals in Clinical Psychiatry* 12:131–135.

Whitlock, J.A. (1999) Brain injury, cognitive impairment and donepezil. *The Journal of Head Trauma Rehabilitation* 14:424–427.

Whyte, J., Hart, T., Schuster, K., Fleming, M., Polansky, M., Coslett, H.B. (1997) Effects of methylphenidate on attentional function after traumatic brain injury: A randomized, placebo-controlled trial. *American Journal of Physical Medicine & Rehabilitation* 76:440–450.

Whyte, J.W., Vaccaro, M., Grieb-Neff, P., Hart, T. (2002) Psychostimulant use in the rehabilitation of individuals with traumatic brain injury. *The Journal of Head Trauma Rehabilitation* 17:284–299.

Whyte, J., Hart, T., Bode, R.K., Malec, J.F. (2003) The Moss attention rating scale for traumatic brain injury: Initial psychometric assessment. *Archives in Physical Medicine & Rehabilitation* 84:268–276.

Whyte, J., Hart, T., Vaccaro, M., Grieb-Neff, P., Risser, A., Polansky, M., Coslett, H.B. (2004) Effects of methylphenidate on attention deficits after traumatic brain injury. A multidimensional, randomized, controlled trial *American Journal of Physical Medicine & Rehabilitation* 83:401–420.

Williams, D.B., Annegers, J.F., Kokmen, E., O'Brien, P.C., Kurland, L.T. (1991) Brain injury and neurologic sequelae: A cohort study of dementia, parkinsonism and amyotrophic lateral sclerosis. *Neurology* 41:1554–1557.

Wilson, S.A.K. (1924) Some problems in neurology. II: pathological laughter and crying. *The Journal of Neurology and Psychopathology* 4:299–333.

Wilson, S.L., Powell, G.E., Brock, D., Thwaites, H. (1996) Vegetative state and responses to sensory stimulation: An analysis of 24 cases. *Brain Injury* 10:807–818.

Woodman, C.L., Noyes, R. (1994) Panic disorder; Treatment with valproate. *Journal The Clinical Psychiatry* 55:134–136.

Wroblewski, B.A., Joseph, A.B., Cornblatt, R.R. (1996) Antidepressant pharmacotherapy and the treatment of depression in patients with severe traumatic brain injury: A controlled, prospective study. *Journal of Clinical Psychiatry* 57:582–587,

Wroblewski, B.A., Joseph, A.B., Kupfer, J., Kalliel, K. (1997) Effectiveness of valproic acid on destructive and aggressive behaviors in patients with acquired brain injury. *Brain Injury* 11:37–47.

Zafonte, R.D., Watanabe, T., Mann, N.R. (1998) Amantadine: A potential treatment for the minimally conscious state. *Brain Injury* 12:617–621.

Zasler, N.D., Martelli, M.F. (2005) Sexual dysfunction. In Silver, J.M., McAllister, T.W., Yudofsky, S.C., (eds.): *Textbook of Traumatic Brain Injury.* Washington DC: American Psychiatric Press Inc, pp. 437–450.

Zhang, L., Plotkin, R.C., Wang, G., Sandel, M.E., Lee, S. (2004) Cholinergic augmentation with donepezil enhances recovery in short-term memory and sustained attention after traumatic brain injury. *Archives in Physical Medicine & Rehabilitation* 85:1050–1055.

Zeilig, G., Drubach, D.A., Katz-Zeilig, M., Karatinos, J. (1996) Pathological laughter and crying in patients with closed traumatic brain injury. *Brain Injury* 10:591–597.

Zencius, A., Wesolowski, M., Burke, W., Hough, S. (1990) Managing hypersexual disorders in brain-injured clients. *Brain Injury* 4:175–181.

7
Neuropsychological Rehabilitation
Evaluation and Treatment Approaches

DEBORAH M. BENSON AND MARYKAY PAVOL

The Role of the Neuropsychologist

Clinical neuropsychologists are professionals within the field of psychology with special expertise in applying the principles of brain–behavior relationships to individuals with various neurological injuries or illnesses, as well as other medical, developmental, and/or psychiatric conditions (National Academy of Neuropsychology [NAN], 2001). Using various tests, techniques, and principles, neuropsychologists evaluate individuals' cognitive, behavioral, and emotional strengths and weaknesses, and the impact of these on the person's ability to function. This information, combined with information from other professionals (physician, occupational, speech-language, physical therapists, etc.) and families/significant others, is utilized to develop, recommend, and implement treatment interventions.

Neuropsychologists hold a doctoral degree in psychology, and are licensed in their state to practice psychology. In addition to their doctoral degree, recent guidelines (NAN, 2001), suggest that neuropsychologists have at least two full-time years of supervised experience and specialized training in the study and practice of clinical neuropsychology and neurosciences, at least one of which is postdoctoral. As further evidence of advanced training, board certification in neuropsychology can be obtained through the American Board of Professional Psychology (ABPP; www.abpp.org) or the American Board of Clinical Neuropsychology (ABCN; www.theabcn.org). Neuropsychologists working in rehabilitation settings may also be board certified through the ABPP in rehabilitation psychology, a specialty area within professional psychology which focuses on assisting the individual with an injury or illness and his or her family in achieving optimal physical, psychological and interpersonal functioning. Rehabilitation psychology emphasizes interdisciplinary teamwork and a holistic, integrated approach, integrating medical, psychological, social, environmental, and political considerations in order to achieve optimal rehabilitation goals.

Neuropsychologists serve in varied roles in neuro-rehabilitation settings. They often function as team leaders or directors of neuro-rehabilitation programs, providing both clinical and administrative supervision and oversight of program functions. They may serve as consultants, called in to evaluate cognitive and emotional functioning in patients with brain injury and to provide further insight to the rest of the interdisciplinary team regarding barriers to participation and make recommendations regarding potential treatment interventions. Often, neuropsychologists are directly involved in educating and counseling patients and families regarding the nature of the injury, effects on cognition/behavior/emotion, expectations for recovery, and recommendations for management of ongoing impairments. Given their background training as research scientists, neuropsychologists are often involved in clinical research activities, as well, utilizing the wealth of information obtained by patients and families to contribute to a greater understanding of the principles, processes and factors underlying rehabilitation outcomes.

Neuropsychological Evaluations in Rehabilitation

A neuropsychological evaluation is used to provide insights into the presence and nature of cognitive impairment. If, for example, a patient complains of memory problems, the neuropsychological assessment will indicate whether the memory failure is due to a primary memory deficit or, instead, to impairments in attention, language, or executive skills that are leading to memory problems. Finding the source of a cognitive problem will have direct implications for treatment and may help to refine a diagnosis. A neuropsychological evaluation consists of paper-and-pencil, question and-answer, and/or computer-administered tests. The examiner, either a neuropsychologist or qualified technician working under the supervision of a neuropsychologist, will prefer to work with the patient in a quiet environment. Results of a recent survey indicate that 76% of neuropsychologists use a flexible battery approach as opposed to a fixed battery, meaning that a majority of neuropsychologists will use a variable but routine group of tests for different types of patients (Sweet et al., 2006).

Prior to beginning testing, the patient should provide consent for the evaluation and should be informed of any limits to confidentiality (American Psychological Association, 2002; NAN, 2003). All tests must be administered and scored in a manner that is consistent with the test publisher's directions; standardized procedures are critical to valid interpretation. The areas assessed might include orientation, attention, memory, language, visual perception/construction, executive function, academic, sensory motor and intellectual skills.

Estimates of premorbid function may also be performed. These estimates of pre-injury ability may be derived from demographic characteristics or from performances on measures believed to be relatively resistant to change (such as reading ability). Examples of methods that use demographic characteristics include those created by Barona et al. (1984) and Krull et al. (1995). These estimation methods have been found to have limited accuracy, especially in the highest and lowest ranges of intellectual function (Basso et al., 2000). An example of an estimation method that uses reading ability is the North American Adult Reading Test (NAART or NART-R), in which the patient is asked to read irregularly pronounced words (Blair & Spreen, 1989). There is evidence that estimates of IQ based on reading skill perform as well or better than estimates based on demographics (Blair & Spreen, 1989; Bright et al., 2002). Johnstone and colleagues provided data suggesting that another test of reading ability (Wide Range Achievement Test-Revised or WRAT-R) provides an even better estimate of low-range verbal IQ, although both the NAART and WRAT-R were best at estimating average IQ, with tendencies to underestimate high-range IQs and overestimate low-range IQs (Johnstone et al., 1996). These estimates based on reading may not perform well at predicting cognitive domains *other* than IQ (Schretlen et al., 2005). Yet another method of estimating IQ comes from combining demographic characteristics with Wechsler Adult Intelligence Scale-III subtests to create algorithms (Schoenberg et al., 2003). Some researchers recommend using different estimation methods for patients in different IQ ranges (Griffin et al., 2002).

The nature and length of the evaluation will differ according to the setting and the patient. A patient in an acute rehabilitation setting who is medically ill, highly confused, perhaps lethargic or agitated, will not be appropriate for lengthy, complicated assessments. In fact, the attempt to assess such a patient with sophisticated instruments will likely result in an invalid profile that does not provide useful information. Instead, this type of patient will require brief, bedside assessments. These evaluations may include assessments of arousal, behavior, orientation, basic language, thought content, visual-fields, simple memory, insight, and mood (Guy & Cummings, 2003). Formal instruments are used whenever possible. Available measures include the Galveston Orientation and Amnesia test (Levin et al., 1979), the Orientation Log (Jackson et al., 1998), the Cognitive Log (Alderson et al., 2003), the Temporal Orientation Test (Benton et al., 1964), Mini Mental Status Examination (Folstein et al., 1975), the Short Test of Mental Status (Kokmen et al., 1991), the Executive Interview (EXIT) (Royall et al., 1992), and the Confusion Assessment Protocol (Sherer et al., 2005). Rating scales such as the Agitated Behavior Scale may also be useful (Corrigan, 1989). The reader is referred to the website provided by the Center for Outcomes Measurement in Brain Injury for additional suggestions for brief assessment and rating scales (Santa Clara Valley Medical Center, 2006). For patients emerging from coma, some commonly used tests include the Coma/Near Coma Scale (Rappaport et al., 1992) and the Coma Recovery Scale-Revised (Kalmar & Giacino, 2005). The following vignette describes a patient who was appropriate for this limited type of cognitive assessment.

JD, a 65-year-old male, was admitted for inpatient rehabilitation for treatment of deficits due to a right frontal hemorrhage. He was known to have had a left frontal hemorrhage 2 years earlier. In the initial evaluation the patient was pleasant and alert but highly distracted, touching and commenting on everything around him. The Cognitive Log was administered and he obtained a score of 3 (out of 30 possible points). He was oriented to his name only. He did not attempt responses to most structured questions. Severe motor perseveration was evident in a writing sample. In a follow-up assessment 4 days later, the patient showed slight improvement in his ability to benefit from cues for orientation to place; he was able to begin a mental sequencing task but could not complete it and again obtained a score of 3. He appeared less distracted by his environment. In the final session prior to discharge, attention appeared to improve further (3-5 minutes). He had severe difficulty initiating and persisting on a simple sequencing task, but, after much prompting, he completed the sequence. His total score was 7. His poor attention and initiation was evident in his other therapies as well.

For patients with sufficient attention and endurance, somewhat longer tests may be used such as the Repeatable Battery for the Assessment of Neuropsychological Status (Randolph et al., 1998), the Dementia Rating Scale-2 (Jurica et al., 2001), and the Neurobehavioral Cognitive Status Examination (Kiernan et al., 1987). These tests offer the advantage of relative brevity (approximately 30 minutes) while assessing a range of cognitive areas. These screening instruments may also be used when the suspicion of cognitive deficit is low but there remains an interest in ruling-out impairment. These tests do not, however, represent a thorough assessment of cognition, particularly in the area of executive function.

When a patient appears to have sufficient stamina and attention to tolerate at least 1 hour of assessment, he or she is appropriate for the more complex and sophisticated measures. These types of assessments tend to occur in post-acute and outpatient settings. These comprehensive evaluations are lengthy and provide the most detailed information about the nature and extent of any cognitive dysfunction. The specific contents of the test battery will vary depending on the clinician, the setting and the referral question. As was noted earlier, the majority of neuropsychologists use a flexible battery as opposed to a firmly fixed battery approach, but this flexible battery may contain a fixed battery. One of the best-known fixed batteries is the Halstead–Reitan Neuropsychological Test Battery (Reitan & Wolfson, 1993). These extended evaluations will include assessment of a wide range of skills and each skill area may include assessments of more specific skills: assessments of attention may include tests of sustained and divided attention; assessments of memory may include tests of verbal, visual, free recall, forced choice, and recognition memory; assessments of language may include tests of naming, comprehension, reading and writing; assessments of visual skill may include tests of visual-spatial and visual-constructional skill; assessments of executive function may include tests of problem-solving, verbal fluency, response inhibition, and mental flexibility. Evaluations of motor skill, personality, malingering, and psychiatric status will frequently be included. Muriel Lezak has published the fourth edition of her widely respected and referenced text on neuropsychological assessment (Lezak et al., 2004) and Spreen and colleagues have recently published a new edition of their detailed test descriptions (Strauss et al., 2006). These are among the many publications describing the specific contents and interpretation of comprehensive test batteries. The following vignette describes a patient who received brief assessment during his inpatient admission followed by a more lengthy assessment after his discharge to home.

MH, a 50 year-old carpenter, fell from a ladder at work and sustained a traumatic brain injury. He underwent inpatient rehabilitation and showed improved attention and memory during his inpatient admission. His score on the Galveston Orientation and Amnesia Test (GOAT) improved to the normal range shortly before discharge to his home, at which time he was typically oriented to self, place, date, and event. He was deemed inappropriate for more advanced cognitive assessment during the time his GOAT score was impaired. After discharge he was seen in the outpatient clinic and completed a full cognitive assessment. The outpatient evaluation showed impairments in memory and visuospatial organization. In particular, immediate learning was generally below expectation and delayed recall showed more significant deficits. His delayed recall was characterized by a tendency to make intrusion errors with information from similar semantic categories. In other words, he used category groupings to guide his recall but was inaccurate in recalling the exact information to be remembered. Errors of this nature are common following traumatic brain injury. Regarding visuospatial skill, his performances on measures of visual construction and ability to judge line angles were impaired and the quality of the errors was suggestive of right hemisphere dysfunction. Scores on tests of language, auditory attention, mental flexibility, and reasoning were within normal limits. Although these performances were not impaired compared to normative samples, they possibly represented a slight decline relative to premorbid function based on one estimate of premorbid IQ and on his wife's report of his abilities prior to the fall. The patient and wife reported that he cried much more frequently following the injury but his self-report did not indicate significant symptoms of depression. He did report mild symptoms of anxiety, including increased fears of death. Increased lability is commonly reported after traumatic brain injury and the anxiety was attributed to his recent serious injury.

When all testing is completed, the examiner scores the results according to the published guidelines. The scores are then compared to normative samples. Normative samples from the test manual or from published studies may be used. These normative samples provide data that may vary according to the demographic characteristics of the patient (age, gender, education, race), and a judgment about a patient's performance will be made according to how that patient compares to others with similar characteristics. Accurate interpretation of a patient's performance relies heavily on the use of appropriate normative samples but should not stop there. In addition, the performance should be interpreted according to estimates of a patient's pre-injury abilities. In other words, findings in the average range may not appear problematic but, if the patient typically performed in the superior range prior to injury, the average findings may actually indicate cognitive decline (Lezak et al., 2004). Lezak also recommends using the *pattern* of cognitive strengths and weaknesses to identify characteristics of particular disorders and to understand the specific nature of poor performances (Lezak, 2003; Lezak et al, 2004). Assessment of strengths and weaknesses is particularly important in a rehabilitation setting, where cognitive strengths may be used to compensate for weaknesses. In addition to the quantitative data derived from test scores, qualitative information (test-taking behavior) can also provide important insight into the nature and source of cognitive impairment (Lezak et al, 2004). These qualitative observations may relate to the patient's affect, frustration tolerance, arousal, speech, emotional state, or the particular nature of the impaired response. Conclusions based on all of these perspectives will provide the most balanced and meaningful information for the patient, family, and treatment team. Once the test performances are thoroughly evaluated, they must be integrated with the patient's social and medical histories in order to develop the diagnoses. The following vignette illustrates the situation where the scores are not frankly impaired compared to normative samples but nonetheless suggest a decline from the patient's premorbid function.

RR, a 40-year-old, right-handed woman with a bachelor's degree, was working overseas as an architect. She and her family report that she was intelligent and successful in her career. She developed sinus-type complaints and reduced hearing in the left ear that was misdiagnosed. On a visit to the United States she was diagnosed with an acoustic neuroma. She underwent surgery for resection but recovery was complicated by a cerebellar bleed. After completing inpatient rehabilitation for gait ataxia and cranial nerve abnormalities, the patient had an outpatient neuropsychological assessment. Verbal IQ was found to be High Average and Performance IQ was Average. Verbal memory was Average, visual memory was High Average, and untimed problem-solving was High Average. Mild impairments were found in auditory attention, visual-motor attention, and visual-motor sequencing. This pattern was believed to suggest mildly decreased information processing speed. Although verbal memory was Average, the test findings, and information from the patient's family, suggested that this represented a decline relative to her premorbid skills. Overall, the assessment findings and family reports indicated reduced performances in timed conditions or when attempting to manage large amounts of information, most likely as a consequence of the cerebellar hemorrhage. The implications of these findings regarding her return to work were discussed with the patient, family, and treatment team.

Once the patient's performances have been evaluated, the findings are included in a report. Strauss et al. (2006) provide a useful chapter on neuropsychological reports, with detailed descriptions and recommendations. The report will typically contain relevant medical and social information as well as the reason for the evaluation. A listing of the tests administered may be provided. All reports should include a comment on whether the findings are believed to be a valid and reasonable reflection of the patient's cognitive status. The validity may be reduced by various factors, including sensory impairment, fatigue, language barrier, pain, or psychiatric difficulties. The report should contain specific information about the test findings. There will also be an interpretation or summary section that provides the examiner's conclusions and diagnoses. Recommendations based on the conclusions should be offered. The recommendations may include directions for treatment (medication, psychotherapy, cognitive rehabilitation), supervision/assistance needs, environmental modifications/accommodations, or recommendations for additional evaluations. Lastly, but perhaps most importantly, a feedback session should be held with the patient (and significant other) to review the findings and recommendations. The feedback session is critical to helping the patient and family understand the nature and severity of any deficits and therefore create an ideal environment for the patient. The feedback may also improve the patient's insight into his or her deficits. Thus, providing feedback represents good clinical practice and, moreover, is mandated by the American Psychological Association (American Psychological Association, 2002). The next vignette illustrates a situation in which the patient's complaints appear to be related to anxiety and poor coping skills as opposed to cognitive impairment per se. This finding has direct implications for treatment recommendations.

JK, a 21-year-old female, underwent brief inpatient rehabilitation after being struck by a car while she was walking. At the time of her injury she was a full-time college student and worked for the city transit authority. She reportedly managed this busy schedule well. The inpatient rehabilitation team found no evidence of dysphagia, cognitive impairment, or coping difficulty and she was sent home after a few days. An outpatient neuropsychological assessment done soon after revealed no evidence of cognitive deficits but indicated mild anxiety complaints. The patient, however, denied any anxiety. Two months later she returned to the physiatrist complaining of difficulty swallowing, impairments in attention and memory, and inability to return to work or school as a result of her injuries. She was deemed neurologically stable. The report of decreasing function in a neurologically stable patient was inconsistent with the expected recovery course. She was referred back to the neuropsychologist who discovered elevated symptoms of anxiety. The patient began psychotherapy and was also referred to a psychiatrist for psychotropic medication management.

Referral Questions

In the earlier years of neuropsychology, patients were referred for cognitive assessment in order to determine the presence and location of a lesion in the brain. With the advent of sophisticated imaging techniques (CT, MRI) a neuropsychological evaluation is no longer needed to ascertain the location of a stroke, tumor, or other structural abnormality. The indications for neuropsychological assessment have thus changed to some degree. Of course, if imaging results are inconclusive the neuropsychological exam continues to serve as part of a medical work-up to determine the cause of identified behavioral changes. When a lesion has been identified, a neuropsychological evaluation may be useful in determining the functional consequences, as the imaging techniques can tell *where* a lesion is located but not *what* effect that lesion may have on behavior. In a rehabilitation context, the neuropsychological findings are important in identifying the cognitive strengths and weaknesses that will influence the patient's ability to benefit from the rehabilitation program. The findings may be used to suggest therapeutic approaches or medication management. The assessment may be important in justifying treatment to insurance companies. Following the treatment, a repeat evaluation may be useful in assessing treatment efficacy, although it is recognized that a patient may make functional improvements that are not reflected in neuropsychological test scores (see discussion below regarding ecological validity). Further, the specific tests and timing of administration must be considered to avoid practice effects that may cloud interpretation. Repeat evaluations are also used to assess the recovery or decline from a medical condition. The evaluation should provide meaningful recommendations regarding supervision needs, capacity for decision-making and readiness for return to work or school. An area of increasing referrals is the forensic setting in which neuropsychological assessments are being used to support or refute legal claims. The following vignette describes a patient who was referred for evaluation of memory complaints.

LQ, a 75-year-old woman, was referred by her neurologist for assessment of memory complaints. The patient and her son reported that she had fallen and hit her head 6 months prior. She denied loss of consciousness and had no post-traumatic confusion. She was evaluated in an emergency department and was sent home, but her memory had become progressively worse since the fall. Results of cognitive testing revealed impairments in memory, naming, and visual-motor sequencing. Recognition memory was better than free recall but not intact. The patient appeared to have some difficulty hearing the examiner. Although this performance pattern may occur in traumatic injuries, the severity of deficits was inconsistent with the mild head injury and the worsening of deficits was inconsistent with recovery from traumatic injury. Given her medical history and specific cognitive profile, the neuropsychologist concluded that Alzheimer's disease was the most likely diagnosis. Recommendations included reassessment in 12 months, hearing screening, additional medical workup to rule-out treatable causes of dementia, genetic or ApoE testing to strengthen the diagnosis, treatment with dementia medications, supervision of complex activities, and use of a memory book.

The next vignette describes a patient for whom the cognitive assessment was useful in making treatment and discharge recommendations.

WM, a 57-year-old male, was admitted for inpatient rehabilitation following a right thalamic hemorrhage. He worked as a phlebotomist in a clinic and lived alone prior to admission. He had few supports in the community and was eager to return to home and work. The patient complained of word-finding and memory deficits, but the results of the brief initial evaluation were equivocal. The rehabilitation team later reported signs of left neglect and impulsivity in therapies. Results of an inpatient cognitive examination revealed mild to severe impairments in immediate memory, attention, visual-spatial skills, and trial and error learning. A left neglect was noted on one task. Language, delayed memory, and hypothetical problem-solving were within normal limits (Average to Low Average). His delayed memory (Low Average) was possibly reduced by poor initial learning. These findings, coupled with the reports from his therapists (impulsivity, reduced safety awareness, poor insight), suggested significant decline from pre-injury levels of function. The patient was educated about the findings and was advised to have supervision for complex activities (medications, finances, cooking, appointments). He was advised against traveling in the community alone and was recommended to live with a friend or family member until his function improved. He was advised to refrain from driving and returning to work immediately after discharge. Additional outpatient cognitive testing and a formal driving assessment were recommended. The patient's inpatient treatment team used these findings to set treatment goals for the remainder of his admission, with focus on complex activities and travel in the community. The patient was referred to a Medicaid waiver program for brain-injured individuals living in the community

Strengths of Neuropsychological Evaluations

As is noted in other chapters of this text, the neuropsychologist is not the only member of the rehabilitation team who will assess cognition. In fact, in many rehabilitation settings, all staff have a role in the assessment and treatment of cognitive deficits. Guidelines to improve the collaboration between neuropsychologists and speech-language pathologists were recently published and highlighted the degree of overlap in these assessments (Brown & Ricker, 2003). So what distinguishes the neuropsychologist from the other team members? Whereas the various therapy areas (physical, occupational, speech-language, and recreation) will tend to be focused on cognition that relates to their specialty, the neuropsychologist will assess a broad range of behavior. Moreover, the therapists will often assess cognition from a functional perspective while the neuropsychologist will utilize a broader array of paper-and-pencil instruments. As described above, these instruments will be administered in a standardized manner and the findings will be interpreted according to normative data. This allows the neuropsychologist to make adjustments for the specific demographic characteristics of a patient. The strength of the neuropsychological approach lies in the fact that it relies on objective measurements and interpretations across a breadth of behaviors. This is not to say that other disciplines don't perform any standardized assessments or that the neuropsychologist does not include any functional assessments. The difference lies in degree of emphasis on standardized and objective techniques and the wide range of behaviors assessed.

Limitations of Neuropsychological Evaluations

While neuropsychological evaluations can provide much useful information, limitations and shortcomings exist. The findings can be influenced by poor motivation, anxiety, depression, pain, sensory problems, medication side effects, and a host of other factors. Presence of confounding factors may reduce the validity of the results and should be noted in the report. It is the neuropsychologist's responsibility to recognize, minimize, and interpret how much the findings are affected by these factors. The assessments themselves tend to be time-consuming and costly. Obtaining insurance approval for neuropsychological assessments and treatments can be challenging and often requires education on the purpose of the evaluation or treatment.

One perceived limitation of neuropsychological assessment is the fact that the findings may not reflect functional improvement in a patient. For example, a patient who has sustained an injury may return for re-assessment of cognition after a period of months or years after an initial evaluation. Since the first evaluation, this patient may have made significant life-style improvements (e.g., improved independent function in the home, participation in volunteer or part-time work, increased social interaction). The neuropsychological findings may, however, not show significant improvement on standardized measures. One might be tempted to conclude that the neuropsychological assessment is invalid, but this would be inaccurate. Rather, this example may reflect a situation in which the assessment reveals continued *impairment* and the functional status reveals that the patient has more *activity* (or less *disability*) because he/she has compensated for the impairment. This interpretation is consistent with the latest definitions from the World Health Organization's (WHO) International Classification of Functioning, Disabilities and Health (World Health Organization, 2002). From this perspective, the neuropsychological assessment is not invalid but instead reflects *impairment* as opposed to *activity* in the same way that a test of motor strength may reveal *impairment* in a hemiparetic leg for a patient who is nonetheless able to use a walker to go to the store (*activity*).

An issue closely related to the topic of functional status is ecological validity. Ecological validity refers to the degree to which a formal test of cognition accurately predicts or correlates with behavior in natural settings. To phrase the issue in WHO terms, as was done by Odhuba et al. (2005), if a neuropsychological evaluation can provide a valid indication of *impairment*, how well does it reflect a patient's ability to perform a task in the "real" world (i.e., *disability* or *activity*)? In recent years there has been increased interest in this question. The data from studies of executive function, driving, and memory skill suggest modest relationships between neuropsychological test findings and measures of everyday functioning (Brown et al., 2005; Burgess et al., 1998; Chaytor & Schmitter-Edgecombe, 2003; Odhuba et al., 2005; Kalechstein et al., 2003; Grace et al., 2005; Higginson et al., 2000; Silver, 2000). The lack of strong correlations between standardized testing, measures of everyday function, and/or clinician ratings suggests that these assessments are sensitive to different skills and are all necessary to obtain a well-rounded evaluation of a patient. In fact, the WHO distinction between *impairment* and *activity* suggests that an imperfect correlation is to be expected when comparing the neuropsychological measures (*impairment*) and the functional assessments (*activity*). Therefore, we need the functional measures to see **what** the patient cannot do and we need the neuropsychological testing to know **why** (and thus know what to treat). While we may agree that both formal and functional measurements are useful, valid measurements of adaptive function are difficult to obtain for several reasons: difficulty re-creating real-life scenarios, differences between methods of evaluating function (formal functional assessments vs. clinician/family ratings), and lack of available instruments with large normative samples (Chaytor & Schmitter-Edgecombe, 2003; Moritz et al., 2004; Silver, 2000). Nonetheless, tests which are believed to have reasonable ecological validity (and which rely more on measures of *function*) include the Multiple Errands Test –Simplified Version (Alderman et al., 2003), the Rivermead Behavioural Memory Test-II (Cockburn & Keene, 2001; Wilson et al., 2003), the Behavior Rating Inventory of Executive Function (BRIEF) (Gioia & Isquith, 2004; Gioia et al., 2000), and the Behavioral Assessment of the Dysexecutive System (Wilson et al., 1996). Burgess and colleagues provide a detailed account of how more "function-led" tests of executive function may be developed (Burgess et al., 2006). For questions of driving safety, the best approach is multidisciplinary including input from physicians, occupational therapists, and neuropsychologists and includes cognitive assessment followed, if the patient performs sufficiently well, by an on-road evaluation (Brown et al., 2005; Grace et al., 2005; Schanke & Sundet, 2000; Whelihan et al., 2005).

Assessment of Malingering

The assessment of malingering or suboptimal performance has become increasingly common, particularly in forensic settings (Slick et al., 2004). According to a survey of board-certified neuropsychologists, these assessments have revealed high base rates of malingering in personal injury and disability cases (Mittenberg et al., 2002). In the fourth edition of the Diagnostic and Statistical Manual of Mental Disorders (DSM-IV), malingering has been defined as "the intentional production of false or grossly exaggerated physical or psychological symptoms, motivated by external incentives such as avoiding military duty, avoiding work, obtaining financial compensation, evading criminal prosecution, or obtaining drugs." (American Psychiatric Association, 1994, p. 739). It is seen as distinct from Factitious Disorder in which external incentives are absent and there instead appears to be a need to maintain a sick role. Malingering is also distinguished from Conversion Disorder, in which the behavior is believed *not* to be under conscious control of the patient and the symptoms appear to be related to psychological stressors. Limitations of the DSM-IV diagnostic criteria have been noted and alternative definitions have been offered, the most influential of these coming from Slick and colleagues (Slick et al., 1999). They proposed diagnostic criteria and practice standards designed to improve objectivity and standardization in the assessment of malingering. Their diagnostic system distinguishes between "Definite," "Probable," and "Possible" malingering. This system also outlines specific criteria for malingering: (A) presence of substantial external incentive, (B) evidence from neuropsychological testing, (C) evidence from self-report, (D) behaviors meeting necessary criteria from groups B or C are not fully accounted for by psychiatric, neurological or developmental factors. The authors note that alternative explanations for what appears to be malingering behavior must be carefully excluded and the consequences of diagnostic error must be considered.

Neuropsychological assessment of malingering may be done through a variety of methods, some of which rely on "conventional" tests and others which were designed specifically for detection of suboptimal effort (Strauss, et al., 2006). A thorough review of the many measures and methods of assessing malingering is beyond the scope of this chapter; the interested reader will find a wealth of research articles and an increasing number of texts addressing this topic such as those by Heilbronner (2005), Larrabee (2005), and Strauss et al. (2006). Examples of commonly used tests that may be employed in the assessment of malingering include the Minnesota Multiphasic Personality Inventory-2 (Larrabee, 2003; Lees-Haley et al., 1991), the California Verbal Learning Test-II (Curtis et al., 2006), and the Wechsler Adult Intelligence Scale-III (Iverson & Tulsky, 2003). These performances may be judged according to established cut-off scores or new indices developed to detect particular patterns of responding. Other measures that were designed specifically for the assessment of effort (also known as Symptom Validity Tests) include the Test of Memory Malingering (Tombaugh, 1996, 1997), 21-Item Test (Iverson et al., 1991), and the Victoria Symptom Validity Test (Slick et al., 1995; Slick et al., 1996). The tests from this latter group fall into one of two categories: (1) Tests which rely on the production of errors that are uncommon in patients with legitimate cognitive deficit; (2) tests that rely on a forced-choice format with probabilistic analysis of performance (Strauss et al., 2006). The use of *multiple* measures of malingering is recommended to enhance diagnostic accuracy (Bianchini et al., 2001). Bianchini et al. also noted the benefit of increasing the apparent difficulty and reducing "transparency" of the various measures.

In summary, the assessment of malingering or feigned impairment is becoming more common, especially in medico-legal settings. The most accurate diagnoses include consideration of multiple factors (medical history, presenting symptoms, secondary gain, neuropsychological findings, thorough differential diagnosis) and should include input from the entire treatment team. A malingering diagnosis should not be made on the basis on one finding or factor alone.

Neuropsychological Treatment

As indicated earlier, providing feedback to patients, families, and other members of the interdisciplinary team is one of the most important elements of the evaluation process. Recommendations generated from the evaluation may include referral to other specialists (e.g., neuropsychiatrist for medication management of depression or attentional disturbance; neuro-optometrist for further evaluation and treatment of vision impairment identified on neuropsychological evaluation). They may include recommendations to external parties such as employers and/or schools regarding strategies or accommodations (e.g., job coach, extended time on exams) that will enable the patient to re-integrate successfully into that setting. Most importantly, recommendations for cognitive or behavioral interventions can serve as a springboard for the development of appropriate and effective treatment interventions. These may include specific cognitive rehabilitation strategies, individual, family or group counseling, and are critical to integrate within the overall rehabilitation treatment plan (Gordon & Hibbard, 2005).

In many neuro-rehabilitation programs, neuropsychologists perform individual, group and family counseling. Other disciplines that may also render these services include social workers and certified rehabilitation counselors. Counseling survivors of brain injury and their families requires specialized experience and training. Due to the cognitive and behavioral challenges often posed by the brain injury, traditional psychotherapeutic techniques may be inappropriate or ineffective with this population, or require modification in order to be beneficial. Incorporation of cognitive rehabilitation techniques into psychotherapeutic work with brain injury survivors can enable the survivor to experience and process complex, abstract information and utilize the counseling session in a way that facilitates positive changes (Laatsch, 1999). Working with the family to understand family dynamics and goals/needs and to provide education and support, is also essential (Sander, 2005). Neuropsychologists are in a unique position within the interdisciplinary team, having the training and knowledge-base needed to address both emotional and cognitive changes and challenges, including family education and support, in order to develop integrated approaches to treatment. Such holistic approaches have been advocated by many (Ben-Yishay et al., 1985; Gordon & Hibbard, 2005; Laatsch, 1999; Mateer et al., 2005; Prigatano, 1999; Wilson, 1997; Uzzell, 2000). Specific psychotherapeutic issues and interventions for survivors and families are covered in subsequent chapters of this text, so will not be reviewed further here.

While neuropsychologists may incorporate cognitive rehabilitation techniques in counseling with brain injury survivors, in many interdisciplinary neuro-rehabilitation programs both occupational and speech-language therapists are trained and competent in integrating cognitive rehabilitation techniques into their practice, as well. Nevertheless, with their training in the fundamentals of research and critical analysis, it is the neuropsychologist who typically serves as educator and sets the model for the interdisciplinary team regarding the utilization of evidence-based approaches to cognitive rehabilitation.

Cognitive Rehabilitation

Cognitive rehabilitation has been defined as a "systematic, functionally oriented service of therapeutic cognitive activities, based on an assessment and understanding of the person's brain-behavior deficits" (Harley et al., 1992). Cognitive rehabilitation services are often differentiated into two approaches; "restorative" approaches, in which the goal is to achieve functional improvements by "reinforcing, strengthening, or reestablishing previously learned patterns of behavior," and "compensatory" approaches, in which the goal is to enable functional improvement by "establishing new patterns of cognitive activity or compensatory mechanisms for impaired neurological systems" (Harley et al., 1992). Mateer and Raskin (1999) have further differentiated approaches to cognitive rehabilitation by including "environmental modifications" as a distinct intervention, with a focus on altering the external environment, rather than the individual themselves (Mateer & Raskin, 1999).

The case of JD, the 65-year-old male whose status post right (and older left) frontal hemorrhage was described earlier in the chapter, illustrates the combined use of restorative, compensatory, and environmental approaches to facilitate improvement in cognitive functioning. Based on the neuropsychological assessment, the certified nursing assistant (who also had certification as a Brain Injury Specialist) was instructed to perform daily orientation exercises, designed to provide repetitive stimulation and cuing re: basic autobiographical and environmental information. When he did not respond to open-ended questions, a multiple-choice format was used. To compensate for his severe attentional impairments, treatment sessions were broken down into 15-minute increments spaced over the course of the day. Environmental modifications included room placement away from high-traffic, noisy areas of the unit (e.g., nurses station), working with his family to reduce visual stimulation in his room (e.g., minimizing room decorations) and providing 1:1 treatment in smaller treatment areas.

In 1998, the National Institutes of Health (NIH) convened an expert panel to critically review practices, principles, and efficacy critically in the area of rehabilitation following traumatic brain injury (TBI), including a review of therapeutic interventions for cognitive and behavioral sequelae of traumatic brain injury. At that time, after reviewing available evidence to date, the panel reported that "despite many descriptions of specific strategies, programs and interventions, limited data on the effectiveness of cognitive rehabilitation programs are available because of heterogeneity of subjects, interventions, and outcomes studied" (NIH, 1998). Nevertheless, they concluded that "evidence supports the use of certain cognitive and behavioral rehabilitation strategies for individuals with TBI in particular circumstances. These interventions share certain characteristics in that they are structured, systematic, goal-directed, and individualized and they involve learning, practice, social contact and a relevant context." The panel recommended that "rehabilitation of persons with TBI should include cognitive and behavioral assessment and intervention". Since that time, a number of reviews of research and literature in the field of cognitive rehabilitation have concluded that available evidence exists to support the use of a number of cognitive rehabilitation strategies/techniques to alleviate impairments and improve the functioning of individuals with brain injuries (Carney et al., 1999; Cicerone et al., 2000, 2005; Malia et al., 2004; Teasell et al., 2003).

In their review of the effectiveness of cognitive rehabilitation on outcomes following TBI, Carney et al. (1999) found very few controlled studies on the effects of cognitive rehabilitation on health or employment outcomes, though they noted that several studies demonstrated improvements on intermediate measures (e.g., neuropsychological test scores) following cognitive rehabilitation. They concluded that "based on the evidence found in this review, we recommend the application of compensatory cognitive strategies, adapted to patient groups and to individuals, to improve the functional ability of persons with TBI." They noted that additional, well-designed, research was needed, which should include standard definitions of interventions and relevant outcome measures.

The case of MH, the 50-year-old carpenter who sustained a work-related TBI from a fall from a ladder, illustrates the use of compensatory memory strategies to improve functional memory abilities following brain injury. Since his language and auditory attention abilities were relative strengths, MH was deemed a good candidate for use of a memory notebook. He was trained to use the notebook to record pertinent to-be-remembered information, such as appointments, phone numbers, and phone messages. The memory book was organized into sections, including structured daily pages, contacts, and a "thoughts and feelings" section, where he was encouraged to record episodes of heightened emotion and thoughts related to these feelings. Written instructions for breathing/relaxation exercises served as a cue to assist him in managing his emotional lability. In weekly counseling sessions, he reviewed this section and worked with the neuropsychologist to identify triggers and develop more adaptive coping strategies for anxiety/stress. Due to his visuospatial deficits, he had some difficulty maintaining the organization of the notebook, and his occupational therapist worked with him to simplify the structure of the notebook and set up a structured weekly routine for "clean up and organization" of the book. MH continued to use a smaller, less elaborate version of notebook/planner long after completion of his rehabilitation, and served as a model for others in this regard during monthly survivor support group meetings.

In a meta-analysis of 30 studies of the effectiveness of attention training after acquired brain injury (subjects included those with TBI, stroke or surgical lesion), Park and Ingles (2001) concluded that "specific-skills training significantly improved performance of tasks requiring attention" and that "acquired deficits of attention are treatable using specific-skills training." However, they also noted that "the methods included in the meta-analysis did not significantly affect outcomes" and suggested that "the learning that occurs as a function of training is specific and does not tend to generalize or transfer to tasks that differ considerably from those used in training". They challenged rehabilitationists to develop training procedures and programs structured to the needs (and cognitive limitations) of individuals with brain injury, including breaking down complex skills into simpler components, providing repetitive practice, and straightforward performance feedback.

In the most comprehensive reviews to date, the Brain Injury Interdisciplinary Special Interest Group (BI-ISIG) of the American Congress of Rehabilitation Medicine (ACRM) conducted evidence-based reviews of the cognitive rehabilitation literature from 1966 through 1997 (Cicerone et al., 2000) and 1998 through 2002 (Cicerone et al., 2005). These reviews incorporated meta-analyses of published literature on the effectiveness of cognitive rehabilitation for individuals with TBI or stroke. One hundred and seventy-one articles were reviewed through 1997, and an additional 87 articles for the updated review. For these reviews, the group evaluated and classified each study with respect to the strength of their methods. Class I studies consisted of prospective, randomized controlled designs; Class II studies included prospective, nonrandomized, cohort studies; retrospective, case-control studies; or clinical series with well-designed controls. Clinical series without concurrent controls and those with appropriate single-subject methodology were classified as Class III. Practice recommendations were then generated based on the relative strengths of the evidence across designated areas of intervention. Practice Standards included those interventions for which there existed at least one well-designed, large Class I study, with supporting Class II or III evidence. Practice Guidelines included interventions with limited Class 1 or well-designed, large Class II studies; and practice options, those interventions with only Class II or Class III evidence substantiating them. Recommendations were generated for the remediation of attention and memory deficits, visuospatial deficits, apraxia, language and communication deficits, and deficits in executive function, problem-solving, and awareness. To summarize, the authors concluded that "support exists for the effectiveness of several forms of cognitive rehabilitation for persons with stroke and TBI" (Cicerone, et al., 2000). More specifically, they found that "there is substantial evidence to support cognitive-linguistic therapies for people with language deficits with left hemisphere stroke... new evidence supports training for apraxia after left hemisphere stroke... evidence supports visuospatial rehabilitation for deficits associated with visual neglect after right hemisphere stroke... substantial evidence to support cognitive rehabilitation for people with TBI, including strategy training for mild memory impairment, strategy training for post-acute attention deficits, and interventions for functional communication deficits" (Cicerone et al., 2005). They found an overall differential benefit of cognitive rehabilitation over other or no treatments in 78.7% of Class I studies included in both reviews.

The case of RR, the 40-year-old architect who sustained a cerebellar bleed following resection of an acoustic neuroma, illustrates the benefits of strategy training for attention deficits, as well as the interaction between cognitive rehabilitation and counseling/psychotherapy.

RR's cognitive rehabilitation treatment included systematic attention process training (Sohlberg & Mateer, 1987), which over time helped increase the amount of information she was able to manage, as well as the speed at which she was able to process this information. She was able to return to her pre-injury job, but revealed in ongoing supportive counseling sessions that she was experiencing significant stress during busy periods when she was handling multiple projects at one time. Working with her therapist and her employer (direct supervisor), she was able to problem-solve how to re-structure and delegate some of her responsibilities during these times, enabling her to manage her work demands successfully.

Of note, the area of computer-based cognitive rehabilitation has had a relatively long history within the cognitive rehabilitation field, though conclusions regarding the effectiveness of this approach have been mixed (Cicerone et al., 2005; Gontkovsky et al., 2002; Lynch, 2002). While the evidence supporting computer-based cognitive rehabilitation interventions is equivocal, newer approaches, including those utilizing computers and/or web-based applications for compensatory purposes, such as cuing or structuring tasks/activities (Jinks et al., 2004), or for receipt of support and information/education (Rotondi et al., 2005) hold promise. This may be true particularly for those survivors and families in rural areas, or who are homebound, with limited access to rehabilitative services. Relevant to these situations, there is some evidence indicating that home based cognitive rehabilitation can be effective (Boman et al., 2004; Warden et al., 2000), though not as effective as intensive cognitive rehabilitation received in an inpatient hospital setting for patients with more severe brain injuries (Salazar et al., 2000).

In summary, while a considerable amount of research now exists to guide cognitive rehabilitation practice, it has been pointed out that there is still a need for more research to further define and tailor cost-effective cognitive rehabilitation interventions (Ricker, 1998).

Effectiveness of Specialized Neuro-Rehabilitation Programs and Interventions

Recent studies provide evidence demonstrating the relative effectiveness of specialized neuro-rehabilitation programs which incorporate neuropsychologically based treatment components (e.g., cognitive rehabilitation, psychotherapy), on functional outcomes (e.g., community integration) for individuals with TBI, stroke, and other acquired brain injuries. Cicerone (2004) performed a selective literature review of TBI rehabilitation programs, concluding that "a small number of studies suggest that post-acute TBI rehabilitation can produce improvements in participation and community integration." One such study compared an "intensive cognitive rehabilitation program" (ICRP), consisting of a highly structured program integrating cognitive and psychosocial interventions, including group, individual, and vocational or educational training, with a "standard neuro-rehabilitation" program (SRP), consisting of a less intensive, less structured program of physical, occupational, speech therapies and neuropsychological treatment, in outpatients with

TBI. The study found that while both groups showed significant improvement in community integration (as measured by the Community Integration Questionnaire), the ICRP group demonstrated greater improvement than the SRP group. Interestingly, the participants' perceived satisfaction with community functioning was unrelated to their level of community integration (Cicerone et al., 2004). Another study comparing TBI survivors participating in outpatient neuropsychological rehabilitation (including psychotherapy and cognitive rehabilitation) with a wait-listed control group, found that the treatment group demonstrated significant improvements in emotional functioning (including less anxiety and depression) and attention, although no changes were found in community integration scores (Tiersky et al., 2005). High Jr., et al. (2006) examined the impact of an outpatient community re-entry program (with emphasis on compensatory strategy training, environmental modification, counseling and education, and transition from clinic to community-based activities) on three groups of persons with TBI that differed in terms of their length of time post-injury (ranging from within 6 months of injury to over 1 year post-injury). They found that all groups demonstrated improvements on measures of overall disability, independence, home competency and productivity. The early-entry group (those injured less than 6 months prior) continued to improve after discharge from the program. The authors concluded that this type of post-acute rehabilitation can be effective "in improving functional outcome after TBI even for persons who have reached stable neurologic recovery at 12 or more months postinjury."

WM, the 57-year-old gentleman who sustained a right thalamic hemorrhage, was unable to return to his prior work as a phlebotomist due to the severity of his cognitive impairments, which persisted (albeit to a lesser degree) even after months of intensive cognitive rehabilitation. Predicting that he would need long-term supports, and given that he had few natural supports (e.g., family, friends) in his life, he was enrolled in the state's brain injury waiver program. He progressed to the point where he was able to travel independently using public transportation along familiar routes, though it was not recommended that he return to driving. As his insight improved, he accepted the recommendation that he not live alone, and joined a group of other individuals with brain injury to live in a supervised home in the community. He developed a routine of attending a structured day program for brain injury survivors 2 days per week, and was able successfully to obtain and hold a volunteer position within a local hospital, with the initial assistance of a life skills trainer accompanying him and providing cuing/coaching until he was able to accomplish the tasks with only intermittent supervision provided by the volunteer coordinator.

The positive impacts of specialized neuro-rehabilitation programs or specific interventions have been demonstrated for stroke survivors, as well. In a systematic review of randomized controlled studies of inpatient stroke rehabilitation, Foley et al. (2003) found that "improved functional outcomes and reduced length of hospital stays were reported among patients receiving specialized rehabilitation" in the majority of studies reviewed, though no differences in mortality or institutionalization were reported between the groups. The heterogeneity of subjects (ranging from mild to severe injuries) as well as treatment interventions (not always well-specified) in this study renders the conclusions less clear. In a study of occupational therapy (OT) interventions for inpatients receiving stroke rehabilitation, Richards et al. (2005) found that patients who spent more OT time in instrumental activities of daily living (such as home management, community integration) versus basic activities of daily living, demonstrated greater improvements in functioning. In a similar population, Hatfield et al. (2005) examined speech-language therapy outcomes, and found that participation in cognitively and linguistically complex activities (e.g., problem-solving, executive function skill training) early on during the rehabilitation stay resulted in better outcomes, regardless of the level of severity of functional communication on admission.

Summary and Conclusions

The rehabilitation neuropsychologist may wear a number of hats within a neuro-rehabilitation program, including maintaining responsibility for administrative functions—providing clinical supervision/oversight; education and training of staff, students, patients, and families and neuropsychological assessment and therapeutic intervention. It has been suggested that graduate academic curriculums be expanded to include neuropsychological rehabilitation (in addition to the greater emphasis typically found on assessment), in order to prepare clinical neuropsychologists better to assess and treat individuals with brain injuries (Uzzell, 2000). The neuropsychologist also serves a key role in assisting the interdisciplinary team in managing reactions to patients/families/each other, maintaining a creative and flexible, yet evidence-based approach to treatment, examining outcomes, and striving for ongoing performance improvement (Prigatano, 1999). By utilizing this holistic approach, the neuro-rehabilitation team can achieve the most coordinated and effective patient care and outcomes.

References

Alderman, N., Burgess, P.W., Knight, C., Henman, C. (2003) Ecological validity of a simplified version of the multiple errands shopping test. *Journal of the International Neuropsychological Society* 9:31 44.

Alderson, A.L., Novack, T.A., Dowler, R. (2003) Reliable serial measurement of cognitive processes in rehabilitation: The cognitive-log. *Archives of Physical Medicine and Rehabilitation* 84:668–672.

American Board of Clinical Neuropsychology. http://www.theabcn.org/.

American Board of Professional Psychology. http://www.abpp.org/.

American Psychiatric Association. (1994) *Diagnostic and Statistical Manual of Mental Disorders*, 4th ed. Washington, DC: American Psychiatric Association.

American Psychological Association. (2002) Ethical principles of psychologists and code of conduct. *American Psychologist* 57:1060–1073.

Barona, A., Reynolds, C.R., Chastain, R. (1984) A demographically based index of premorbid intelligence for the WAIS-R. *Journal of Consulting and Clinical Psychology* 52:885–887.

Basso, M.R., Bornstein, R.A., Roper, B.L., McCoy, V.L. (2000) Limited accuracy of premorbid intelligence estimators: A demonstration of regression to the mean. *Clinical Neuropsychology* 14:325–340.

Benton, A.L., Van Allen, M.W., Fogel, M.L. (1964) Temporal orientation in cerebral disease. *Journal of Nervous and Mental Disease* 139:110–119.

Ben-Yishay, Y., Rattok, J., Lakin, P., Piasetsky, E.D., Ross, B., Silver, S., Zide, E., Ezrachi, O. (1985) Neuropsychological rehabilitation: quest for a holistic approach. *Seminars in Neurology* 5:252–258.

Bianchini, K.J., Mathias, C.W., Greve, K.W. (2001). Symptom validity testing: A critical review. *The Clinical Neuropsychologist* 15:19–45.

Blair, J.R., Spreen, O. (1989) Predicting premorbid IQ: A revision of the National Adult Reading Test. *The Clinical Neuropsychologist* 3:129–136.

Boman, I.-L., Lindstedt, M., Hemmingsson, H., Bartfai, A. (2004). Cognitive training in home environment. *Brain Injury* 18(10):985–995.

Bright, P., Jaldow, E., Kopelman, M.D. (2002) The National Adult Reading Test as a measure of premorbid intelligence: A comparison with estimates derived from demographic variables. *Journal of the International Neuropsychological Society* 8:847–854.

Brown, P., Ricker, J.H. (2003) Evaluating and treating communication and cognitive disorders: Approaches to referral and collaboration for Speech-Language Pathologists and Clinical Neuropsychology. Technical report. *American Speech-Language-Hearing Association, Supplement* 23:47–57.

Brown, L.B., Stern. R.A., Cahn-Weiner, D.A., Rogers, B., Messer, M.A., Lannon, M.C., Maxwell, C., Souza, T., White, T., Ott, B.R. (2005) Driving scenes test of the Neuropsychological Assessment Battery (NAB) and on-road driving performance in aging and very mild dementia. *Archives of Clinical Neuropsychology* 20:209–215.

Burgess, P.W., Alderman, N., Evans, J., Emslie, H., Wilson, B.A. (1998) The ecological validity of tests of executive function. *Journal of the International Neuropsychological Society* 4:547–558.

Burgess, P.W., Alderman, N., Forbes, C., Costello, A., Coates, L. M.-A., Dawson, D.R., Anderson, N.D., Gilbert, S.J., Dumontheil, I., Channon, S. (2006). The case for the development and use of "ecologically valid" measures of executive function in experimental and clinical neuropsychology. *Journal of the International Neuropsychological Society* 12:194–209.

Carney, N., Chestnut, R.M., Maynard, H., Mann, N.C., Petterson, P., Helfond, M. (1999) Effect of cognitive rehabilitation on outcomes for persons with traumatic brain injury: A systematic review. *Journal of Head Trauma Rehabilitation* 14:277–307.

Chaytor, N., Schmitter-Edgecombe, M. (2003) The ecological validity of neuropsychological tests: A review of the literature on everyday cognitive skills. *Neuropsychological Review* 13:181–197.

Cicerone, K.D. (2004) Participation as an outcome of traumatic brain injury rehabilitation. *Journal of Head Trauma Rehabilitation* 19(6):494–501.

Cicerone, K.D., Dahlberg, C., Kalmar, K. Langenbahn, D.M., Malec, J.F., Bergquist, T.F., Felicetti, T., Giacino, J.T., Harley, J.P., Harrington, D.E., Herzog, J., Kneipp, S., Laatsch, L., Morse, P.A. (2000) Evidence-based cognitive rehabilitation: Recommendations for clinical practice. *Archives of Physical Medicine and Rehabilitation* 81:1596–1615.

Cicerone, K.D., Dahlberg, C., Malec, J.F., Langenbahn, D.M., Felicetti, T., Kneipp, S., Ellmo, W., Kalmar, K., Giacino, J.T., Harley, J.P., Laatsch, L., Morse, P.A., Catanese, J. (2005) Evidence-based cognitive rehabilitation: Updated review of the literature from 1998 through 2002. *Archives of Physical Medicine and Rehabilitation* 86:1681–1691.

Cicerone, K.D., Mott, T., Azulay, J., Friel, J.C. (2004) Community integration and satisfaction with functioning after intensive cognitive rehabilitation for traumatic brain injury. *Archives of Physical Medicine and Rehabilitation* 85:943–950.

Cockburn, J., Keene J. (2001) Are changes in everyday memory over time in autopsy-confirmed Alzheimer's disease related to changes in reported behavior? *Neuropsychological Rehabilitation,* 11:201–271.

Corrigan, J.D. (1989). Development of a scale for assessment of agitation following traumatic brain injury. *Journal of Clinical and Experimental Neuropsychology* 11:261–277.

Curtis, K.L., Greve, K.W., Bianchini, K.J., Brennan, A. (2006) California Verbal Learning Test indicators of malingered neurocognitive dysfunction: Sensitivity and specificity in traumatic brain injury. *Assessment* 13:46–61.

Foley, N.C., Teasell, R.W., Bhogal, S.K., Doherty, T., Speechley, M.R. (2003) The efficacy of stroke rehabilitation: A qualitative review. *Topics in Stroke Rehabilitation* 10(2):1–18.

Folstein, M.F., Folstein, S.E., McHugh, P.R. (1975) "Mini-Mental state." A practical method for grading the cognitive state of patients for the clinician. *Journal of Psychiatric Research* 12:189–198.

Gioia, G.A. Isquith, P.K. (2004) Ecological assessment of executive function in traumatic brain injury. *Developmental Neuropsychology* 25:135–158.

Gioia, G.A., Isquith, P.K., Guy, S.C., Kenworthy, L. (2000) *Behavior Rating Inventory of Executive Function.* Lutz, FL: Psychological Assessment Resources.

Gontkovsky, S.T., McDonald, N.B., Clark, P.G., Ruwe, W.D. (2002). Current directions in computer-assisted cognitive rehabilitation. *NeuroRehabilitation* 17:195–199.

Gordon, W., Hibbard, M.R., (2005) Cognitive rehabilitation. In Silver, M., McAllister, T., Yudofsky, S. (eds.): *Textbook of Traumatic Brain Injury.* Virginia: American Psychiatric Publishing, Inc, pp. 655–660.

Grace, J., Amick, M.M., D'Abreu, A., Festa, E.K., Heindel, W.C., Ott, B.R. (2005) Neuropsychological deficits associated with driving performance in Parkinson's and Alzheimer's disease. *Journal of the International Neuropsychological Society* 11:766–775.

Griffin, S.L., Mindt, M.R., Rankin, E.J., Ritchie, A.J., Scott, J.G. (2002) Estimating premorbid intelligence: Comparison of traditional and contemporary methods across the intelligence continuum. *Archives of Clinical Neuropsychology* 17:497–507.

Guy, S.K., Cummings, J.L. (2003) The mental status exam. In Feinberg T.E., Farah M.J. (eds.): *Behavioral Neurology & Neuropsychology,* 2nd ed. New York: McGraw-Hill, pp. 23–32.

Harley, J.P., Allen, C., Braciszewski, T.L., Cicerone, K.D., Dahlberg, C., Evans, S., Foto, M., Gordon, W.A., Harrington, D., Levin, W., Malec, J.F., Millis, S., Morris, J., Muir, C., Richert, J., Salazar, E., Schiavone, D.A., Smigelski, J.S. (1992) Guidelines for cognitive rehabilitation. *NeuroRehabilitation* 2:62–67.

Hatfield, B., Millet, D., Coles, J., Gassaway, J., Conroy, B., Smout, R.J. (2005) Characterizing speech and language pathology outcomes in stroke rehabilitation. *Archives of Physical Medicine and Rehabilitation* 86(2):S61–S72.

Heilbronner, R.L. (ed.). (2005) *Forensic Neuropsychology Casebook.* New York:Guilford Publications, Inc.

Higginson, C.I., Arnett, P.A., Voss, W.D. (2000) The ecological validity of clinical tests of memory and attention in multiple sclerosis. *Archives of Clinical Neuropsychology* 15:185–204.

High, W., Roebuck-Spencer, T., Sander, A.M., Struchen, M.A., Sherer, M. (2006) Early versus later admission to postacute rehabilitation: Impact on functional outcome after traumatic brain injury. *Archives of Physical Medicine and Rehabilitation* 87:334–342.

Iverson, G.L., Tulsky, D.S. (2003) Detecting malingering on the WAIS-III: Unusual Digit Span performance patterns in the normal population and in clinical groups. *Archives of Clinical Neuropsychology* 18:1–9.

Iverson, G.L., Franzen, M.D., McCracken, L.M. (1991) Evaluation of an objective assessment technique for the detection of malingered memory deficits. *Law and Human Behavior* 15:667–676.

Jackson, W.T., Novack, T.A., Dowler, R.N. (1998) Effective serial measurement of cognitive orientation in rehabilitation: The orientation log. *Archives of Physical Medicine and Rehabilitation* 79:718–720.

Jinks, A., Kellinger, F., Garber, H.J. (2004) Handheld pc/web-based task reminder for brain-injured adults [Abstract]. *Rehabilitation Engineering & Assistive Technology Society of North America* http://www.resna.org/ProfResources/Publications/Proceedings/2004/Papers/Research/CAC/.

Johnstone, B., Callahan, C.D., Kapila, C.J., Bouman, D.E. (1996) The comparability of the WRAT-R reading test and NAART as estimates of premorbid intelligence in neurologically impaired patients. *Archives of Clinical Neuropsychology* 11:513–519.

Jurica, P.J., Leitten, C.L., Mattis, S. (2001). *Dementia Rating Scale-2*. Odessa, FL: Psychological Assessment Resources.

Kalechstein, A.D., Newton, T.F., van Gorp, W.G. (2003). Neurocognitive functioning is associated with employment status: A quantitative review. *Journal of Clinical and Experimental Neuropsychology* 25:1186–1191.

Kalmar, K., Giacino, J.T. (2005) The JFK coma recovery scale-revised. *Neuropsychological Rehabilitation* 15:454–460.

Kiernan, R.J., Mueller, J., Langston, J.W., Van Dyke, C. (1987) The neurobehavioral cognitive status examination: A brief but differentiated approach to cognitive assessment. *Annals of Internal Medicine* 107:481–485.

Kokmen, E., Smith, G.E., Petersen, R.C., Tangalos, E., Ivnik, R.C. (1991) The short test of mental status. *Archives of Neurology* 48:725–728.

Krull, K.R., Scott, J.G., Sherer, M. (1995) Estimation of premorbid intelligence from combined performance and demographic variables. *The Clinical Neuropsychologist* 9:83–88.

Laatsch, L. (1999) Application of cognitive rehabilitation techniques in psychotherapy. In Langer, K.G., Laatsch L., Lewis L. (eds.): *Psychotherapeutic Interventions for Adults with Brain Injury or Stroke: A Clinician's Treatment Resource*. Connecticut: Psychosocial Press, pp. 131–148.

Larrabee, G.J. (2003) Exaggerated MMPI-2 symptom report in personal injury litigants with malingered neurocognitive deficit. *Archives of Clinical Neuropsychology* 18:673–686.

Larrabee, G.J. (ed.). (2005) *Forensic Neuropsychology: A scientific approach*. New York: Oxford University Press.

Lees-Haley, P.R., English, L.T., Glenn, W.G. (1991) A fake-bad-scale for personal injury claimants. *Psychological Reports* 68:203–210.

Levin, H.S., O'Donnell, V.M., Grossman, R.G. (1979) The galveston orientation and amnesia test: A practical scale to assess cognition after head injury. *Journal of Nervous and Mental Disease* 167:675–684.

Lezak, M.D. (2003) Principles of neuropsychological assessment. In Feinberg, T.E., Farah M.J. (eds.): *Behavioral Neurology and Neuropsychology,* 2nd ed. New York: McGraw-Hill.

Lezak, M.D., Howieson, D.B., Loring, D.W. (2004) *Neuropsychological assessment,* 4th ed. New York: Oxford University Press.

Lynch, B. (2002) Historical review of computer-assisted cognitive retraining. *Journal of Head Trauma Rehabilitation* 17(5):446–457.

Malia, K., Law P., Sidebottom, L., Bewick, K., Danziger, S., Schold-Davis, E., Martin-Scull, R., Murphy, K., Vaidya, A. (2004) Recommendations for best practice in cognitive rehabilitation therapy: Acquired brain injury. The Society for Cognitive Rehabilitation, Inc. (pp. 1–57).

Mateer, C.A., Raskin, S. (1999) Cognitive rehabilitation. In Rosenthal, M., Griffith, E., Kreutzer, J.S., Pentland, B. (eds.): *Rehabilitation of the Adult and Child with Traumatic Brain Injury.* Philadelphia: FA Davis, pp. 254–270.

Mateer, C.A., Sira, C.S., O'Connell, M.E. (2005) Putting humpty dumpty back together again: The importance of integrating cognitive and emotional interventions. *Journal of Head Trauma Rehabilitation* 20(1):62–75.

Mittenberg, W., Patton, C., Canyock, E.M., Condit, D.C. (2002) Base rates of malingering and symptom exaggeration. *Journal of Clinical and Experimental Neuropsychology* 24:1094–1102.

Moritz, S., Ferahli, S., Naber, D. (2004) Memory and attention performance in psychiatric patients; Lack of correspondence between clinician-rated and patient-rated functioning with neuropsychological test results. *Journal of the International Neuropsychological Society* 10:623–633.

National Academy of Neuropsychology. (2001) NAN definition of a clinical neuropsychologist.*Official Position of the National Academy of Neuropsychology.*

National Academy of Neuropsychology. (2002) Cognitive rehabilitation. *Official Statement of the National Academy of Neuropsychology.*

National Academy of Neuropsychology. (2003) Informed consent in clinical neuropsychology practice. *Official Statement of the National Academy of Neuropsychology.*

National Institutes of Health. (1998, October 26–28) Rehabilitation of persons with traumatic brain injury. *NIH Consensus Statement 1998* 16(1):1–41.

Odhuba, R.A., Van der Broek, M.D., Johns, L.C. (2005) Ecological validity of measures of executive functioning. *British Journal of Clinical Psychology* 44:269–278.

Park, N.W., Ingles, J.L. (2001) Effectiveness of attention: Rehabilitation after an acquired brain injury: A meta analysis. *Neuropsychology* 15(2):199–210.

Prigatano, G.P. (1999) *Principles of Neuropsychological Rehabilitation.* New York: Oxford University Press.

Prigatano, G.P. (1999). The outcome of neuropsychological rehabilitation programs that incorporate cognitive rehabilitation and psychotherapeutic intervention. In Prigatano, G.P., (ed.): *Principles of Neuropsychological Rehabilitation.* New York: Oxford University Press, pp. 244–262.

Randolph, C., Tierney, M.C., Mohr, E., Chase, T.N. (1998) The Repeatable Battery for the Assessment of Neuropsychological Status (RBANS): Preliminary clinical validity. *Journal of Clinical and Experimental Neuropsychology* 20:310–319.

Rappaport, M., Dougherty, A.M., Kelting, D.L. (1992) Evaluation of coma and vegetative states. *Archives of Physical Medicine and Rehabilitation* 73:628–634.

Reitan, R.M., Wolfson, D. (1993) *The Halstead-Reitan Neuropsychological Test Battery: Theory and clinical interpretation,* 2nd ed. South Tucson, AZ: Neuropsychology Press.

Richards, L.G., Latham, N.K., Jette, D.U., Rosenberg, L., Smout, R.J., De Jong, G. (2005) Characterizing occupational therapy practice in stroke rehabilitation. *Archives of Physical Medicine and Rehabilitation* 86(2):S51–S60.

Ricker, J.H. (1998) Traumatic brain injury rehabilitation: Is it worth the cost? *Applied Neuropsychology* 5:184–193.

Rotondi, A.J., Sinkule, J., Sprig, M. (2005) An interactive web-based intervention for persons with tbi and their families. Use and evaluation by female significant others. *Journal of Head Trauma Rehabilitation* 20(2):173–185.

Royall, D.R., Mahurin, R.K., Gray, K.F. (1992) Bedside assessment of executive cognitive impairment: The executive interview. *Journal of the American Geriatrics Society* 40:1221–1226.

Salazar, A.M., Warden, D.L., Schwab, K., Spector, J., Braverman, S., Walter, J., Cole, R., Rosner, M.M., Martin, E.M., Ecklund, J., Ellenbogen, R.G. (2000) Cognitive rehabilitation for traumatic brain injury: A randomized trial. *The Journal of the American Medical Association* 283(23):3075–3081.

Sander, A. (2005) Interventions for Caregivers. In High Jr., W.M., Sander, A.M., Struchen, M.A., Hart, K.A. (eds.): *Rehabilitation for Traumatic Brain Injury*. New York: Oxford University Press. pp. 156–175.

Santa Clara Valley Medical Center (2006). *The Center for Outcome Measurement in Brain Injury.* http://www.tbims.org/combi.

Schanke, A.K., Sundet, K. (2000) Comprehensive driving assessment: Neuropsychological testing and on-road evaluation of brain injured patients. *Scandinavian Journal of Psychology* 41:113–121.

Schretlen, D.J., Buffington, A.L.H., Meyer, S.M., Pearlson, G.D. (2005) The use of word-reading to estimate "premorbid" ability in cognitive domains other than intelligence. *Journal of the International Neuropsychological Society* 11:784–787.

Schoenberg, M.R., Duff, K., Scott, J.G., Adams, R.L. (2003) An estimation of the clinical utility of the OPIE-3 as an estimate of premorbid WAIS-III FSIQ. *Clinical Neuropsychology* 17:308–321.

Sherer, M., Nakase-Thompson, R., Yablon, S.A., Gontkovsky, S.T. (2005) Multidimensional assessment for acute confusion after TBI. *Archives of Physical Medicine and Rehabilitation* 86:896–904.

Silver, C.H. (2000) Ecological validity of neuropsychological assessment in childhood traumatic brain injury. *Journal of Head Trauma Rehabilitation* 15:973–988.

Slick, D.J., Hoop, G., Strauss, E. (1995) *The Victoria Symptom Validity Test.* Odessa, FL: Psychological Assessment Resources.

Slick, D.J., Hoop, G., Strauss, E., Spellacy, F. (1996) Victoria symptom validity test: Efficiency for detection of feigned memory impairment and relationship to neuropsychological tests and MMPI-2 validity scales. *Journal of Clinical and Experimental Neuropsychology* 18:911–922.

Slick, D.J., Sherman, E.M.S., Iverson, G.L. (1999) Diagnostic criteria for malingered neurocognitive dysfunction: Proposed standards for clinical practice and research. *The Clinical Neuropsychologist* 13:545–561.

Slick, D.J., Tan, J.E., Strauss, E.H., Hultsch, D.F. (2004) Detecting malingering: A survey of experts' practices. *Archives of Clinical Neuropsychology* 19:465–473.

Sohlberg, M.M., Mateer, C.A. (1987) Effectiveness of an attentional training program. *Journal of Clinical and Experimental Neuropsychology* 9:117–130.

Strauss, E., Sherman, E.M.S., Spreen, O. (2006) *A Compendium of Neuropsychological Tests: Administration, Norms and Commentary*, 3rd ed. New York: Oxford University Press.

Sweet, J.J., Nelson, N.W., Moberg, P.J. (2006) The TCN/AACN 2005 "Salary Survey": Professional practices, beliefs, and incomes of U.S. neuropsychologists. *The Clinical Neuropsychologist* 20:325–364.

Teasell, R.W., Foley, N.C., Bhogal, S.K., Speechley, M.R. (2003). An evidence-based review of stroke rehabilitation. *Topics in Stroke Rehabilitation* 10(1):29–58.

Tiersky, L.A., Anselmi, V., Johnston, M.V., Kurtyka, J., Roosen, E., Schwartz, T., Deluca, J. (2005) A trial of neuropsychologic rehabilitation in mild-spectrum traumatic brain injury. *Archives of Physical Medicine and Rehabilitation* 86:1565–1574.

Tombaugh, T.N. (1996) *Test of Memory Malingering (TOMM)*. North Tonawanda, NY: Multi Health Systems.

Tombaugh, T. (1997) Test of Memory Malingering (TOMM): Normative data from cognitively intact and cognitively impaired individuals. *Psychological Assessment* 9:260–268.

Uzzell, B.P. (2000) Neuropsychology and vascular dementia. *Topics in Stroke Rehabilitation* 7(3):29–37.

Uzzell, B.P. (2000). Neuropsychological rehabilitation. In Christensen, A.-L., Uzzell, B.P. (Eds.): *International Handbook of Neuropsychological Rehabilitation*. (pp. 353–369). New York: Kluwer Academic/Plenum Publishers.

Warden, D.L., Salazar, A.M., Martin, E.M., Schwab, K.A., Coyle, M., Walter, J. (2000) A home program of rehabilitation for moderately severe traumatic brain injury patients. *Journal of Head Trauma Rehabilitation* 15(5):1092–1102.

Whelihan, W.M., DiCarlo, M.A., Paul, R.H. (2005) The relationship of neuropsychological functioning to driving competence in older persons with early cognitive decline. *Archives of Clinical Neuropsychology* 20:217–228.

Wilson, B.A. (1997) Cognitive rehabilitation: How it is and how it might be. *Journal of the International Neuropsychological Society* 3:487–496.

Wilson, B.A., Alderman, N., Burgess, P.W., Emslie, H., Evans, J.J. (1996) *Behavioral Assessment of the Dysexecutive Syndrome*. Bury St. Edmunds, England: Thames Valley Test Company.

Wilson, B.A., Cockburn, J., Baddeley, A., Hiorns, JR. (2003) *The Rivermead Behavioral Memory Test-II Supplement Two*. Bury St. Edmunds, England: Thames Valley Test Company.

World Health Organization. (2002) *International Classification of Functioning, Disability and Health*. Geneva, Switzerland: World Health Organization.

8
The Role of the Neuro-Rehabilitation Optometrist

M.H. ESTHER HAN

Introduction

The multidisciplinary management of the patient with acquired brain injury (ABI) is critical in addressing all of the functional needs of the patient. It is often difficult to determine why a patient is reporting a specific difficulty. In such circumstances it is important that all members of the rehabilitation team be able to recognize when to make referrals to the appropriate professional. One of the main purposes of this chapter is to inform rehabilitative professionals about the components of the evaluation and management of ABI patients with vision dysfunctions. A study by Sabates et al. (1991) found that patients can report vision difficulties for months or even several years post-injury. They also found that appropriate referrals were typically recommended by family members or rehabilitation personnel rather than physicians. Several sources have stated that many rehabilitation professionals are not familiar with the vision evaluation and management options available for the ABI patient (Richter, 2001; Wainapel, 1995). Other than for low-vision management, the field of vision rehabilitation is relatively new. Abnormal vision function can interfere with the rehabilitative process, as it will affect a patient's ability to integrate visual input with their kinesthetic, proprioceptive, and vestibular input. When such a sensory mismatch occurs, balance and coordination are negatively affected. A secondary purpose of this chapter is to present case reports describing the optometric management and outcome of specific vision diagnoses seen in the types of ABI patients typically referred to neuro-rehabilitation optometrists, also called neuro-optometrists in the optometric literature.

ABI patients with vision problems may see different providers who specialize in the treatment of vision and/or ocular conditions but may not be as knowledgeable in the management of the specific problem that the patient is experiencing. A neuro-rehabilitation optometric evaluation is uniquely indicated for patients experiencing symptoms related to binocular (strabismic and nonstrabismic), oculomotor, accommodative, and visual perceptual dysfunction as will be further discussed in this chapter. In addition to the correction of refractive error with lenses, and contact lenses, neuro-rehabilitation optometrists are also specially trained to manage visual field defects using prisms and vision rehabilitation. Often during the acute stages of the patient's rehabilitation process or when neurological changes are associated with a sudden onset of vision symptoms, a neuro-ophthalmological evaluation is necessary, particularly when management of the patient requires blood work, brain imaging, prescription medications, or hospitalization.

Assessment

The vision rehabilitation case history (See Table 8.1 for a list of the common elements of the vision rehabilitation case history) involves a comprehensive investigation of the nature of the brain injury, referral source, types of rehabilitation services received, visual problems affecting activities of daily living, personal and family medical history, and personal and family ocular history. The case history continues throughout the evaluation and can often be the most revealing part of the examination for both the patient and the evaluator. This occurs when the patient is relieved to discover that an undiagnosed vision disorder may be contributing to his or her difficulties. During the case history, the examiner also gains a better picture of the patient's visual needs, and how he/she typically responds to vision challenges, e.g., avoidance, trying harder, or frustration.

The nature of the injury reveals the location of the brain injury and the possible areas of function that may be affected. In addition, vision deficits will arise from damage to areas of the brain other than the occipital lobe, within which the primary visual cortex resides (Gianutsos et al., 1998). The number of years post injury provides an indication of the acute versus chronic nature of the vision symptoms. A patient evaluated in the first 6 months after an ABI may experience a sudden decrease in his or her visual symptoms within one year of the injury (Suter, 1995). However, there are some patients who chronically experience visual symptoms several years after the incident. Clinically, it is known that ABI patients are prone to suffer from multiple head injuries and each incident is highly likely to exacerbate an existing vision dysfunction. Therefore it is important to know whether a patient has suffered from multiple head injuries.

The source and the specific reason for the referral are significant. For instance, a vestibular therapist may refer a patient experiencing intermittent diplopia, or double vision, during a gaze stabilization task. The patient's diplopia now becomes

TABLE 8.1. Elements of the vision rehabilitation case history

1. Nature of the injury including the type of injury, date of injury, number of injuries, length of hospitalization
2. Referral source
3. Rehabilitation history including in-patient or outpatient rehabilitation services received to date
4. Current vision problems or complaints that affect overall performance and/or the progress of other types of rehabilitation
5. Personal and family medical history, including medications and allergies
6. Personal and family ocular history
7. Social history which includes occupation, mobility, driving history, and support resources

TABLE 8.2. Common vision symptoms following ABI

Intermittent blurred vision (distance, near, or both)
Dulling of vision
Eyestrain
Diplopia
Headaches
Light sensitivity
Depth perception problems
Reading efficiency and reading comprehension problems
Dizziness, loss of balance, or vertigo
Visual neglect
Loss of peripheral vision

an obstacle in his/her progress in the vestibular therapy. Regular communication is also necessary between the referral source and the treating optometrist to evaluate progress in therapy. This is particularly the case for patients with cognitive deficits who may not be able to adequately judge their progress in therapy.

The rehabilitation history reveals the levels of function affected by the ABI and whether a physiatric evaluation was performed in the past. Often patients with mild traumatic brain injury (TBI) are examined and may report significant cognitive difficulties. A physiatric evaluation would be indicated for this patient so that the physiatrist can make further recommendations.

The chief goal of the vision rehabilitation evaluation is to determine the current vision needs of the patient. This requires a lengthy discussion of the functional difficulties a patient may be experiencing in daily life. This may range from bumping into people when walking, shaving only one side of the face, driving challenges, or poor multitasking abilities in the work setting. The evaluating optometrist will incorporate the case history and the vision findings to determine if a vision deficit is contributing to the patient's reported difficulties.

The main vision complaints that are elicited during the case history include the following: blurred vision, eyestrain, diplopia, light sensitivity, poor depth perception, reading inefficiency, poor reading comprehension, dizziness, visual neglect, and loss of peripheral vision (See Table 8.2). The possible etiologies of these symptoms will be discussed in more detail in the balance of the chapter.

The personal and familial medical and ocular history is important to ensure that the patient is being routinely managed for other systemic conditions. Patients are often inundated with medical appointments, and will benefit from being reminded to follow-up with their other medical providers. ABI patients are also prescribed numerous medications; some have vision side effects that may affect an ABI patient more than a non-brain injured patient. In such cases, the optometrist attempts to decrease the severity of the symptoms maximally using visual hygiene strategies, lenses, and/or vision rehabilitation. The patient is informed that complete remediation may not occur, but rather the goal is to maximize vision function by decreasing the frequency and severity of the symptoms.

The social history gives the examiner an idea of how the patient functioned in the pre-injury state. The difficulty of coping with functional losses as a result of the injury is often greater in higher functioning individuals. Mobility and driving needs also are extensively reviewed to determine necessary recommendations.

Refractive Status

One of the main elements of the vision rehabilitation examination is the determination of the refractive status. The patient may manifest emmetropia, myopia, hyperopia, astigmatism, or presbyopia (See Appendix A for definitions of terms). These conditions are corrected using spectacles, or contact lenses. Refractive surgery has also been recently used for the correction of refractive error. Recommendations regarding this treatment option should be done on a case-by-case basis, as poor fixation, poor binocular status, and accommodative fluctuations may negatively affect surgical outcomes.

Myopia is corrected by minus or concave lenses, and hyperopia with plus or convex lenses (see Fig. 8.1). Astigmatism exists when refractive error differs in orthogonal meridians of the eye. Presbyopia is characterized by the need for additional plus lenses for near-point tasks, and it generally manifests in patients older than 40 years.

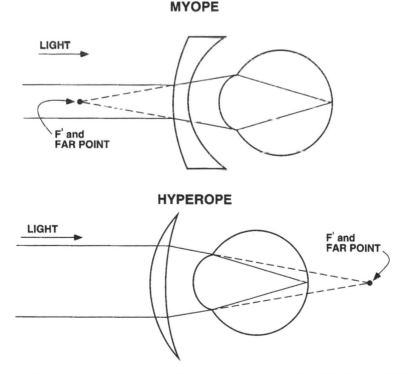

FIGURE 8.1. Correction of myopia and hyperopia with lenses (Cho & Benjamin, 1998).

Symptoms related to refractive status may include blurred vision at a distance or near, shadows or halos around images, and eyestrain under sustained viewing conditions. One study indicated that 46% of patients with closed-head injury report some form of blurred or decreased vision (Sabates, 1991). Decreases in contrast sensitivity may also contribute to the quality of their vision and not significantly affect their visual acuity. This is particularly true in cerebrovascular (CVA) patients. Contrast sensitivity deficits were reported in 62% of patients with ischemic events affecting the posterior visual pathways (Warren, 1993). This is further exacerbated in elderly patients who often have cataracts that will also contribute to decreased contrast sensitivity and visual acuity levels.

Suchoff et al. (1999) found that 50% of ABI patients in their study required a prescription for spectacles. These patients included those who needed glasses for the first time, those who needed a replacement for lost glasses, and those requiring a change in their prescription. In a study by Sabates et al. (1991), 88% of patient's eyes were correctable to 20/20. This reinforces the fact that most of the patients' vision complaints can be resolved with the appropriate refractive correction. This is particularly true since changes in refractive status are observed post-injury and will typically include increases in myopia, fluctuating prescriptions in hyperopic patients, and/or decreases in the degree of hyperopia (Padula, 1988a).

A consideration when determining the refractive status in an ABI patient is that some patients experience a significant degree of vision fluctuation. During the examination, these fluctuations will be observed when measuring acuity and when determining the patient's prescription. Careful monitoring of visual acuities is necessary after one to two months of wearing the new prescription. Upon follow-up, it is possible that a change in the prescription will be indicated as vision continues to stabilize. In addition, some ABI patients report significant improvement in clarity and comfort with very small refractive changes that would typically not be noticeable by the non-brain-injured individual.

Recommendations regarding choice of lens design are very important and patients may require several pairs of glasses for different needs. Mobility is one of the main issues that must be considered when writing the spectacle prescription. Progressive (no-line multifocal lenses) and bifocals are strongly not advised for patients with poor mobility. Single-vision lenses made of polycarbonate material are recommended for distance use when walking. Progressive lenses have defocus and distortion at the periphery of the lenses that may contribute to the patient's unsteadiness (see Fig. 8.2). The patient, wearing either progressive or bifocal lenses, often views through the reading portion and will experience blurred vision when looking down at their feet when walking. This may occur when going up or down steps or during physical therapy sessions when patients will inevitably look at their feet. Single-vision near or single-vision intermediate glasses are typically advised for sustained visual activities such as reading or computer use.

ABI patients who have not worn glasses prior to the injury have clinically been noted to be poorly compliant with spectacle wear despite a significant increase in acuity because the patient prefers "soft" vision that is not crisp. The improved clarity increases the amount of visual stimulation they experience, particularly in busy and crowded environments. Another obstacle to compliance with spectacle

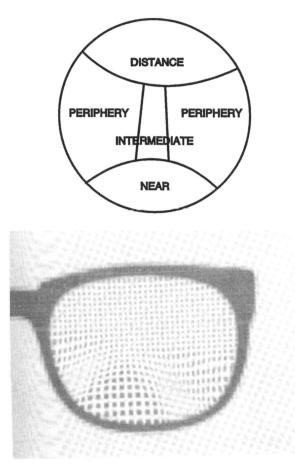

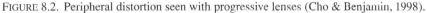

FIGURE 8.2. Peripheral distortion seen with progressive lenses (Cho & Benjamin, 1998).

wear is the presence of cognitive deficits. These patients may consistently forget or lose their glasses, and may not remember or understand which pair of glasses to use for a specific task. A multifocal (bifocal or progressive) lens design would be optimal for such patients who do not have mobility issues.

Prescribing for the dizzy patient is challenging because of aberrations inherent to any type of spectacle lenses. For instance, rotational magnification can magnify or minify the effect of head movement depending on the power of the lens (Weiss, 2002). Slight decreases in the amount of minus given to a myope may stabilize vision enough to improve peripheral awareness and posture (Weiss, 2002).

Sensorimotor Status

Evaluation of sensorimotor status includes the assessment of oculomotor, binocular, and accommodative function. The neural network contributing to these areas of function encompasses the frontal, parietal, and cerebellar regions of the brain (Ciuffreda et al., 2001). A single locus of damage or diffuse damage from a TBI can lead to multiple levels of deficits in visual function. Suter (1995) stated that 71% of TBI patients in an acute rehabilitation center were diagnosed with either an oculomotor or binocular dysfunction, suggesting that a vision rehabilitation evaluation is strongly indicated post-injury.

Oculomotor, binocular, and accommodative functions are directly responsible for the efficient input of visual information to the brain. When these systems are not functioning adequately, excess cognitive effort is exerted in an attempt to keep vision clear and single enough to take in visual information. This excess effort takes away from the cognitive processes of attention and comprehension during a task such as reading. In ABI patients with cognitive deficits and vision deficits, performing near-vision tasks can be physically and mentally exhausting.

Oculomotor or versional function includes fixation, pursuit, and saccadic eye movement abilities (See Appendix A for definitions). This involves horizontal and vertical eye movements. Evaluation of binocular or vergence function includes the assessment of ocular alignment, measurement of stereopsis, and determination of fusion (convergence and divergence) ranges at distance and near. Binocular tasks involve eye movements related to depth determination. Accommodative testing is typically performed in pre-presbyopic patients (younger than 45 years) and includes the measurement of amplitude and facility (monocularly and binocularly).

Most of the literature is based upon studies in only the TBI or CVA population. Ciuffreda et al. (2001) briefly review the possible etiology for the vision deficits observed in whiplash patients. Whiplash results in musculoligamentous strain or sprain of the cervical region. They propose that damage to the following areas in the neck may affect vision function: (1) damage to small blood vessels supplying specific vision-related areas of the brain (i.e., brain stem); (2) damage to nerve roots or peripheral nerves affecting cranial nerves III, IV, and VI; (3) cervical sympathetic irritation, (4) vertebrobasilar artery insufficiency; and (5) disturbance of neck proprioceptive information related to the sense of head position, neck reflexes and postural porcesses, and the vestibular system.

Oculomotor Function

Deficits of oculomotor (versional) function in the ABI population include deficits of fixation, pursuits, and saccades. Abnormal findings in oculomotor function will involve the ability to initiate a necessary eye movement, latency, accuracy or gain, and visual attention involved in the required eye movement task (Warren, 1993; Ciuffreda & Tannen, 1995).

Oculomotor dysfunctions were observed in 39.7% (Suchoff et al., 1999) of TBI patients and 15% (Ciuffreda et al., 2001) in CVA patients. Attention deficits associated with eye movements are unique to CVA patients particularly those with hemispheric involvement and a corresponding hemianopic visual field defect (Ciuffreda et al., 2001). With respect to fixation, saccadic intrusions are abnormally large saccades that interrupt accurate fixation and are associated with cerebellar

TABLE 8.3. Visual symptoms
associated with oculomotor deficits

Loss of place, skipping lines when reading
Poor reading efficiency
Reading comprehension problems
Dizziness, loss of balance, or vertigo

disease (Ciuffreda & Tannen, 1995). Nystagmus, another fixation abnormality, is the involuntary and rhythmic oscillation of the eye (Ciuffreda & Tannen, 1995). Acquired nystagmus is associated with myelin disease, brain stem strokes, cerebellar disease, and vestibular dysfunction (Ciuffreda & Tannen, 1995).

Oculomotor function is controlled by the following structures: superior colliculus, frontal eye fields, parietal lobe, temporal lobe, reticular system, and the cerebellum (Warren, 1993; Ciuffreda & Tannen, 1995). Injury at any level may interfere with the quality of oculomotor activity. Ciuffreda and Tannen (1995) extensively reviewed the neurophysiology of fixation, saccade, and pursuit eye movements as well as the effects of specific neurological lesions on oculomotor function. For instance, parietal lesions lead to increased latency with respect to initiating a saccadic eye movement into the affected field of a patient with unilateral neglect (Warren, 1993; Ciuffreda & Tannen, 1995). Damage to the frontal eye fields affects direct voluntary visual searching abilities. A patient may also exhibit reduced awareness of the environment and increased latency of saccade initiation towards the affected field (Warren, 1993). Deficits in the pathways involving the superior colliculus affect peripheral awareness and eye movements towards unanticipated or new stimuli in the environment (Warren, 1993). Deficits in oculomotor function can significantly affect the ABI patient's activities of daily living (ADLs). Table 8.3 lists typical symptoms of patients with deficits in oculomotor function.

The main treatment option for deficits in oculomotor function is vision rehabilitation with the goal of developing more systematic or organized eye movement patterns. Warren (1993) described that patients with visual field defects will often scan the intact field first and will also spend less time searching in the affected field. She also stated that patients with expressive or receptive aphasia demonstrated a more simplistic visual scanning pattern. These patients will report more fatigue and stop searching for further details within a complex visual pattern thereby further limiting their ability to verbally express what was seen (Warren, 1993).

A more specialized area within vision rehabilitation is oculomotor auditory biofeedback typically administered in conjunction with traditional vision rehabilitation. Auditory biofeedback helps to increase awareness further and improves the voluntary control of one's eye movements through auditory reinforcement. The efficacy of auditory biofeedback has been documented in the optometric literature for the treatment of nystagmus, saccadic intrusions, and reading eye movement inefficiencies (Ciuffreda & Tannen, 1995; Fayos & Ciuffreda, 1998; Ciuffreda & Tannen, 1999).

Binocular Function

Deficits of binocular (vergence) dysfunction include strabismic and nonstrabismic dysfunctions. Nonstrabismic dysfunctions can be categorized into distance- and near-vision disorders. The two common distance disorders are divergence excess (DE) and divergence insufficiency (DI). In ABI patients, the DI condition is clinically more observed of the two distance disorders. At near, the two nonstrabismic disorders are convergence insufficiency (CI) and convergence excess (CE). CI is the most common binocular vision diagnosis seen after a brain injury. The literature consistently states an incidence of 40% in the TBI population (Suter, 1995; Cohen et al., 1989). When a patient exhibits binocular dysfunctions at both distance and near, the two possible diagnoses are basic esophoria and basic exophoria. There are currently no studies, determining the prevalence of these latter conditions in individual with ABI.

The strabismic conditions that can be seen after a brain injury are esotropia, exotropia, and hypertropia. The strabismus can be characterized as being constant or intermittent, and can occur at distance, near or both. A patient may prefer to consistently fixate with one eye while the other is turned or the patient may alternate fixation from one eye to the other. Another characteristic of the strabismus that needs to be assessed is the comitancy or whether the size of the eye turn changes in different positions of gaze. A patient with a non-comitant deviation may report diplopia only when looking in one direction. Noncomitant deviations will occur concurrently with a palsy of a cranial nerve that affects the extraocular muscles, such as cranial nerves III, IV, and VI.

Sabates et al. (1993) found that 75% of closed-head trauma patients with cranial nerve palsies resolved without surgical intervention within six months to a year. At times, surgical correction of an acquired strabismus is indicated to decrease the size of the turn. This is often recommended when the angle of deviation has been stable. The patient should also be advised of the possible surgical outcomes. One study stated that third and fourth nerve palsies generally require surgical correction, and 25% of the patients in the study required some form of surgical correction (Sabates et al., 1993). Some patients may require multiple surgeries: in another study of TBI patients who required surgical correction, 50% required more than one surgery, and 30% required more than two (Suter, 1995). It is strongly proposed that surgical intervention in conjunction with vision rehabilitation will improve the outcome of postsurgical vision function (size of the turn, frequency of double vision, visual comfort, and possibly decreases the need for multiple surgeries) (Suter, 1995).

A study by Sabates et al. (1991) found 30% of patients with closed-head trauma (n = 181) reported diplopia and 33% manifested cranial nerve palsies. A study by Gianutsos et al. (1988) showed that 73% (n = 26) of patients with severe head trauma exhibited some degree of binocular dysfunction. Suchoff et al. (1999) stated that 41.9% of ABI patients show an exo-deviation as compared to an occurrence of 2.11% in the normal population. Vertical deviations (greater than 1 prism diopter) were seen in 9.7% as compared to an occurrence of 1.6% in normals. The prevalence of eso-deviations (1.6%) is not very different from that seen in

TABLE 8.4. Symptoms associated with binocular deficits

Diplopia (double vision) at distance, near, or both; horizontal, vertical, or diagonal.
Intermittent or constant eye turn at distance, near, or both; Can be horizontal, vertical, or both.
Neck or shoulder discomfort (Padula, 1988a)
Poor object localization (Padula, 1988a)
Poor depth perception
Head turn or head tilt (Suter, 1995)
Poor body posture (Suter, 1995)

normal individuals (1.28% occurrence). Ciuffreda et al. (2001) stated that 40% of CVA patients manifest reduced binocular abilities. Prevalence rates of cranial nerve palsies in TBI patients are as follows: 16.2% to 25% for third nerve palsies, 16.7% for sixth nerve palsies, 32.0% to 36% for fourth nerve palsies, and 25% for multiple nerve involvement (Suter, 1995; Falk & Aksionoff, 1992). Table 8.4 lists the common symptoms reported by patients with deficits in binocular function.

The treatment options for the above binocular vision dysfunctions include one or a combination of the following: fusional prism to correct for the double vision, a form of occlusion (binasal or partial occlusion), surgical correction and vision rehabilitation (Suter, 1995; Padula, 1988b). The main goal is to decrease the severity and frequency of the patient's symptoms. In patients experiencing constant double vision and who are unable to undergo a vision rehabilitation evaluation, it is recommended to patch the eyes on a daily alternating schedule to allow for visual information to enter each eye, to provide peripheral visual cues for each eye, to prevent suppression, and to increase the chances for spontaneous recovery of fusion (Suter, 1995).

Accommodative Function

The main types of accommodative dysfunctions include (1) Accommodative insufficiency, (2) accommodative infacility, and (3) accommodative excess. Accommodative dysfunction is more commonly seen in TBI patients as opposed to CVA patients because a TBI results in more diffuse damage as opposed to the more discrete lesions that occur in a CVA (Leslie, 2001). However, damage to the brain stem area will result in more damage to the areas controlling accommodative, binocular, and oculomotor function (Leslie, 2001; Chan & Trobe, 2002). Leslie (2001) stated that accommodative dysfunctions should be viewed as disturbances or loss of learned ability to appropriately change accommodation for an object of regard.

The reported prevalence of deficits in accommodative function differs depending on the study. Accomodative dysfunctions were noted in 36% to 69% (Gianutsos et al., 1988) of head injured patients, and 20% (Leslie, 2001) in mid-facial trauma patients. Table 8.5 lists the common symptoms reported by patients with accommodative dysfunction. Sabates et al. (1991) stated that 13% of patients with closed head trauma experienced headaches, and 6% reported difficulties with reading.

TABLE 8.5. Visual symptoms associated with accommodative deficits

Frontal headaches or brow aches
Intermittent or constant blurred vision (distance, near, or both), worsening later in the day
Pain around the eyes during visual activities
Limited ability to read or use computer for long periods (Leslie, 2001)
Limited progress in other rehabilitation therapies involving near-vision work (Leslie, 2001)

However, it must be noted that 29% of the patients also reported a history of post-concussive migraines. It was once thought that visual and ocular side effects of medications may exacerbate deficits on accommodation. A retrospective study by Han et al. (2005) found that commonly prescribed medications (antihypertensives, antidepressants, antianxiolytics, and anticonvulsants) taken by either TBI or CVA patients do not appear to severely exacerbate accommodative dysfunctions.

The common treatment options of accommodative dysfunctions include a near-vision spectacle prescription, and/or vision rehabilitation. The goal of therapy is to develop flexibility between the accommodative and binocular systems to maximally stabilize vision function. Additionally, some pre-presbyopic patients may require a near-vision prescription at an earlier age then would be expected due to the difficulties in initiating or sustaining accommodation (Cohen & Rein, 1992).

Visual Processing: Central Versus Peripheral

Vision is made up of central and peripheral processing systems (Rosen et al., 2001). The central visual processing has been called focal processing and is said to be attributed to the parvocellular (P) visual pathways, while peripheral visual processing has also been called ambient processing and mediated by the magnocellular (M) visual pathways (Rosen et al., 2001). ABI patients demonstrate poor peripheral awareness, which results in poor spatial organization (Padula, 1988b). The function of peripheral visual processing is to match visual information with other sensorimotor systems at the level of the midbrain (Padula, 1988b). An individual with poor peripheral visual processing pays attention to visual details rather than the gestalt, resulting in variable visual abilities. For example, some patients report stationary objects appearing to move, and overstimulating settings such as supermarkets, airports, and shopping malls to be very visually unsettling. An ABI patient in the supermarket tends to be overwhelmed by the visual details of the items on the shelf instead of seeing the aisle as a gestalt. This individual is not required to process all of the specific details when shopping but is unable to ignore unimportant visual information.

Literature regarding the treatment options for deficits in peripheral processing is limited but may include binasal occlusion or low amounts of base-in prism to improve peripheral awareness and thus help stabilize vision (Padula, 1988a,b) One of the indications of prescribing either occlusion or prism is the subjective response of the patient, who may report that print is clearer and not moving as much, and that vision is more comfortable (Padula, 1988a). Clinically, treatment options need to be patient specific since patients respond to their injuries differently and will manifest unique symptoms. Their specific visual difficulties and rehabilitation expectations also need to be considered in conjunction with their pre-injury functional levels. Generally, compensatory strategies are recommended after each evaluation to help minimize the effects of their vision deficits while they are receiving rehabilitation services, and may include the need to limit exposure to visually stimulating environments. This is especially the case in crowded public settings. For instance, appointments should be scheduled after or before commuter rush hours. When a patient must be in a visually overstimulating environment (i.e., watching a movie or a theater performance), he or she must know to take a visual break as they may often feel physically and cognitively drained, even 1 to 2 days after the event. In the early stages of rehabilitation, the patient must be careful to avoid performing visual tasks in cluttered, or visually overstimulating situations. Vision efficiency and fatigue will occur sooner when a patient attempts to perform vision activities while doing other tasks requiring processing via other sensory (verbal, motor, or auditory) modalities. For such patients, some of the goals of vision rehabilitation is to eventually maximize their ability to process sensory (visual, auditory, verbal, or motor) information simultaneously, or to visually attend to two or more things at once or to rapidly switch visual attention from one object to another. The main objective of therapy is not necessarily to be able to perform the given visual activity, but rather the discussion of how to process and eventually apply the strategies while performing the activity. Also, therapy sessions are critical opportunities for patients to describe specific difficulties they are experiencing and for the optometrist to guide them with task-specific strategies.

Visual Perceptual Function

Approximately 70% of the afferent sensory input to the brain is vision related and vision information is processed, either directly or indirectly, in every lobe of the brain (Suter, 1995). Cortical fibers participate in integrative functions and connect the different associative areas of the brain. These associative areas often mediate and process the sensory and motor input from different areas of the brain. Suter (1995) stated that there are over 90 intracortical pathways that involve an area of the brain that processes visual input. Before attempting to treat visual perceptual deficits, the refractive and sensorimotor status (oculomotor, binocular, and accommodative, if indicated) need to be extensively assessed to determine whether the patient can efficiently and clearly input visual information before he/she can process the information. For example, a patient seeing constant double vision may show some of the symptoms listed in Table 8.6 only because he/she sees two images. This individual may have trouble walking or picking up objects and would have significant trouble with higher level cognitive processing.

A visual perceptual evaluation or certain subtests of a comprehensive neuro-psychological evaluation is used to determine areas that require remediation. Some

TABLE 8.6. Visual symptoms associated with visual perceptual deficits

Confuses similarly shaped objects
Difficulty recognizing objects in different orientations
Difficulty recognizing objects close to or overlapping other objects
Visual memory problems
Difficulty following verbal directions
Often asks to repeat instructions

areas that are evaluated include: visual discrimination, visual spatial relations, form perception, form constancy, figure/ground perception, visual pattern recognition, visual-motor integration, visual perceptual speed, and visual memory (spatial and sequential).

Visual attention is also an important aspect in successfully performing visual tasks. Warren (1993) summarized the process of visual attention as a three-step process in which the first step involves a disengaging operation, in which the eye ceases to attend to an object, then there is a moving operation in which attention is shifted to a new object, and finally there is a comparing operation, in which the previous object is compared with the new one for similarities and differences. These steps all require adequate sensorimotor function and intact visual perceptual abilities.

Clinically, prognosis is guarded for visual perceptual therapy in patients with severe forms of ABI. The goal of therapy is therefore to create strategies that maximize performance. Auditory strategies, repetition strategies, and different viewing perspectives are practiced and the patient's initial visual symptoms are carefully monitored for decreases in frequency.

Visual-Vestibular Function

This area of vision rehabilitation is relatively new. Poor balance occurs when there is a mismatch in the inputs received from the vestibular, visual, and proprioceptive systems. In the presence of a vestibular dysfunction, inputs from the other two systems become more critical in maintaining balance. In visually busy environments (i.e., supermarkets, crowded streets, and moving trains) patients may experience extreme forms of dizziness because they are unable to suppress the excessive visual movements occurring in the background (Hellerstein & Freed, 1994).

Many of the visual-vestibular dysfunctions relate to the phenomenon of the vestibulo-ocular reflex (VOR). The VOR depends on a stable bifoveal retinal image during high-frequency head movements (greater than 2 Hz) while the cervico-ocular reflex (COR) stabilizes vision during low frequency head movements based upon sensory inputs from the neck and facet joints (Rosen et al., 2001). Patients with VOR deficits experience oscillopsia, blurred vision, decreased dynamic visual acuity, poor depth perception, and/or diplopia (Weiss, 2002). Therefore, deficits in

TABLE 8.7. Visual symptoms associated with
visual-vestibular deficits

Light-headedness or heavy-headedness
Headache
Vertigo
Motion sickness
Swimmy, fuzzy, and foggy vision during head movement
Feeling disoriented
Sensation that the world is moving
Fullness in the ears
Floating feeling
Nausea
Fatigue
Avoidance of movement or changes in head posture
Jumpy, bouncing, or jerking vision
Blurred vision with head movement

oculomotor, binocular, and accommodative function are associated with symptoms
of vestibular dysfunction due to a mismatch of visual and vestibular inputs creating
a sense of imbalance. Visual problems will often exacerbate a vestibular problem
as evidenced clinically when some patients complete their vision rehabilitation
and report a decrease in the severity in their vestibular symptoms.

Patients with vestibular dysfunction, as stated by Rosen et al. (2001), often use
other sensory modalities such as the cervico-ocular reflex (COR), pursuit and saccadic eye movements to obtain vestibular information. This suggests the need for
optimal levels of vision function in the presence of a vestibular dysfunction. Similarly, patients with vestibulospinal reflex (VSR) dysfunction experience postural
instabilities that worsen with movement or in areas of poor lighting or uneven surfaces (Rosen et al., 2001). In either VOR or VSR dysfunction, the goal of vision
rehabilitation would be to strengthen the patient's ability to rely more on visual
input rather than vestibular input. Some commonly associated vision symptoms
reported by patients having a vision-vestibular dysfunction are listed below in
Table 8.7.

Visual Field Status

The prevalence of visual field defects ranges from 32.5% (Sabates et al., 1991;
Suchoff et al., 1999) to 65% (Zihl, 2000) in ABI patients. Zihl (2000) authored a
comprehensive review of visual field deficits and categorized most visual field defects as unilateral (88.8%) and 11.2% as bilateral defects. With respect to etiology,
61.5% of visual field defects were found to be associated with stroke, 14.6% with
cerebral hemorrhage, and 11.3% with closed head trauma (Zihl, 2000). In patients
with visual field defects, 50–90% report difficulties with reading, and 17–70%
report difficulties with activities that require visual exploratory abilities (Mueller

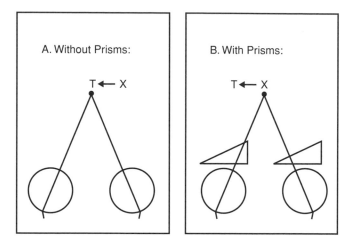

FIGURE 8.3. Schematic representation of yoked prism effect on spatial localization with the subject instructed to gaze straight ahead (top view): A. Without the yoked prisms, where T = a midline object, X = an object to the right of midline. B. With the yoked prisms, where objects T and X are not optically displaced laterally to the left by the prisms without any change in eye position (Kapoor et al., 2001).

et al., 2003). Patients also report inability to safely drive a car (Julkunen et al., 2003).

Visual fields can be assessed using a variety of conventional methods. A gross estimate of the visual field can be performed using confrontational visual fields. Clinically, it is often subject to significant inter-examiner differences. The automated visual field can be performed using a screening or a threshold method. Functional visual fields are measures of practical vision and may be performed in conjunction with a yoked prism trial. The base of the prism is prescribed in the same direction as the affected field. For example, a patient with a right homonymous hemianopia will be prescribed base-right yoked prisms (see Fig. 8.3).

Special considerations regarding visual field deficits are visual neglect and midline shift syndrome. Suchoff and Ciuffreda (2004) stated that 12% to 49% of right-brain stroke patients demonstrate visual neglect and it occurs more frequently in stroke than in TBI patients. Some patients may experience the Riddoch Phenonmenon in which they detect moving objects in the affected field but not stationery objects (Gerner, 1993). Patients with visual neglect lean away from the area of loss, while patients with a visual field defect without inattention lean or turn toward the area of loss (see Fig. 8.4) (Padula, 1988b). Yoked prisms using magnitudes of 5 to 20 prism diopters will bring about observable changes (Suchoff & Ciuffreda, 2004). Since significant improvement in visual neglect can be observed within six months of the incident, these patients may benefit from being monitored rather than prescribing the yoked prisms early in the rehabilitative process (Suchoff & Ciuffreda, 2004).

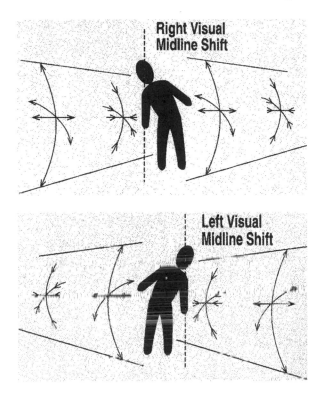

FIGURE 8.4. Visual midline shift to the right and left (Padula, 1988b).

Midline shift syndrome is observed in some patients with visual field deficits, and these individuals demonstrate postural deficits with the patient leaning away from the affected side, complaining that the floor looks tilted, and that the wall or floor may be appearing to shift or move. Hemiparetic patients will posture their bodies as though there was an expansion of space on the affected side and a corresponding contraction of space on the unaffected side. The two types of shift are the left-right shift and the anterior-posterior shift (Padula, 1988b).

Efficacy of yoked prisms in ABI patients with midline shifts has been founded on alterations in body posture noted upon clinical observations as well as upon quantitative assessments (Padula et al., 2001; Kapoor et al., 2001). Center of gravity changes have been documented in young, healthy subjects without history of an ABI using dynamic posturography (Gizzi et al., 1997). Adaptive neurological changes have also been observed after 2 hours of wear in patients with right hemispheric lesions (Rosetti et al., 1998). Interestingly, yoked prisms were found to improve higher cognitive levels, particularly with respect to "mental space representation." Rode et al. (2001) found that patients with visual neglect showed improved performance on tasks related to mental imagery. About 24 hours after discontinuing the yoked prism, the patients' improvements decreased but not to previous levels, indicating that the prisms also facilitated the learning process during the mental imagery task. The authors suggested that yoked prisms influence plasticity of multi-sensory integration processes as well as cognitive processes related to mental representation of visual space.

Additional treatment options for visual field defects include mirrors attached to spectacles, similar to the side mirrors used by cyclists (Suter, 1995; Suchoff et al., 2004). Partial or half-field Fresnel prisms are also used to increase peripheral awareness (Suter, 1995; Suchoff et al., 2004). However, some patients do not respond well as they tend to report diplopia peripherally. Clinically, this option is most effective in cognitively intact patients. Compensatory strategies should be routinely recommended and may include using a finger or brightly colored ribbon on the affected side of a book while the patient is reading. Typoscopes or rulers are helpful in keeping their place when reading. Despite adequate visual acuity, large print reading material will often improve reading speed while the patient is receiving vision rehabilitation. Alternatively, the patient can be prescribed a magnifier to enlarge normal-sized print and thereby improve reading fluency.

Rehabilitation of visual field defects mainly involves teaching compensatory strategies which incorporate the active training of exploratory saccadic eye movements into the area of field loss (Nelles et al., 2001; Reinhard et al., 2005). Optometric vision rehabilitation and occupational therapy follow this model of treatment, and it has been shown both in the literature and in the clinic setting that improvement in visual scanning and visual searching abilities, as well as when performing functional activities, are notably observed (Nelles et al., 2001).

The literature also describes a new treatment modality called "visual restoration therapy" or "visual restitution therapy" (VRT), which is purported to restore and expand the visual field in patients with optic nerve disease and post-chiasmal brain lesions through binocular stimulation of areas adjacent to the visual field defect that have residual vision, for example in patients with homonymous hemianopic defects (Reinhard et al., 2005; Sabel & Kasten, 2000; Poggel et al., 2004). It involves a computer-based program incorporating two half hour home training sessions daily for six months (Sabel & Kasten, 2000). Patients with severe binocular, accommodative (for patients under 45 years of age), and/or oculomotor dysfunctions may not be able to perform the training due to the onset of visual symptoms that may occur after 15 to 20 minutes of sustained near-vision activity. These conditions should be treated prior to starting a VRT treatment program to ensure maximum benefit from the therapy.

Most studies using VRT indicate subjective improvements in activities of daily living, such as reading, visual response time, visual attention, visual confidence with mobility, and temporal visual processing (Mueller et al., 2003; Reinhard et al., 2005). Objective improvements were variable with an average visual field increase of 5 degrees and a range of 0 to 20 degrees (Sabel & Kasten, 2000). One study which controlled for fixation showed no change in absolute visual field defect (Reinhard et al., 2005). However, small increases in the visual field subjectively appear to improve visual function with near activities such as reading (Mueller et al., 2003).

Clinically, both treatment modalities (compensatory or VRT) will produce subjective improvement in activities of daily functioning that require visual attention and visual processing speed (Mueller et al., 2003; Nelles et al., 2001). As with any rehabilitation program, the patient's goals and expectations should be carefully discussed when making treatment recommendations. Some patients are motivated to do home-based therapy while others require constant more attention and counseling through a formal office-based program.

Photosensitivity

Patients with photosensitivity are not photophobic, which is typically an indication of an ocular inflammatory condition. Specifically for TBI patients, discomfort associated with normal illumination includes the following: atypical light sensitivity, photic-driven headache, and reduced or prolonged dark adaptation (Jackowski, 2001). Photosensitive patients clinically report sensitivity to indoor lighting, in addition to outdoor sunlight. They may be more sensitive to only fluorescent or only to incandescent lighting. Fluorescent lighting emits light at different wavelengths (Smith, 1999). Some of the emitted light is in the UV spectrum and is normally undetectable to the eye but ABI patients, especially TBI patients, report more sensitivity to fluorescent as opposed to incandescent lighting. Jackowski (2001) summarized that 44% of TBI patients report discomfort to bright illumination and a greater frequency showed a decreased threshold for illumination tolerance. Zihl and Kerkhoff (1990) also showed that 39% of TBI patients reported symptoms related to impaired light adaptation. A retrospective study showed that 30–60% of TBI and 18–30% of CVA patients report symptoms of light sensitivity (Han et al., 2005).

Other factors associated with photosensitivity include altered or tonic pupillary diameters or highly fluctuating pupillary responses. Patients with abnormal pupillary responses report sensitivity to all types of intense lighting (Jackowski, 2001). Anomalous patterns of dark adaptation and deficits in peripheral processing systems possibly exist in TBI patients with photosensitivity (Rosetti et al., 1998). Other sources also confirm a post-retinal explanation rather than a retinal etiology for symptoms of photosensitivity in TBI patients with normal retinal functioning (Zihl & Kerkhoff, 1990; Du et al., 2005).

The most basic form of management for these patients is a lightly tinted lens for indoor use. Patients with a general sensitivity to light will clinically respond best to a 30% to 40% brown or gray tint while the patients with sensitivity to fluorescent lighting may respond better to 30% to 40% light blue or gray tint. The outdoor tint should be 85% to 90% dark using the colors described above. Patients with abnormal pupillary responses and photosensitivity respond best to neutral gray filters (Jackowski, 2001). Studies using CPF-450-S (yellow) filters demonstrated increased contrast sensitivity, improved reading rates (not to normal levels), and elimination of hypersensitive responses to light under certain conditions (Jackowski, 2001).

Special lens coatings or lenses such as antireflective coatings or polarizing lenses will reduce the effects of glare and excessive reflections. For some patients, polarizing sunglasses significantly decreases the effects of glare from light reflecting off windshields, water, snow, and wet highway surfaces (Brooks & Borish,

1996). Polarized lenses only permit light waves oriented in a specific direction to pass through the lens and enter the eye resulting in reduction of glare and improved comfort for the photosensitive patient (Brooks & Borish, 1996). For antireflective coatings, a manufacturing difficulty that occurs when prescribing the anti-reflective coating and a tint is that the tinting process must be done before the antireflective coating is applied. As most lenses are already coated before they are cut to fit the spectacle frame, a delay may occur when making up the prescription. Clip-on sunglasses and brimmed hats are also very helpful in increasing patient comfort in brightly lit environments.

Contrast Sensitivity Status

Almost 62% of patients with ischemic brain lesions affecting the posterior visual pathways have poor contrast sensitivity (Warren, 1993). Occipital or occipitotemporal lesions are associated with a loss of the ability to discriminate medium to high spatial frequencies (smaller-sized targets), while temporal or parietal lesions affect low-spatial-frequency (larger-sized targets) discrimination.

Poor contrast sensitivity is also reported in patients with visual field defects and in elderly individuals (Warren, 1993). Deficits in contrast sensitivity will affect how a patient functions under foggy and dark conditions (Suter, 1995). Elderly patients with cataracts already have decreased contrast sensitivity that potentially worsens when they sustain a brain injury. Additional symptoms related to poor contrast sensitivity are complaints of poor vision despite normal visual acuity. Treatment options may involve contrast-enhancing colored tints or filters, high contrast reading material, and task specific lighting (Suter, 1995).

Ocular Health Status

Only the diagnoses most commonly seen in patients receiving vision rehabilitation are going to be discussed in this section. For an extensive description of ocular sequelae associated with ABI, see Gerner (1993), Suchoff, et al. (1999), Vogel (1992), and Sabates et al. (1991). The most common conditions seen are dry eyes and blepharitis. A study by Suchoff et al. (1999) found 22.6% of ABI patients were diagnosed with some form of dry eye or external eye pathology (blepharitis, keratitis, pterygium, and corneal degeneration). Etiology is unknown at this time. The prevalence of dry eyes or similar conditions, as listed above, is 11.2% to 13% in the normal population (Suchoff, et al., 1999).

Management options typically include lid hygiene which involves warm compresses with gentle lid massage with closed eyes for several minutes typically twice daily and instillation of one to two drops of artificial tears afterwards. Artificial tears can be used as needed throughout the day. Severe dry eye cases may require the use of an ophthalmic gel or ointment formulation to provide longer lasting lubrication when sleeping. The main disadvantage of the gel or ointment is the temporary blurring of vision upon instillation in the eye. More recently, very severe dry eyes associated with poor corneal integrity have been treated with Restasis (cyclosporine ophthalmic emulsion 0.05%) twice daily. Patients typically report symptomatic improvement one to four months after initiation of treatment.

Case Reports

The following cases are examples of the visual functional outcomes of patients who received conventional optometric vision rehabilitation therapy as part of their overall treatment recommendations. Optometric vision rehabilitation therapy is a modality that treats deficits of binocular, accommodative, oculomotor, and perceptual functions by gradually conditioning a patient's vision capabilities in each of the areas listed above and then training the client to integrate these areas to perform activities of daily living more effectively. This is accomplished through the use of lenses, prisms, mirrors, occlusion, filters (polarized, anaglyphic, and colored), computer programs, and other visual-motor and perceptual-motor activities which incorporate basic physiological and optical principles that are inherent to the training of normal vision processes (Scheiman & Wick, 2002; Ciuffreda, 2002).

Optometric vision rehabilitation therapy typically involves a combination of in-office therapy and home-based therapy activities. Generally, patients receive an individualized program of training activities specific to their abilities and to their progress. Therapy can be performed on an individual basis or in a group setting as recommended by the evaluating provider. The activities may be done directly with the optometrist or with a trained vision therapist in a session supervised and programmed by the optometrist.

MB is a 58-year-old male who was referred for vision rehabilitation evaluation by his vestibular therapist for the following vision-related complaints: intermittent blurred vision, reading difficulties, poor attention when reading, difficulty distinguishing lines and spaces between lines, experiencing eyestrain after 3 to 4 pages of reading, words appearing to swim and overlap when reading, double vision when watching television, fronto-temporal headaches when reading, eyes tearing with sustained reading, difficulty keeping left eyelid open, light sensitivity to indoor lighting and sunlight, and difficulty using laptop computer for sustained periods. MB also reported difficulty progressing with his vestibular therapy, anxiety and severe dizziness in crowded situations, dizziness and nausea when viewing moving objects, frequent loss of balance, and inability to look at a moving train.

Etiology

MB was diagnosed with a pituitary microadenoma in 2000 that was carefully being monitored and treated with medications. He reported a long-standing central vestibular dysfunction.

Pertinent Visual Findings

1. Refractive status: MB manifested a moderate hyperopic and astigmatic prescription in each eye and was also found to be presbyopic. Best-corrected distance visual acuities were 20/20 in the right and left eyes.
2. Sensorimotor status

    Oculomotor function: Fixation abilities in the left eye revealed an intermittent jerk nystagmus. His left eye also demonstrated poorer quality of movement with more losses of fixation noted during pursuit and saccadic eye movement testing.

    Binocular function: MB manifested esophoria and a right hyperphoria at distance. At near, testing revealed a convergence insufficiency and right hyperphoria at near. His compensatory fusion reserves at both distance (base-in or divergence ranges) and near (base-out or convergence ranges) were found to be restricted and inadequate for his needs.
3. Visual field status: MB did not show the typical bitemporal visual field defects associated with pituitary tumors. He did exhibit scattered visual field defects.

Assessment

1. Convergence insufficiency
2. Deficits of pursuit and saccades
3. Photosensitivity
4. Hyperopia, astigmatism, and presbyopia

Recommendations

1. Vision rehabilitation was strongly advised to remediate deficits in his oculomotor and binocular function. Additional goals included increasing the flexibility of his oculomotor and binocular abilities to more comfortably respond to complex visual and moving stimuli. MB's progress in vestibular therapy will be carefully monitored to determine the presence of visual obstacles to his progress.
2. Four pairs of spectacles were advised: (i) polarized prescription sunglasses with a progressive multifocal lens design for outdoor use, (ii) progressives with a 35% gray tint and anti-reflective coating for indoor use, (iii) single-vision spectacles with 35% gray tint and anti-reflective coating for computer use, and (iv) single-vision spectacles with 35% gray tint and anti-reflective coating for prolonged near-vision use, such as reading.
3. Until his visual skills improve, a referral for a low vision magnifier (4×) was advised so that he will be more comfortable when reading his smaller print books during the early stages of his vision rehabilitation.

Outcome

After completing his vision rehabilitation, MB reported that he was able to read for much longer periods without the use of his magnifier, use his computer for sustained periods of time, drive confidently at night and in poor weather conditions (snow, rain, and overcast days), and continues to progress in his vestibular therapy program. MB is currently being followed every three months to monitor his visual symptoms. His complicated systemic health history and changes in medications or medical health significantly affects his vestibular and vision function. His refractive status frequently changes, requiring a new prescription for all four pairs of glasses. In addition, there are times when he requires horizontal and vertical fusional prism for his intermediate and distance diplopia and there are periods when he does not require it for optimal visual function. MB is a unique case that was successfully treated with vision rehabilitation. However, his complicated medical health requires frequent follow-up evaluations to monitor his visual function.

ID is a 76-year-old woman who was referred by an occupational therapist at the inpatient rehabilitation center she attended immediately after her stroke. She experienced the following visual complaints: difficulty reading, poor awareness to the left side (not noticed by patient), decreased peripheral vision to the left, poor visual scanning abilities, bumping into things on the left side, past pointing, and sitting with body shifted to the right. ID also reported that she was unable to write after the stroke because she wrote with her left hand.

Etiology

A stroke in November 2004 with in-patient rehabilitation and transferred to an outpatient facility. ID demonstrated weakness of the upper and lower extremities on the left side. Initially, ID was wheelchair bound.

Pertinent Visual Findings

1. Refractive status: ID manifested a very high myopic prescription with poor visual acuities due to the presence of dense cataracts in each eye. Her best-corrected distance acuities ranged from 20/80 to 20/100 in each eye. Her ophthalmologist followed ID every 6 months for the cataracts. ID was apprehensive about the surgery and chose to have the cataracts monitored.
2. Sensorimotor status
   Oculomotor function: ID demonstrated increased latency in the initiation of her pursuit and saccadic eye movements, particularly to the left side. Standardized testing revealed slow speed, poor accuracy, and difficulty in finding the beginning of the line.
   Binocular function: ID showed restricted fusion ranges at both distance and near. She also exhibited poor awareness of double vision, which can also be attributed to her poor visual acuities.
3. Visual field status: Left homonymous hemianopia with neglect. Yoked prism (6^Δ base left) were trialed and ID was able to read faster and subjectively reported she was able to see more to the left. Objectively, ID's body posture immediately

improved and she did not lean to the right while wearing the yoked prisms. Her improved posture was maintained at her one-month follow-up examination.

Assessment

1. Visual field defect
2. Oculomotor dysfunction
3. Cataracts
4. Myopia and presbyopia

Recommendations

1. The yoked prisms were prescribed and incorporated into her distance prescription. She was advised to keep her old lenses as patients sometimes report less comfort with the yoked prisms with time as they progress in their other therapies (physical and occupational). A one-month follow-up was advised to monitor her symptoms and vision findings.
2. Vision rehabilitation was advised at the follow-up visit to improve oculomotor abilities, specifically visual scanning, and accuracy.
3. Large-print reading material was advised as a compensatory strategy because of her decreased acuities, oculomotor deficits and visual field deficits.

Outcome

ID attended ten vision rehabilitation sessions twice a month with good compliance with home vision therapy. She reported the following improvements: improved eye-hand coordination, improved ease with reading, less symptoms of visual neglect, increased visual awareness and less past-pointing. ID was discharged with maintenance home vision therapy activities as she indicated that she was scheduled for cataract surgery. A progress vision evaluation was scheduled for six months to allow for her eyes to adequately recover from the surgery. Vision rehabilitation will be continued if indicated at that point.

NP is an 11-year-old girl who was evaluated for the following vision complaints: constant blurred distance vision, intermittent near-vision blur, severe headaches, loss of place when reading, using her finger to read, intermittent double vision when reading, dizziness when experiencing headaches and fatigue after 30 minutes of schoolwork. Academically, NP was strong prior to the TBI and grades worsened afterward. She also reported that her vision worsened since the accident.

Etiology

TBI in June of 1999 due to a ceiling collapse.

Pertinent Visual Findings

1. Refractive status: NP initially did not bring her distance glasses, which she first received 3 months prior to this evaluation. She manifested a low myopic and

astigmatic prescription. Best-corrected distance visual acuities were 20/20 in each eye.

2. Sensorimotor status

Oculomotor function: NP exhibited saccadic intrusions in the left eye with fixation, and increased latency with pursuit movements in the left eye. NP also showed poor performance on standardized tests of oculomotor function.

Binocular function: NP manifested an intermittent exotropia at near with severely low fusion ranges at both distance and near. She also exhibited a right hyperdeviation at both distance and near.

Accommodative function: NP showed severe deficits in her accommodative function, particularly with respect to her sustaining ability.

Assessment

1. Intermittent exotropia
2. Oculomotor dysfunction
3. Accommodative insufficiency
4. Myopia

Recommendations

1. Single-vision distance prescription should be worn for distance use only. Prolonged near-vision work should be done without spectacles.
2. Vision rehabilitation was strongly advised to decrease frequency of visual symptoms.

Outcome

NP attended 20 sessions of vision rehabilitation with the following improvements noted: less double vision when reading, fewer headaches, less loss of place when reading, and no mention of dizziness. Overall, she was more confident academically. Upon reevaluation, her vision dysfunctions were fully resolved.

Conclusion

The literature strongly emphasizes the need for ABI patients to undergo a comprehensive vision evaluation (Sabates et al., 1991; Suchoff et al., 1999). These authors indicate that most vision symptoms can be resolved with the appropriate refractive correction at distance and near. Additionally, lightly tinted lenses, prisms, and occlusion recommendations are management options for ABI patients who may be experiencing poor progress in their rehabilitation programs as a direct consequence of their undiagnosed vision dysfunctions. Sabates et al. (1991) stated that many patients with vision problems may go undiagnosed for months to years after

TABLE 8.8. Post-Traumatic Vision
Syndrome (Padula, 1988b)

Post-traumatic vision syndrome (PTVS)
Eyestrain Headaches
Double vision
Focusing inability
Poor fixation and tracking
Decrease in color function
Staring behavior
Poor visual memory
Glare sensitivity
Balance, coordination, and postural deficits

their injury. Those working in the rehabilitation field should be readily able to recognize those patients suffering from vision dysfunctions secondary to their brain injury. Recognizing vision dysfunction is very difficult for those not specializing in vision because there is no visible sign, such as a broken limb or a red eye, for the provider to see and then make the appropriate referral. In most cases, vision deficits can be only be detected based upon direct complaints from the patient, neuropsychological or occupational therapy assessments, or subtle observations made by those working regularly with the patients. Consequently, a brief history questioning vision function should routinely be a part of every evaluation of an individual post acquired brain injury since most patients may not consider the importance of their vision in the rehabilitative process. Table 8.8 above summarizes the common vision symptoms reported by ABI patients. The common diagnoses and findings that will be reported to the referring provider may include accommodative dysfunction, convergence insufficiency or exotropia, low blink rate, poor fixation, poor pursuit and saccadic eye movements, and unstable peripheral processing abilities.

Efficacy of vision rehabilitation for ABI patients in the optometric literature is limited to studies with small sample sizes or case reports. These studies clearly demonstrate improvements in oculomotor and binocular function and elimination of symptoms associated with deficits in these areas of function (Ciuffreda et al., 2001; Padula, 1992; Berne, 1990; Hellerstein & Winkler, 2001; Ciuffreda et al., 1996). Further studies describing the efficacy of vision rehabilitation in the ABI population need to be conducted to document the prognosis of vision rehabilitation. Depending on the nature of the injury, therapy is typically initiated and specifically tailored with the goal of maximizing visual function in each individual. Each case is unique and it is often difficult to estimate prognosis in brain-injured patients as compared to noninjured patients. Literature and clinical experience reiterates the benefits of cortical redundancy when performing a specific task and neural plasticity when considering rehabilitation therapies that maximize the overall function of the ABI patient (Suter, 1995). As in all rehabilitative fields, such considerations form the basis in developing individual treatment recommendations for our patients with brain injury and vision dysfunctions.

References

Berne, S.A. (1990) Visual therapy for the traumatic brain-injured. *Journal of Optometric Vision Development* 21:13–16.

Brooks, C.W. & Borish, I.M. (1996) *System for Ophthalmic Dispensing*, 2nd ed. Boston: Butterworth-Heinemann.

Chan, R.P., Trobe, J.D. (2002) Spasm of accommodation associated with closed head trauma. *Journal of Neuro-Ophthalmology* 22(1):15–17.

Cho, M.H., Benjamin, W.J. (1998) Correction with multifocal spectacle lenses. In Benjamin W.J. (ed.): *Borish's Clinical Refraction*. Philadelphia: W.B. Saunders Company, pp. 888–927.

Ciuffreda, K.J. (2002) The scientific basis for and efficacy of optometric vision therapy in nonstrabismic accommodative and vergence disorders. *Optometry* 73:735–762.

Ciuffreda, K.J., Tannen, B. (1995) *Eye Movement Basics for the Clinician*. St. Louis: Mosby.

Ciuffreda, K.J., Tannen, B. (1999) Training of nystagmus: A multi-sensory approach. *Journal of Behavioural Optometry* 10(3):63–66.

Ciuffreda, K.J., Suchoff, I.B., Marrone, M.A., Ahmann, E. (1996) Oculomotor rehabilitation in traumatic brain-injured patients. *Journal of Behavioural Optometry* 7(2): 31–38.

Ciuffreda, K.J., Han, Y., Kapoor, N., Suchoff, I.B. (2001) Oculomotor consequences of acquired brain injury. In Suchoff, I.B., Ciuffreda, K.J., Kapoor, N (eds.): *Visual & Vestibular Consequences of Acquired Brain Injury*. Santa Ana: Optometric Extension Program, 77–88.

Cline, D., Hofstetter, H.W., Griffin, J.R. (1989) *Dictionary of Visual Science*. Radnor: Chilton Trade Book Publishing.

Cohen, A.H., Rein, L.D. (1992) The effect of head trauma on the visual system: The doctor of optometry as a member of the rehabilitation team. *Journal of American Optometry Association* 32(8):530–536.

Cohen, M., Groswasser, Z., Barchadski, R., Appel, A. (1989) Convergence insufficiency in brain-injured patients. *Brain injury* 3(2):187–191.

Du, T., Ciuffreda, K.J., Kapoor, N. (2005) Elevated dark adaptation threshold in traumatic brain injury. *Brain injury* 19(13):1125–1138.

Falk, N.S., Aksionoff, E.B. (1992) The primary care optometric evaluation of the traumatic brain injury patient. *Journal of American Optometry Association* 63(8):547–553.

Fayos, B., Ciuffreda, K.J. (1998) Oculomotor auditory biofeedback training to improve reading efficiency. *Journal of Behavioural Optometry* 9(6):143–152.

Fox, R.S. (2005) The rehabilitation of vergence and accommodative dysfunctions in traumatic brain injury. *Brain Injury Professional* 2(3):12–15.

Gerner, E.W. (1993) Visual sequelae of closed head trauma. In Mandel, S., Sataloff, R.T., Schapiro, S.R. (eds.): *Minor Head Trauma: Assessment, Management, and Rehabilitation*. New York: Springer-Verlag, pp. 235–244.

Gianutsos, R., Ramsey, G., Perlin, R.R. (1988) Rehabilitative optometric services for survivors of acquired brain injury. *Archives of Physical Medicine & Rehabilation* 69: 573–578.

Gizzi, M., Khattar, V., Eckert, A. (1997) A quantitative study of postural shifts induced by yoked prism. *J Optom Vis Dev* 28:200–203.

Han, M.E., Bell, S.B., Rutner, D., Kapoor, N., Ciuffreda, K.J., Suchoff, I.B. (2005) Medications prescribed to brain injury patients: A retrospective analysis. *Investigative Ophthalmology & Visual Science* 46:E-Abstract 5038.

Hellerstein, L., Freed, S. (1994) Rehabilitative optometric management of a traumatic brain injury patient. *Journal of Behavioural Optometry* 5(6):143–148.

Hellerstein, L., Winkler, P.A. (2001) Vestibular dysfunction associated with traumatic brain injury: Collaborative optometry and physical therapy treatment. In Suchoff, I.B., Ciuffreda, K.J., Kapoor, N. (eds.): *Visual & Vestibular Consequences of Acquired Brain Injury*. Santa Ana: Optometric Extension Program, pp. 220–235.

Jackowski, M.M. (2001) Altered visual adaptation in patients with traumatic brain injury. In Suchoff, I.B., Ciuffreda, K.J., Kapoor, N. (eds.): *Visual & Vestibular Consequences of Acquired Brain Injury*. Santa Ana: Optometric Extension Program, pp. 145–173.

Julkunen, L., Tenovuo, O., Jääskeläinen, S., Hämäläinen, H. (2003) Rehabilitation of chronic post-stroke visual field defect with computer-assisted training. *Restorative Neurology and Neuroscience* 21:19–28.

Kapoor, N., Ciuffreda, K.J. (2005) Vision problems. In Silver, J.M., McAllister, T.W., Yudofsky, S.C. (eds.): *Textbook of Traumatic Brain Injury*, 1st ed. Washington DC: American Psychiatric Publishing, Inc., pp. 405–417.

Kapoor, N., Ciuffreda, K.J., Suchoff, I.B. (2001) Egocentric localization in patients with visual neglect. In Suchoff, I.B., Ciuffreda, K.J., Kapoor, N. (eds.): *Visual & Vestibular Consequences of Acquired Brain Injury*. Santa Ana: Optometric Extension Program, pp. 131–144.

Leslie, S. (2001) Accommodation in acquired brain injury. In Suchoff, I.B., Ciuffreda, K.J., Kapoor, N. (eds.): *Visual & Vestibular Consequences of Acquired Brain Injury*. Santa Ana: Optometric Extension Program, pp. 56–76.

Mueller, I., Poggel, D.A., Kenkel, S., Kasten, E., Sabel, B.A. (2003) Vision restoration therapy after brain damage: Subjective improvements of activities of daily life and their relationship of visual field enlargements. *Visual Impairment Research* 5(3):157–178.

Nelles, G., Esser, J., Eckstein, A., Tiede, A., Gerhard, H., Diener, H.C. (2001) Compensatory visual field training for patients with hemianopia after stroke. *Neuroscience Letters* 306:189–192.

Padula, W.V. (1988a) Chapter VI: The neuro-optometric rehabilitation examination. In Padula, W.V. (ed.): *Neuro-Optometric Rehabilitation*, 3rd ed. Santa Ana: Optometric Extension Program, pp. 78–87.

Padula, W.V. (1988b) Chapter XIV: Post-trauma vision syndrome caused by head injury. In Padula, W.V. (ed.):*Neuro-Optometric Rehabilitation*, 3rd ed. Santa Ana: Optometric Extension Program, pp. 179–193.

Padula, W.V. (1992) Neuro-optometric rehabilitation for persons with TBI or CVA. *Journal of Optometric Vision Development* 23:4–8.

Poggel, D.A., Kasten, E., Sabel, B.A. (2004) Attentional cueing improves vision restoration therapy in patients with visual field defects. *Neurology* 63:2069–2076.

Richter, E.F. (2001) Interdisciplinary management and rehabilitation of acquired brain-injured patients. In Suchoff, I.B., Ciuffreda, K.J., Kapoor, N. (eds.): *Visual & Vestibular Consequences of Acquired Brain Injury*. Santa Ana: Optometric Extension Program, pp. 10–31.

Rode, G., Rossetti, Y., Boisson, D. (2001) Prism adaptation improves representational neglect. *Neuropsychologia* 39:1250–1254.

Rosen, S.A., Cohen, A.H., Trebling, S. (2001) The integration of visual and vestibular systems in balance disorder—a clinical perspective. In Suchoff, I.B., Ciuffreda, K.J., Kapoor, N. (eds.): *Visual & Vestibular Consequences of Acquired Brain Injury*. Santa Ana: Optometric Extension Program, pp. 174–200.

Rosetti, Y., Rode, G., Pisella, L., Farne, A., Li, L., Boisson, D., Perenin, M.T. (1998) Prism adaptation to a rightward optical deviation rehabilitates left hemispatial neglect. *Nature* 395:166–169.

Reinhard, J., Schreiber, A., Schiefer, U., Kasten, E., Sabel, B.A., Kenkel, S., Vonthein, R., Trauzettel-Klosinski, S. (2005) Does visual restitution training change absolute homonymous visual field defects? A fundus controlled study. *British Journal of Ophthalmology* 89:30–35.

Sabates, N.R., Gonce, M.A., Farris, B.K. (1991) Neuro-opthalmological findings in closed head trauma. *Journal of Clinical Neuroophthalmology* 11(4):273–277.

Sabel, B.A., Kasten, E., (2000) Restoration of vision by training of residual functions. *Currunt Opinion in Ophthalogy* 11:430–436.

Scheiman, M., Wick, B. (2002) *Clinical Management of Binocular Vision*. 2nd ed. Philadelphia: Lipponcott Williams and Wilkins.

Smith, N.A. (ed.): *Lighting for occupational Optometry*. IIIISC Handbook No. 23. Leeds: H and H Scientific Consultants Ltd.

Suchoff, I.B., Ciuffreda, K.J. (2004) A primer for the optometric management of unilateral spatial inattention. *Optometry* 75(5):305–318.

Suchoff, I.B., Kapoor, N., Waxman, R., Ference, W. (1999) The occurrence of ocular and visual dysfunctions in an acquired brain-injured patient sample. *Journal of American Optometry Association* 70(5):301–309.

Suter, P.S. (1995) Rehabilitation and management of visual dysfunction following traumatic brain injury. In Ashley, M.J., Krych, D.K. (eds.): *Traumatic Brain Injury Rehabilitation* Boca Roton: CRC Press, pp. 187–219.

Vogel, M.S. (192) An overview of head trauma for the primary care practitioner: Part II— Ocular damage associated with head trauma. *Journal of American Optometry Association* 63(8):542–546.

Wainapel, S.F. (1995) Vision rehabilitation: An overlooked subject in physiatric training and practice. *American Journal of Physical Medecine & Rehabilation* 74:313–314.

Warren, M. (1993) Hierarchical model for evaluation and treatment of visual perceptual dysfunction in adult acquired brain injury, part I. *The American Journal of Occupational Therapy* 47(1):42–54.

Weiss, L.M. (2002) Visual-vestibular interaction in the acquired brain injured patient. *Journal of Optometric Vision Development* 33:33–41.

Zihl, J. (2000) *Rehabilitation of Visual Disorders After Brain Injury*. East Sussex: Psychology Press Ltd, pp. 11–90.

Zihl, J., Kerkhoff, G. (1990) Foveal photopic and scotopic adaptation in patients with brain damage. *Clinical Vision Sciences* 5(2):185–195.

Glossary of Clinical Terms (Cline et al., 1989; Kapoor & Ciuffreda, 2005)

Accommodation: The ability to change focus and maintain a clear image of an object (when looking from far to near and vice versa), using the eye's crystalline lens-based mechanism.

Accommodative Amplitude: The closest point of clear vision that is typically measured monocularly.

Accommodative Infacility: A condition in which slow or difficult accommodative responses are observed in response step changes in lens power.

Accommodative Insufficiency: A condition in which the measured amplitude of accommodation is less than expected given the patient's age.

Astigmatism: Unequal refractive error in orthogonal meridians of the eye. Rays of light from infinity come to a focus at two different distances relative to the retina, with accommodation minimally stimulated.

Binocular: Viewing with two eyes at the same time.

Contrast Sensitivity: The ability to detect threshold contrast targets. Measuring contrast sensitivity measures the ability to resolve spatial properties across a range of spatial frequencies and levels of contrast (Warren).

Convergence: The turning inward of the eyes toward each other.

Convergence Excess: A condition in which esophoria is greater at near than far.

Convergence Insufficiency: The condition in which exophoria is greater at near than far, with a receded near point of convergence and reduced relative fusional convergence at near.

Diplopia: The condition in which a single object is perceived as two objects rather than one; double vision.

Divergence: A deviation or relative movement of the two eyes outward from parallelism.

Divergence Excess: A condition in which exophoria is greater at distance than near and often associated with an exotropia.

Divergence Insufficiency: A condition in which there is greater esophoria at distance than near and is often associated with esotropia.

Emmetropia: Essentially no refractive error present.

Esophoria: A condition in which the two eyes intersect in front of the plane of regard when fusion is disrupted.

Exophoria: A condition in which the two eyes intersect beyond the plane of regard when fusion is disrupted.

Exotropia: A type of strabismus in which the non-fixating eye is turned outwards.

Fixation: Ocular alignment with the image of the fixated target falling on the fovea; may be performed one eye at a time (i.e., monocularly) or with both eyes at the same time (i.e., binocularly).

Fusion: Single, cortically integrated vision under binocular viewing conditions

Fusional Prism: The amount of prism an individual can fuse.

Fusional Range: The range over which the vergence system can be stimulated by the addition of prisms binocularly and still maintain single, binocular vision at both distance (6 m) and near (40 cm). Three parameters are recorded: the first is the amount of prism at which the patient reports blurred vision; the second is the amount of prism at which the patient reports diplopia; and, the third is the amount of prism at which the patient regains fusion.

Hemianopia: Hemi-field visual field defect, which may be unilateral or bilateral (i.e., homonymous or bitemporal).

Hyperopia: Far-sightedness; when rays of light from infinity come to a focus behind the eye, with accommodation minimally stimulated.

Monocular: Viewing with one eye at a time.

Myopia: Near-sightedness; when rays of light from infinity come to a focus in front of the eye, with accommodation minimally stimulated.

Nystagmus: Rapid involuntary oscillation or movement of the eyes, the presence or absence of which may be diagnostic of neurological and vision disorders.

Oscillopsia: Illusory movement of the world generally related to vestibular dysfunction.

Presbyopia: Normal age-related, physiological loss of focusing ability.

Pursuit: Slow, continuous, and conjugate eye movement used when the eyes follow an object as it is moved slowly and smoothly.

Prism: A lens that deviates the path of light as it passes through it. An image will move towards the apex of the lens.

Refractive Status: The degree to which images on the retina are not focused.

Saccade: Rapid, step-like conjugate eye movement that redirects the line of sight from one position to another.

Strabismus: An anomaly of binocular vision in which one eye fails to intersect an object of regard.

Stereopsis: Relative depth perception based on horizontal retinal image disparity

Vergence: When the two eyes move to track targets moving in depth.

Versional Eye Movements: When the two eyes move (includes fixation, pursuit, and saccade) to follow targets moving laterally, vertically, or obliquely in one plane, with no change in depth.

Vestibulo-Ocular Reflex (VOR): Rapid, reflex movement of the eyes which functions to counteract head movements and maintain stable gaze on an object.

Yoked Prism: Prisms with bases oriented in the same direction.

9
Nursing Care of the Neuro-Rehabilitation Patient

ANTHONY APRILE AND KELLY REILLY

The Role of Rehabilitation Nurses

Rehabilitation nurses are licensed professionals (registered nurses) with additional training and experience in rehabilitation. Training typically consists of an orientation to the hospital followed by a didactic component related to care of the rehabilitation patient and a preceptorship of varying lengths dependent on previous experience. Rehabilitation nurses can become credentialed through certification in rehabilitation nursing through the Association of Rehabilitation Nurses (ARN) or further credentialed in neuro rehabilitation nursing by obtaining certification in Neuroscience Nursing through the American Association of Neuroscience Nurses (AANN). Appendix 1 lists a number of professional associations of interest to the rehabilitation nurse. Clinical judgment, skills and an evidence-based approach to practice must be maintained through continuing education, training, and the ongoing evaluation of neuro-specific competencies to validate proficiency of care of the neuro rehabilitation patient. These are continuous processes that must be sought by nurses to maintain expertise in the rapidly advancing fields of neuroscience and neurorehabilitation. Professional associations, like the ARN and AANN, provide professional development through education, advocacy, collaboration and research within the specialty (Doble et al., 2000).

Nursing rehabilitation of the neurological patient begins in the acute phase of the injury or illness (Barker, 2002, pp. 477–500), and can extend beyond acute care, through various phases (acute, subacute) of inpatient rehabilitation and into the home or other long-term care setting. The rehabilitation nurse must integrate specialized knowledge, skills, experience, and a compassionate attitude, in order to meet the needs of the patient and family. The application of these skills and expertise can occur through administrative and/or clinical roles and functions.

Administratively, rehabilitation nurses can function as case managers, especially common in acute care and acute rehabilitation settings. In this role, nurses must advocate for patients and families by representing concerns regarding care both within and outside of the clinical setting. The case manager must review each patient's case for the appropriate treatments and services. If expected treatments or services are omitted from the plan of care or denied by the insurance companies, the case manager will appeal the decision in order to try and obtain the care or services the patient requires. The nurse case manager must be involved from the beginning of care, before admission into rehabilitation, to help the patient and family transition from the medical management to rehabilitative phases of care; and then from inpatient to outpatient and/or home-based services, facilitating a smooth transition and adjustment. Nurse case managers also help obtain needed health care and social/financial services. These can include financial assistance, medical benefits, visiting nurse and/or attendant care, independent living arrangements, elder or adult care, transportation, day treatment programs, hospice care, and preventive health care. The needs of the patient and family will guide what services are sought and implemented (Barker, 2002, p. 477–500). A more detailed discussion of the role and responsibilities of the case manager can be found in Chapter 10.

Clinical Neuro-Rehabilitative Nursing Care

From the vantage point of the rehabilitation nurse, the main focus of rehabilitation is to assist the patient to move toward increasing independence in self-care. Dorothea Orem's model of self-care defines a system that includes wholly compensatory systems, partly compensatory systems, and supportive educative systems (Edwards, 2000). A wholly compensatory patient system refers to self-care needs being met solely through help of others. A partially compensatory system includes the patient meeting his or her own self-care needs with the partial support from others. And a supportive educative system includes the patient meeting his or her own self-care needs through the instruction and encouragement of others (Edwards, 2000). Based on the nurse's and other interdisciplinary team members' assessments, an initial plan of care for a neurorehabilitation patient is developed as a partial compensatory system if basic activities are successfully initiated in the acute care setting. The goal for the patient will then be to progress to a supportive educative system enabling self-care in the rehabilitative setting (Edwards, 2000).

Ms. Jones is an 87-year-old female admitted into the neuro rehab unit 3 weeks status post-hemorrhagic stroke. Upon admission, Ms. Jones is noted to have left-sided hemiplegia with self-care deficits secondary to impaired mobility. She has reduced safety awareness and is impulsive. Ms. Jones is able to assist with bathing, toileting, and dressing but lacks the motor skills, endurance, and cognitive abilities to complete these tasks on her own. Through collaborative assessment and training from her occupational therapist, and carryover/reinforcement by nursing staff of skills learned in therapy, Ms. Jones is taught proper body mechanics and encouraged to rest and time her activities to increase her endurance, thus increasing her ability to become more independent in her own care.

The initial rehabilitation nursing assessment must be thorough, valid, and reliable, as it provides the basis for developing the nursing plan of care. It must include a history, as the general health of the patient before the injury or illness must be established in order to determine the patient's capacity to return to an optimal level of functioning. The assessment will span physical, neurological, and functional components, including level of consciousness (LOC), vital signs, visual and pupil evaluation, motor and sensory functioning, cranial nerve functions, cognition, communication, and behavior (Barker, 2002, p. 477–500). The Functional Independence Measure (FIM) provides a standardized, objective way of measuring the patient's current motor and cognitive abilities (Hawley et al., 1999), and is commonly utilized in acute rehabilitation settings to measure outcomes. Subsequent assessments must focus on the areas of deficit from the initial assessment, and can help determine the patient's progress.

Level of Consciousness

Nursing assessment of level of consciousness includes determination of the patient's state of arousal, awareness to person, place and time, and responsiveness to environmental stimuli (Barker, 2002, p. 53). It can be performed by using the Glasgow Coma Scale (GCS), which evaluates eye opening, motor and verbal responses (which can range from spontaneous to responsive to speech, to pain, to no response) and is a reliable measure of consciousness (refer to Chapter 2, Table 2.1).

Vital Signs

Vital sign assessment of the neuro rehabilitation patient can show telltale signs of deterioration of neurological status. Patients with increased intracranial pressure (IICP) present with bradycardia secondary to the stimulation of the brainstem; the presence of bradycardia, hypertension, and widening pulse pressures are considered to be a late finding of IICP (Barker, 2002, p. 77). The pupil evaluation assesses the size, shape, equality and reaction of the pupils. Normal assessment findings include regular-shaped, reactive pupils. Unequal and/or oval pupils are indicators of IICP and as a new assessment finding could indicate a herniation of the brain from an area of higher pressure to lower pressure (Barker, 2002, p. 71).

Motor Function

Motor function and mobility assessments identify deficits in the interactions of muscles, peripheral and central nerve processes, and the impact on mobility. The assessment requires that bilateral extremities be evaluated at the same time. Muscle strength, bulk, and tone are evaluated in the upper and lower extremities. A muscle-strength grading scale rates muscle strength from total paralysis to active movement against full resistance and is a good tool for comparison to determine improvement in the patient's condition (Edwards, 2000). If the patient is unable to understand simple commands, motor function is assessed by the use of a painful stimulus. Central stimulation includes trapezius pinch, sternal rub, supra orbital pressure, and nipple or testicle pinch that stimulates a total body response; however, these are contraindicated in patients with brain injury. Peripheral stimulation can differentiate affected areas of the body and include nail bed pressure and pinching the inner aspect of the arm or leg (Barker, 2002, p. 65–69).

Mobility is assessed through range of motion, balance, bed mobility, transfer ability, wheelchair mobility, ambulation, neuromuscular problems, coordination and sensory function, and the ability to understand and follow instructions. Impaired mobility affects all body systems including the skin, bladder and bowel, respiratory system, and increased contractures of ligaments and muscle atrophy. For mobility-impaired patients, nursing staff need to provide frequent turning and positioning, use pressure relieving surfaces, monitor for incontinence of bladder or bowel, ensure adequate nutrition, monitor lung sounds, provide regular gentle exercise, assess for deep vein thrombosis, assess for postural hypotension, and use recreational therapy to stimulate social interaction (Edwards, 2000).

Based on the initial nursing assessment, Ms. Jones requires moderate assistance to transfer from the bed to a chair or wheelchair. Impaired mobility puts Ms. Jones at risk for potential complications. The nursing care plan includes head to toe skin assessment and risk assessment each shift along with frequent turning and positioning, every two hours with more frequent assessments of the areas at risk for injury (e.g., bony prominences). A pressure relieving mattress is in place to help alleviate areas prone to pressure ulcers. Frequent assessments of bowel and bladder habits help to plan for appropriate intervals of toileting. Ms. Jones will be toileted every 3–4 hours through the day and night. A nutrition consult is ordered to ensure adequate dietary intake for optimal healing. Routine vital signs and monitoring of respiratory or circulatory complications will occur daily to prevent potential complications of impaired mobility.

Sensory Function

Sensory assessments evaluate superficial and deep sensations that may show deficits with regard to the peripheral nerves, spinal roots, spinal cord, brainstem, thalamus and cerebral cortex. All sensory assessments are evaluated bilaterally. Superficial assessments include light touch evaluated by strolling the patient's skin, superficial pain evaluated by the use of a pinprick, and skin temperature assessed with hot or cold water. Evaluation of deep sensations includes assessment of the sensation of vibration, position sense, and deep pain.

The nurse must assess the hearing and visual ability of the patient, including interviewing the family regarding the patient's pre-morbid hearing/visual status, and ensuring the patient has access to necessary devices (e.g., hearing aid, corrective lenses). Deficits in hearing or vision can be a result of injury or illness that can be partial or complete. If a hearing deficit is identified, the nurse must ensure patient safety by validating that the patient understands instructions, and accommodating the patient by using alternative methods of communication, such as written notes or sign language (Edwards, 2000). Visual deficits can include disturbances in the visual fields or reduced visual acuity. The nurse must instruct the patient to scan the visual field and provide a safe environment with adequate lighting and free of obstructions (Edwards, 2000).

Cognitive/Communication Disorders

The patient's cognitive status is a reflection of the resiliency of memory, judgment, reasoning, and problem-solving ability, and will impact his or her ability to utilize/benefit from nursing education and interventions. The nurse's assessment of the cognitive status of patients with ABI includes orientation to person, place, and time as well as their ability to understand and follow directions. The patient must also be observed for confusion, impulsivity, perseveration, memory impairment, emotional lability, disinhibition, and agitation. Nursing interventions include repetitive review and cuing for orientation; use of memory aids (e.g., calendars, notebooks) consistency with the environment, staff, and schedules; use of bed, chair or door alarms; establishing structured supplemental activity routines during nontherapy hours; encouraging family involvement and providing education and guidance. Nursing interventions for communication impairments (e.g., receptive, expressive aphasia) can include repetition, control of the environment, use of short simple sentences, and family education on effective communication techniques. Working with the speech-language pathologist to develop alternative communication strategies (e.g., picture board) to help the patient express basic needs is essential.

For patients with behavioral challenges (e.g., agitation), it is important to maintain a calm and controlled approach to the patient, including giving simple instructions and avoiding scolding. Physical restraints are an intervention of last resort, and can often be avoided by behavioral strategies such as providing verbal redirection, rest periods, limiting visitors, and reducing environmental stimuli (Edwards, 2000). Documentation of type and duration of behavioral challenges will enable appropriate strategies/interventions to be developed by the neuropsychologist and/or medical staff.

Safety

Patients with acquired brain injuries are at risk for many safety related issues, including elopement and falls. Careful monitoring of ambulatory, yet disoriented, patients to prevent inadvertent wandering off or elopement is critical. Staff and family education will help decrease the risk of elopement.

Potential for injury related to falls is assessed initially by review of the patient's history. Patients at risk include those with cognitive impairment, a history of falls, impaired mobility, a history of syncope, or use of an assistive device (Corrigan et al., 1999). A further assessment of sensory function, urinary function, gastrointestinal function, mental status, neurological status, and medication assessment for potential alteration in level of consciousness will help identify risk factors and appropriate interventions. Fall prevention programs should be based on safety related interventions that involve the patient and family. Interventions for risk of falls include a frequent reorientation to person, place, and time, placing the call bell within reach with instructions (visual and/or verbal, as would benefit the patient) on use, assuring that the patient has his/her own assistive device, toileting the patient frequently, assessing recent administration of diuretics, assessing GI function, maintaining the bed in a low position with brakes on, ensuring adequate lighting, and monitoring side effects of medications. Nurses must communicate their assessment findings and any clinical updates to each other when changing shift and to other members of the neurorehabilitation team. Additionally, if the patient is at significant risk of falls, increased supervision by ancillary staff can help maintain patient safety (CDC, 2005).

Ms. Jones is at risk for falls due to her impaired mobility and impulsivity. Both Ms. Jones and family members are educated to her risk for falls and appropriate interventions including use of call bell and ensuring the bed is in the lowest position and brakes are on. Due to memory impairments, a sign is posted in her room reminding her to "Use the call bell if you need assistance." Ms. Jones will be toileted frequently and supervised by ancillary staff when attempting activities of daily living to ensure safety is maintained.

Nutrition

Nutritional assessments can help identify issues that would lead to potential negative complications. A complete nutritional assessment is used to identify the proper protein, carbohydrate, fat, vitamin, and fluid intake to meet the metabolic demands of a healing body. In collaboration with the dietician and/or nutritionist, this should include analysis of weight, dietary history, interest and choices, muscle wasting, fat stores and lab results (Barker, 2002, p. 248). When oral intake is not possible, patients will receive nutrition via a gastrostomy tube (G-tube) and the nurse must perform ongoing assessment of the patient's fluid intake, weight, and serum albumin. Nursing care of the patient with a G-tube includes thorough skin assessments and skin care around the insertion site, and assessing placement of the G-tube by checking for residual stomach contents. The patient's position must be upright greater than 30 degrees for feedings to decrease risk of aspiration. Patient and family education begins with the type, time, and frequency of feedings. Care of the insertion site and initiation and discontinuation of feedings should be taught progressively to validate understanding (Barker, 2002, p. 248–251).

A swallowing assessment is needed to minimize the risk of aspiration in the neuro rehabilitation patient. A patient with impaired swallowing may exhibit drooling, ineffective coughing, need for suctioning, and respiratory difficulty when eating. Related difficulties may include slurred speech, inability to smile, purse lips, presence of facial droop, pocketing of food, inadequate swallowing with first attempt, and increased time to finish a meal (Edwards, 2000). Appropriate interventions for patients at risk for aspiration due to impaired swallowing include a referral for a swallowing evaluation to detect/diagnose the impairment, and the consistent implementation of strategies, typically established by the speech-language pathologist. These may include sitting the patient upright, ensuring foods have proper consistency, nonmixing of solids and liquids, placing food on the unaffected side of the mouth, and using small mouthfuls. Cuing/compensatory strategies include minimizing environmental distractions, teaching the patient to concentrate on chewing and swallowing before taking another mouthful, providing additional time and supervision. Patients should remain upright 20–30 minutes after eating (Barnes, 2003).

Patients who cannot tolerate feedings by mouth will be started on hyperalimentation via a centralized venous catheter. Hyperalimentation gives the patient fluid, protein, carbohydrates, and fats through the veins via total parenteral nutrition (TPN) and lipids to ensure adequate nutrition is maintained. Nursing care of the patient receiving TPN includes central line assessments and dressing changes. The assessment of proper nutritional requirements based on routinely ordered labs are necessary to meet the changing needs of patients and the assessment, monitoring and evaluation of the patient for therapeutic results and signs and symptoms of complications is required on a shift by shift basis. The eventual goal is to slowly introduce feedings by mouth and reduce the need for hyperalimentation (Edwards, 2000).

Bowel and Bladder Function

As described in Chapter 5, changes in continence are common following acquired brain injury. Nurses must ask patients specific questions related to difficulties with continence to help determine their needs in this area. Careful observation and documentation is also necessary, since many patients will be unable to reliably report their needs, due to sensory, cognitive or behavioral impairments. In designing interventions, nurses must take into account cognitive status, ability to participate in interventions, age, mobility, and gastrointestinal disturbance (e.g., constipation) (Barker, 2002, p. 489–490), in addition to the cause of incontinence. It is important to ensure regular toileting during the day and night. Using input/output records to identify fluid intake, time of voiding, sensation of fullness and feeling of emptying the bladder can be beneficial. Intermittent catheterization, condom catheters, and indwelling catheters provide a way to handle and measure urinary drainage (Barker, 2002, p. 489–490). The patient and or family can be taught to plan fluid intake and bladder emptying prior to activities.

Bowel function assessment includes patient history of bowel patterns including time and characteristics of last stool, medications that affect function, and medical or psychological problems that affect function (including infection, trauma or stress). Constipation and diarrhea need to be assessed and treated. Nutritional assessment must include sources of fiber and proper hydration to maintain proper bowel function. Planning for bowel movements after meals often ensures emptying. Patients and families must be taught the importance of regular bowel elimination and the complications of constipation and diarrhea (Barker, 2002, p. 490–493).

Wound Care

A primary goal of nursing care is to prevent and, when necessary, heal pressure ulcers. Risk factors that identify patients at risk for altered skin integrity include age, underlying disease processes, neurological injuries, impaired circulation, impaired mobility, impaired sensation, low serum protein albumin, poor nutrition, and bladder or bowel incontinence. Factors that increase incidence of pressure related injury include sustained pressure from surfaces or devices, and complications of stomas and related equipment. Shearing forces, which are defined as adjacent surfaces moving across each other, and friction, the rubbing of one surface on another, contribute to the increased incidence of pressure related injury and therefore need to be managed (Makelbust & Sieggreen, 2000).

Nursing interventions for the neuro rehabilitation patient at risk for skin related injury include the use of a risk assessment scale to detect if the patient's status is improving or declining. The Braden scale (Brown, 2004) is commonly used to predict pressure ulcer risk in patients. The scale assesses patients' sensory perception, mobility, activity, moisture, nutrition, and friction and sheer. Each section is scored from 1 to 3 or 4 points. The lower the score on the assessment the higher the risk of pressure related injury (Brown, 2004). Additionally, a daily nutritional assessment must be done to ensure adequate metabolic requirements are being met. Patients must be assessed for frequent turning and positioning determined by the heightened risk of the skin assessment. Turning and repositioning schedules are evaluated based on the patient's assessment score and the use of assistive equipment if available. Current technology incorporated into the beds and mattresses have turn and assist functions that support the patient's needs for frequent turning and positioning. Manual turning and positioning should occur at a minimum of every 2 hours and be adjusted according to the nurse's assessment and incorporated into the plan of care. Shear and friction need to be managed by positioning the head of the bed no greater than 30 degrees and a lift sheet or other device should be used to move or reposition the patients to decrease friction and shear. Skin care includes a daily inspection of the skin, keeping the skin clean and dry, minimizing exposure to moisture, and avoiding massage of bony prominences. Patient teaching begins with the nurse's use of the assessment tool, nutrition assessment and care of the skin. If interventions are needed teaching should include treatments, expected course of healing and complications associated with pressure ulcers (Makelbust and Sieggreen, 2000).

Nurses must maintain competency in staging and the treatment of pressure ulcers. Documentation needs to be factual and accurate describing the location and size of the wound, description of the wound base, sinuses and color and consistency of drainage. Staging is based on severity of the injury. Stage I includes changes to the skin color, consistency, and temperature. Stage II includes partial tissue loss of the epidermis and the dermis. Stage III is a full thickness skin loss through the subcutaneous tissue. Stage IV is a full-thickness skin loss through the fascia to the muscle or bone. Any changes noted to the patient's skin need to be reported and evaluated to prevent the extensive complications of pressure ulcers (Makelbust & Sieggreen, 2000).

Pain Management

Pain is a sensory experience that evokes emotional, social, spiritual, and physical responses. The clinical definition of pain is "whatever the person says it is, existing wherever the person says it does" (McCaffery, 1999). Patients at risk for under-treatment of pain include the elderly and the cognitively impaired (Galloway & Turner, 1999). Nurses must assess pain on an ongoing basis. The initiation of the plan of care should occur during the admission process, at regular intervals, and with any new reports of pain. A thorough pain assessment includes location, intensity, timing, quality; a description of what makes the pain worse and what makes it better, the patient's pain goal, and what changes in behavior occur with pain. Pain-assessment scales identify the severity or intensity of pain and include a 0 to 10 scale (Pasero et al., 1999) and a noncommunicative assessment that evaluates behavioral cues (Pasero et al., 1999). Pharmacological interventions should be based on the patient's reports of pain with appropriate score (Pasero et al., 1999). Nonpharmacological interventions and complementary therapies should be based on what decreased the pain as reported by the patient. Reassessment of pain must be done after implementation of an intervention. Effectiveness should be documented and communicated. Breakthrough pain, or transitory episodes of moderate to severe pain, can be a significant barrier to participation and progress in rehabilitation, and must be comprehensively managed. Patients are at risk for breakthrough pain with activity, which usually presents as extreme pain that causes distress. Management involves specific dosing to be included in the medical treatment of pain, and includes coordination with other members of the neurorehabilitation team (e.g., PT, OT), particularly around timing of medication administration. Nurses must anticipate, prevent and treat the side effects of analgesia, which can include constipation, nausea and vomiting, sedation, pruritis (itching), mental status changes, and respiratory depression. Nurses also need to educate the patient and family on pain management (St. Marie, 2002).

Barriers to effective pain management can occur from a knowledge deficit of pain-management theory, inadequacy of the pain-assessment cycle, concern for the side effects of pain medication, and/or fear of addiction. Addiction occurs in less than 0.1% of patients using narcotics for medical purposes (Pasero et al., 1999). To prevent withdrawal, weaning of narcotics should be established in the plan of care. Education regarding tolerance, dependence, and addiction need to be addressed for the patient receiving pain management, in order to alleviate any misconceptions regarding receipt of pain medication (St. Marie, 2002).

Sleep Disturbances

Neuro-rehabilitation patients are at risk for alteration in sleeping patterns related to the brain injury, pain, and/or the effects of medications. The normal progression of traumatic brain injury or stroke can lead to an initial reversal of the day/night cycle (Edwards, 2000). Co-morbidities and medications can also affect sleep. Nursing interventions include helping and teaching patients to keep a routine, use comfort and alternative measures (e.g., music) to relax, toilet before sleep, create a quiet environment, and treat pain timely and effectively (Barker, 2002, p. 258–259).

Sexual Dysfunction

Neuro-rehabilitation patients are at risk for alteration in sexual function and reproduction, and the rehabilitation nurse often takes on the role of educating the patients on the effects of injury, illness, or medications on sexual function and reproduction.

Knowledge of factors that influence the dynamics of a relationship and the physical and psychological aspects of sexual functioning is required. The nurse must create an environment of acceptance and be aware of resources that are available for support in this sensitive area; referral to specialists (neuro-urologist, neuro-psychiatrist, and psychotherapist) may be indicated (Chandler & Brown, 1998).

Family Training

The neurorehabilitation team must provide family-centered care to restore the patient and family to optimal health. Patients and families should be setting goals and be involved in all levels of care planning. As many neurorehabilitation patients will need continued assistance with self-care upon discharge from an inpatient setting, it is vital to include the family in most educational and training interventions. Language and cultural differences need to be evaluated and taken into account (Edwards, 2000) as should the relationships between spiritual beliefs and health and religious practices. The availability and interpersonal dynamics of the patients' social support systems must be assessed (Barker, 2002, p. 477–499).

Discharge training starts upon admission to the neuro rehabilitation unit. Patient and family education is started at the beginning of rehabilitation and progressed to the point at which the patient and family have the ability to manage their own care at home. Patients and families need to understand the compensatory mechanisms that occur after a brain injury and the adaptive devices used to assist motor and sensory functioning. When communication is an issue, families are taught alternative methods for communicating to meet the needs of patient, via a collaborative approach between the speech-language pathologist and nursing staff. Safety interventions are implemented and strategies for applications to the home settings should be discussed prior to discharge so that arrangements can be made in advance. Medication regimens should be adjusted from an inpatient-oriented, around the clock schedule, to a home schedule for ease of compliance. Understanding of the purpose, timing, and side effects of medications needs to be validated prior to discharge. Nutritional requirements and assessments should be understood prior to discharge and arrangements of proper foods, amount and consistency, should be in place at home for the patient to maintain optimal dietary intake. If tube feedings are necessary, the patient or family needs to be competent in initiating and discontinuing feedings, and skin care around the insertion site. Complications of bowel and bladder incontinence, pressure ulcers, pain, sleep disturbances, and sexual dysfunction must also be understood to ensure adequate resources are supplied and optimal transition occurs from the inpatient to outpatient setting.

Ms. Jones' team has been preparing for an anticipated discharge in 1 week. Ms. Jones will require a walker, nutritional supplements, pain and medication management, and continued outpatient therapies upon discharge. Ms. Jones will be going home to her daughter's house so that she will have supervision and assistance. PT and OT review and train the family in equipment usage and transfer techniques. The nutritionist discusses the increased caloric needs of healing and explains to Ms. Jones and her daughter that to meet the increased caloric needs, dietary supplementation will be needed. These supplements are available at most stores and her daughter is able to have them available at the house when Ms. Jones arrives. The R.N. reviews names, times, and side effects of all medications that Ms. Jones takes daily. Both the patient and family verbalize understanding of all medications that Ms. Jones will be going home on, including the use of pain medications before physical therapy. The patient and family are educated to the signs and symptoms of complications from pain, pressure injury, bowel or bladder incontinence, and sleep and sexual dysfunction. Follow-up appointments and contact numbers are given prior to discharge to ensure that the proper resources are in place.

Conclusion

The nurse is an integral part of the interdisciplinary neurorehabilitation team, whose goal is to meet the needs of patients and families by restoring the patient to an optimal level of health and improving his or her quality of life. It is a well-organized team that results in a reduction of deaths, disability, and need for long-term institutions. Teams must communicate regularly to discuss patient's assessments, problem identification, short- and long-term goals, and decision-making (Langhorne & Legg, 2003). The R.N. plays a vital role in the communication of patient status to family members and other members of the health care team. The nursing assessment and plan of care needs to be fully integrated into the interdisciplinary plan of care to ensure holistic management and achievement of the patient and family's goals.

Patients are estimated to spend 8–13 % of time engaging in therapeutic activities throughout the day (Thorn, 2000) leaving them in the care of the R.N. for a majority of the time spent on an inpatient neuro-rehabilitation unit. It is the nursing department that is in the unique position to observe patients and communicate important patient information to the physician when changes in vital signs or responsiveness occur, to the neuropsychologist when changes in cognition or behavior occur, to PT/OT when mobility issues are apparent, and to speech therapy when nutrition/swallowing issues are identified. Nursing can also facilitate carryover of goals established in therapies by other disciplines and communicate back to those disciplines to facilitate adjustments in interdisciplinary rehabilitation management. With the patient and family as the central focus, the neuro-rehabilitation team can maximize the potential for the patient with acquired brain injury to achieve the goals of reducing disability and acquiring new skills and strategies that maximize activity (Barnes, 2003).

References

Barker, E. (2002) *Neuroscience Nursing: A Spectrum of Care,* 2nd ed. St. Louis, Missouri: Mosby (Original work published 1994).

Barnes, M. (2003) Principles of neurological rehabilitation. *Journal of Neurology, Neurosurgery, and Psychiatry* 74:3–7.

Brown, S. (2004) The braden scale: A review of the research evidence. *Orthopedic Nursing* 23(1):30–38.

Centers for Disease Control and Prevention. Web-based Injury Statistics Query and Reporting System (WISQARS) [Online]. (2005) National Center for Injury Prevention and Control, Centers for Disease Control and Prevention (producer). Retrieved June 18, 2006, from www.cdc.gov/ncipc/wisqars.

Chandler, B., Brown, S. (1998) Sex and relationship dysfunction in neurological disability. *Journal of Neurology, Neuroscience, and Psychiatry* 65:877–880.

Corrigan, B., Allen, K., Moore, J. et al. (1999) Preventing falls in acute care. In Abraham, I., Bottrell, M., Fulmer, T., & Mezey, M. (eds.): *Geriatric Nursing Protocols for Best Practice.* New York: Springer Publishing Company, Inc., pp. 77–99.

Doble, Rosemary K., Curley, Martha A.Q., Hession-Laband, Eileen. Marino, Barbara L., Shaw, Susan M. (2000). Using the synergy model to link nursing care to diagnosis-related groups. *Critical Care Nurse* 20(3):XX–XX.

Edwards, P.A. (2000) *The Specialty Practice of Rehabilitation Nursing: A Core Curriculum,* 4th ed. Glenview, IL: Association of Rehabilitation Nurses.

Galloway, S., Turner, L. (1999) Pain assessment in older adults who are cognitively impaired. *Journal of Gerontological Nursing* 25(7):34–39.

Hawley, C.A., Taylor, R., Hellawell, D.J., Pentland, B. (1999) Use of the functional assessment measure (FIM+FAM) in head injury rehabilitation: A psychometric analysis. *Journal of Neurology, Neurosurgery, and Psychiatry* 67:749–754.

Langhorne, P., Legg, L. (2003) Evidence behind stroke rehabilitation. *Journal of Neurology, Neurosurgery, and Psychiatry* 74:18–21.

Makelbust, J. Sieggreen, M. (2000) *Pressure Ulcers: Guidelines for Prevention and Management,* 3rd ed. Pennsylvania: Springhouse.

Pasero, C., Reed, B.A., McCaffery, M. (1999) Pain in the elderly. In McCaffery, M. & Pasero, C., (eds.): *Pain: Clinical Manual for Nursing Practice,* 2nd ed. St. Louis, MO: Mosby, pp. 674–710.

St. Marie, B. (2002) *Core Curriculum for Pain Management Nursing.* Philadelphia, Pennsylvania: WB Saunders.

Thorn, S., RGN, BSc, DipN. (2000) Neurological rehabilitation nursing: A review of the research. *Journal of Advanced Nursing* 31(5):1029–1038.

Professional Nursing References

American Nurses Association	www.nursingworld.org
Association of Rehabilitation Nurses	www.rehabnurse.org
American Pain Society	www.ampainsoc.org
American Association of Critical Care Nurses	www.aacn.org
American Association of Neuroscience Nurses	www.aann.org
American Heart Association	www.aha.org
American Society of Pain Management Nurses	www.aspmn.org
Association of Rehabilitation Nurses	www.rehabnurse.org
National Institute of Nursing Research	www.ninr.nih.gov
National League for Nursing	www.nln.org

10
Case Management in the Neuro-Rehabilitation Setting

ROBIN TOVELL-TOUBAL

Introduction

Case management, as defined by the Case Management Society of America, is a collaborative process that assesses, plans, implements, coordinates, monitors, and evaluates options and services to meet an individual's health needs through communication and available resources to promote quality, cost-effective outcomes (Ahrendt, 2006). The case management profession was initiated in North America in the early 1900s within the field of community mental health. Case management providers were public health nurses who coordinated patient services. After World War II, case managers were employed to help coordinate care for servicemen who required multiple medical specialties to optimize their recovery. In the private sector, insurance companies began to employ nurses to manage health insurance claims for complex cases. As the practice of case management grew, other professionals were brought in to provide neuro-rehabilitation case management (Fitzsimmons, 2003).

Neuro-rehabilitation services grew in demand in the late 1970s and early 1980s, as improved medical care led to increased chances that a patient would survive a catastrophic injury. Neuro-rehabilitation programs responded to this demand by offering a variety of services. The most comprehensive programs offered case management services, also known as service coordination.

Case Management in the Neuro-Rehabilitation Setting

The Brain Injury Association of America states that there is an annual occurrence of 1.4 million traumatic brain injuries (TBI) a year (www.biausa.org). Thurman et al. (1999) estimated that 80,000 to 90,000 of those brain injuries result in long-term disability. The National Institutes of Health (1998) issued recommendations regarding rehabilitation practices for persons with TBI, which included case management as a component of the extended care and rehabilitation available to TBI survivors. Because survivors of brain injury often have complex needs, including physical, cognitive, and emotional challenges, many of which can be life-long, there can be many professionals involved in the rehabilitation and recovery process. It is essential to coordinate the care and services provided, and to have a "point person" who can act as a liaison between the various providers, family members and insurance company representatives. The key staff member responsible for this care coordination is the rehabilitation case manager.

The Difference between Rehabilitation Case Management and Insurance Case Management

Rehabilitation case management differs from insurance case management in a number of ways. Insurance case managers are employed either directly by the insurance company or indirectly through a private case management firm that contracts with the insurance company. For survivors with moderate to severe injuries, families are encouraged to request the assignment of an insurance case manager to monitor care and help ensure the survivor gets all the services he/she is entitled to. It has been demonstrated that individuals whose insurance case managers are able to provide financial assistance and independently authorize rehabilitation treatment will fare better than those whose insurance case managers are not able to autonomously authorize treatment (Ashley et al., 1994). While some insurance case managers are able to visit survivors in their home or at the rehabilitation program, most are dependent upon written and verbal reports to monitor progress.

Rehabilitation case managers are employed by the rehabilitation facility and are the liaison with the insurance company case manager. They are able to interact with and observe the survivor on a daily basis and have the important responsibility of providing as comprehensive a clinical description to the insurance case manager as possible, usually by telephone or written correspondence.

Ideally, both insurance and rehabilitation case managers will work together with the survivor and family to monitor medical needs and utilization of benefits. The goal is to maximize the individual's benefits, by structuring services so that the benefits are utilized over the greatest length of time at the lowest frequency of use (Cesta, 2002).

Qualifications of a Neuro-Rehabilitation Case Manager

Rehabilitation case management is traditionally conducted by certified rehabilitation counselors and certified case managers who hold professional degrees in rehabilitation counseling, nursing or social work. Other professionals such as psychologists, speech/language, and occupational therapists can be trained as case managers. The Commission on Rehabilitation Counselor Certification (www.crccertification.com) is responsible for certification of professional counselors who specialize in rehabilitation. Case management certification is also available through the Commission for Case Manager Certification (www. ccmcertification.org). Neuro-rehabilitation case managers can also become certified as brain injury specialists, through the Academy of Certification for Brain Injury Specialists (www.aacbis.net).

Rehabilitation case management requires many different types of skills. From an interpersonal perspective, case managers must be able to work in an empathetic and supportive manner with survivors and families and possess excellent communication skills (Goodall, et al., 1993). In addition to strong interpersonal skills, it is important for a case manager to have clinical experience in brain injury rehabilitation and to be appropriately credentialed. Clinical experience provides the case manager with a deeper understanding of the complex needs of brain injury survivors. It is also critical for case managers to be familiar with various advocacy organizations, social service agencies, entitlement programs and legal rights of individuals with disabilities. These include the national and state chapters of associations for individuals with neurological illnesses/injuries (e.g., Brain Injury Association of America, American and National Stroke Associations); benefits available through the social security administration (e.g., social security disability insurance, supplemental security income); workers' compensation; state programs/funding for crime victims; housing options; programs for students with disabilities; vocational rehabilitation agencies; medicare, medicaid, and medicaid waiver programs; para-transit services; recreational programs; companies specializing in environmental modifications; the Americans with Disabilities Act (ADA); the Family Medical Leave Act; Individuals with Disabilities Education Act (IDEA) and other pertinent legislation (Goodall et al., 1993).

Funding for Case Management Services

Funding for case management can be obtained through private or public funding streams. Private funding examples include insurance companies that hire case managers to perform utilization review activities and service coordination, comprehensive rehabilitation programs that employ case managers to coordinate clients' services, and families who hire private case managers to help them better coordinate the multiple needs of the survivor.

Public funding for case management can be obtained through those states that offer medicaid waiver programs with specific Home- and Community-Based Services (HCBS) for individuals with acquired brain injury. Medicaid HCBS waiver programs are designed to help survivors live in the least restrictive setting. Participants agree to waive their right to placement in a nursing home. Case management services, usually referred to as service coordination, are provided so that the waiver participants can access various services and therapies outside of the nursing home setting in their own communities. In 2001, Medicaid HCBS waiver programs were offered in 20 states. The programs are funded by tax dollars and/or dedicated fines such as those levied on individuals who are charged with driving while intoxicated (Vaughn & King, 2001). A comparison study across various states demonstrated that traumatic brain injury waiver programs saved various states millions of dollars in Medicaid funding that would have previously been spent on nursing home costs (Spearman et al., 2001). As of 2006, there are 48 states and the District of Columbia that offer Medicaid HCBS waiver programs (www.cms.hhs.gov/MedicaidStWaivProgDemoPGI/05_HCBSWaivers-Section1915(c).asp).

AB was 18 years old when he sustained a traumatic brain injury due to a motor vehicle accident. He was just about to begin college at the time of the injury. Post-injury sequelae included hemi-paralysis, a severe speech impairment, and memory problems. His mother was actively involved in his recovery. She maintained him on her employer's health insurance plan as a disabled adult child. The rehabilitation case manager worked with his mother as relentless advocates when the insurance company frequently denied his treatment. When his insurance was exhausted, she enrolled him in the Medicaid HCBS waiver program, so that he was able to receive structured services that improved his functional status. Over the years of treatment he progressed from using a wheelchair to using a cane for long distances. While his speech remains very difficult to understand, he uses an augmentative communication device. The service coordination of the Medicaid waiver program provided enough structure and support that his mother was able to continue working. Her employer's health insurance also provided AB with the opportunity to access more rehabilitation services than the HCBS waiver program was able to offer. Keeping this young man in the community in the least restrictive setting was clearly beneficial to him. It also saved the taxpayers many thousands of dollars over the course of his lifetime. His mother benefited as well, knowing that her son was receiving excellent treatment in a structured day program as well as the love and care of his home environment each night.

Clinical Case Management Responsibilities

Establishing Rapport, Building Trust, and Empowering Clients

Establishing rapport with survivors and their families is a key component of successful case management. To establish rapport, the case manager should use each point of contact as an opportunity to foster a productive working relationship with the survivor and the family, and reinforce active involvement in the rehabilitation process. Family involvement is an important factor in successful outcomes; although Kreutzer et al. (1997) emphasized that there are many reasons why engaging the family as effective rehabilitation partners is complex and not easily achieved. Challenges in productive family involvement can include cultural differences (Simpson et al., 2000) as well as unstable pre-injury family dynamics magnified post-injury. It is important for the case manager to provide sufficient time, reassurance and resources to overwhelmed families to help them establish trust and reduce tension. It is also helpful to make certain that families receive training on constructive coping skills to deal with the frustration, stress and anger they may be experiencing. Referral for individual, group, and/or family counseling as needed is critical.

During the initial meeting, the rehabilitation case manager should gather a medical, psychosocial and employment history as well as goals for discharge. In addition to information gathering, the case manager should be a provider of information and education to the survivor/family at this time. He/she should educate them about the role of the rehabilitation case manager. In most cases, family members have never worked with a case manager and don't know what to expect (Fitzsimmons, 2003). For families of inpatients, it is important to review program policies, visiting hours, and information about passes. It is also important to provide an overview of what the survivor/family can expect (e.g., estimated length of stay, possible next steps such as homecare or outpatient therapy) over the coming weeks/months. It is always helpful to provide written material, such as an orientation booklet, to supplement verbal information. While it is important to recognize that families will vary on the amount of contact, information, and involvement they expect or desire, it is generally useful to arrange follow-up meetings at regular intervals to discuss progress toward goals, barriers and next steps.

Throughout the entire process of establishing rapport and building trust, a case manager needs to demonstrate effective interpersonal skills. Case managers need to be aware of not only what they say, but also how they say it. Survivors and families need to be treated with respect and dignity, especially as they find themselves in the vulnerable position of requiring the aide of others around them. Mozzoni and Bailey (1996) noted that clinicians who received training on how to effectively give feedback helped to improve the functional outcomes of their clients. Case managers must be attuned to the awareness and motivation levels of survivors. Miller et al. (1999) describe how the transtheoretical model of change (Prochaska et al., 1992), which has been used successfully in the field of addictions, can be applied to the rehabilitation setting. The stages include precontemplation, contemplation, determination, action, maintenance, and relapse. Precontemplation is marked by lack of awareness of deficits. Contemplation is the stage in which the individual has some awareness of difficulties but is ambivalent about making change. The determination stage is when an individual expresses awareness and the desire to change. In the action stage the individual is fully engaged in rehabilitation. Maintenance occurs as the individual attempts to maintain the gains that he or she has made during rehabilitation. Relapse occurs when prior behavior patterns return as the main method of functioning. At this point, the case manager's role is to help the individual move through the early stages of precontemplation, contemplation and determination (Van der Broek, 2005).

It is important to empower survivors and families to become self-advocates versus fostering dependence. Case managers can find themselves involved in performing tasks for survivors and families that they can easily do for themselves. The relationship between the case manager, survivor, and family should be an active partnership. By fostering a mutual partnership, the case manager is assisting the survivor in regaining independence (Fitzsimmons, 2003). One practical way to empower survivors and families is to work with them to set goals for various tasks that can be accomplished from one appointment to the next and to encourage collaboration. The level of collaboration varies depending on the extent to which the survivor can manage his or her own goals. Active problem solving can help engage the survivor in the process of setting goals (Van der Broek, 2005).

A family's coping style can influence how they handle their loved one's injury. Kosciulek (1994) identified two coping styles that were predictive of family adaptation: positive reappraisal and tension management. Positive reappraisal refers to the ability to redefine stressful events to make them more manageable, while tension management is characterized by a family's belief that the problems that they are encountering can be successfully overcome.

Development of Goals

With feedback and input from all members of the interdisciplinary team, the case manager can work with the survivor and family to set short- and long-term goals. The process of goal-setting involves arriving at an overlap between the needs and wants of all who are actively involved. Survivors who are actively involved in their own goal-setting have a higher level of goal attainment than those who are not as actively involved in the process (Webb & Glueckauf, 1994). Goal-setting can be achieved through a sequence of steps, including problem identification, goal definition, option appraisal, and solution selection. For instance, if after undergoing a neuropsychological evaluation, a survivor identifies that he has a memory problem, he and the rehabilitation team may develop a goal of needing to use an external memory aid/device. Working with his family and therapist(s), the survivor can then appraise the various devices available and select one (e.g., daily planner) that best meets his needs. The clinical team facilitates the movement through these different steps by discussing pros and cons of change, removing barriers, emphasizing personal choice, and clarifying details on the use of the chosen assistive device (Van der Broek, 2005).

Monitoring Overall Treatment and Progress

Rehabilitation case managers monitor the survivor's progress through a number of different means. During interdisciplinary meetings, the rehabilitation case manager can gather feedback from the various team members on the survivor's progress. If the individual is making satisfactory progress across all disciplines then the rehabilitation case manager can use the review to help plan for next steps. If the survivor is making less than adequate progress, the case manager and team can discuss ways to overcome obstacles/barriers to progress.

In addition to team meetings, case managers need to review discipline specific progress notes, observe survivors in treatment sessions and communicate regularly with the survivor and family, to obtain information that may not be discussed or available during team meetings. By using all of these tools, the rehabilitation case manager will be able to obtain the most comprehensive picture of the survivor, provide a projected discharge date from the current level of rehabilitation program, and offer guidance regarding future rehabilitation, medical and psychosocial needs.

Discharge Planning

Discharge planning from an inpatient rehabilitation program aims to prepare the survivor and family for a positive transition to home and the surrounding community. With input from various members of the interdisciplinary team, the case manager must address the amount of assistance or supervision needed, and help the survivor/family determine how this can be provided upon discharge (e.g., by hiring a 24-hour aide, or moving into an assisted living facility). Equipment needs (e.g., walker, augmentative communication device), and environmental modifications (e.g., grab bars, ramp) must be determined and completed prior to discharge. Recommendations for continued rehabilitation (e.g., home-based or outpatient therapies) must be ascertained and referrals made to ensure continuity of care. While usually the primary goal for the brain injury survivor, discharge to home can be an overwhelming prospect to families. They may feel their loved one has not progressed enough and needs more therapy before being discharged, or that they are unprepared to manage the burdens of time and care that many survivors will need upon returning home. It is critical that the case manager communicates openly and works collaboratively with the survivor and family from the outset, in order to minimize shock, upset and crises that can occur close to discharge.

Discharge planning in an outpatient setting typically involves assisting the brain injury survivor to develop and achieve realistic goals in areas such as homemaking, caretaking, employment, school and social/leisure activities. A primary goal upon discharge from outpatient rehabilitation is for the survivor to be actively engaged in regular, productive activities, which promote physical, cognitive, and emotional health, and are pleasurable and meaningful to the individual. The transition from a structured to an unstructured environment can be very challenging for the survivor. Discharge planning must help to replace the structure of rehabilitation with the structure of meaningful activities and daily functional tasks. At this level of care, it becomes crucial for the case manager to work with other agencies, organizations, or providers, to develop a broad community-based network that can support the survivor and family. Survivors and families also benefit from follow-up phone calls or meetings to ensure that they are making a smooth transition to home/community activities, and are demonstrating carry-over of the rehabilitation gains into these naturalistic settings.

Interdisciplinary Team–Family Meetings

It is important to provide feedback to survivors and families, to increase awareness of limitations and strengths, discuss progress, and ensure collaborative goal setting. The survivor is much more likely to be open to feedback if family members validate the concerns and recommendations of the treating therapists. The interdisciplinary team–family meeting can be an effective forum for providing feedback, as well as gaining valuable insights that can aid in treatment, and establishing a collaborative relationship between the survivor, family and rehabilitation team. It is important that the case manager meet with the team ahead of time to coordinate the information that is to be communicated, and avoid mixed or conflicting messages. A structured agenda can assure increased productivity and efficiency. Case managers need to be sensitive to the possibility that survivors may feel overwhelmed during family/team meetings and should try and create a comfortable, nonthreatening environment (e.g., open circle versus conference table set-up). Abreu et al. (2002) described a survivor-centered approach to interdisciplinary team meetings, emphasizing the value of concise team meetings with active survivor involvement. Team meetings should include written agendas, summary of goals and the survivor should have the option to audiotape or videotape the meeting. Survivors can be encouraged to take notes at the end of meetings to facilitate recall of the main points reviewed. At the conclusion of the meeting, the case manager should schedule a follow up meeting so the survivor and the family understand that they will have on-going opportunities to provide and receive feedback in a formalized manner.

Administrative Case Management Responsibilities

Case managers are responsible for a wide variety of administrative matters that include obtaining authorizations from funding sources, integrating interdisciplinary progress notes and coordinating treatment. The case manager must ensure early on that the survivor and family understand the benefits and limitations of their particular insurance. In addition to discussing private insurance benefits, case managers must understand and be prepared to talk with survivors and families about accessing public insurance programs such as Medicaid and Medicare very early in the rehabilitation stay, when it is often clear that the survivor may need to access those types of public benefit programs after they exhaust their private benefit plans. The case manager must be able to guide and assist families in taking the necessary steps to apply for the appropriate programs.

In most private insurance plans, primary care physicians play a critical role in helping survivors to access medical benefits of all types. As a result, case managers must work with families to obtain primary care physician (PCP) referrals and inform families when referrals and benefits are about to exhaust. They should encourage families to monitor the referrals and to learn how the appeals process works for their insurance company. The more informed the family, the better advocates they can be.

Insurance Authorizations/Advocacy

One of the most critical administrative tasks for the case manager is to obtain treatment authorization from insurers. It is important for the rehabilitation case manager to learn about policy restrictions and limitations. Whenever possible, the survivor or family can be asked to provide a copy of the insurance policy benefits booklet for the case manager to review. If the policy book cannot be located, then the family and rehabilitation case manager can call the insurance company jointly to verify the level of benefits available. Survivors who are still employed may be able to use the human resources division of their company to locate information about their insurance benefits. Another important factor to consider when obtaining information about a survivor's policy is whether it is "contractual" or "as medically needed." A policy that has contractual limits (e.g., 30 days maximum of acute rehabilitation) is much more limited than one based on medical necessity.

Each insurance company has its own set of requirements and paperwork that must be submitted in order to obtain authorizations. In general, most insurance companies want progress reports to support each request for authorization. The case manager can generate these progress reports by incorporating key information from each member of the interdisciplinary team, or the case manager can simply send each discipline's individual progress report. In either case, progress reports must reflect the details of progress and continued goals across all disciplines, in order to justify additional treatment. Documentation must indicate the medical necessity of continued treatment, and the expectation for significant functional improvement over a reasonable period of time, as most insurance companies do not provide coverage for "maintenance" therapy. If a survivor has not made significant gains during a given reporting period, it is important to provide the reason for the lack of progress, and plans to overcome the barrier(s). If the insurance company denies an authorization for treatment that the interdisciplinary team feels is justified, family members have the option of filing an appeal with the insurance company. This type of appeal is called an internal appeal. If an internal appeal is denied, the family can then file an external appeal (e.g., with the state insurance department). Additionally, families may decide to utilize attorneys, advocacy organizations or local/state representatives to support them in advocating for the survivor to receive continued services.

Coordination with Other Care Providers

Coordinating treatment between the neuro-rehabilitation team and other care providers (e.g., primary care physicians [PCP]) is another responsibility of the rehabilitation case manager. The PCP can be very supportive of the need for rehabilitation and can help advocate for continued care when indicated. Many health maintenance organization (HMO) plans require that the PCP be a "gate-keeper" and write referrals for treatment. This means that the case manager will need to routinely call the PCP's office to obtain referrals if the family member cannot obtain the referrals for treatment. PCPs also have an active role in referring survivors to other specialty physicians when the need arises. Once consent to release information is obtained, case managers can help survivors by calling the new specialty physician in advance of the appointment to describe the relevant issues and forward appropriate medical information. The case manager needs to follow up with the survivor, family and specialty physician to learn the outcome of the visit. The

PCP will often be the one provider who continues to follow the survivor after rehabilitation ends. Keeping the PCP informed of rehabilitation progress and goals, as well as post-discharge recommendations, can help ensure good continuity of care.

Coordination with Attorneys

Rehabilitation case managers must often provide information to attorneys, with the survivor's consent/request. In the field of brain injury rehabilitation there can be multiple attorneys working with one survivor. The most common types of attorneys for this population are personal injury and workers' compensation attorneys. Some survivors may also retain attorneys for social security or for disability insurance matters. In any case, attorneys may call upon the rehabilitation case manager to solicit verbal feedback regarding a survivor's progress, and obtain updated progress/evaluation reports, especially if a court appearance is approaching. Attorneys may ask rehabilitation case managers to project a list of the survivor's current and future needs so as to put a dollar cost on the amount of care that will be needed during the individual's lifetime. While rehabilitation case managers are not expected to be life care planners, it is important to be able to provide estimates of current and future needs.

Coordination with Schools, Vocational, and Social Service Agencies

As discharge approaches, there is often a need to refer survivors to other agencies for supportive services and programs. Generally, each of these services or programs requires an application or exchange of information regarding the survivor's abilities or difficulties. To complete most referrals, rehabilitation case managers must fill out paperwork, submit progress reports, schedule evaluations, and/or medical appointments that will document the survivor's medical condition and level of functioning.

For school-age survivors and those entering or returning to college, there are various considerations that must be addressed. Each student's unique needs must be taken into consideration. Depending on how severe the brain injury, some students may benefit from classification as special education students. This classification process entitles the student to a variety of services and accommodations that are mandated by federal law and documented in an individualized education plan (IEP). Some of these accommodations are as follows: longer time for tests and projects, assigned note-takers, permission to use a tape recorder during lectures, private tutoring, and alternate forms of testing. Rehabilitation case managers can help guide students and their families through the classification process, and work closely with school personnel to provide information regarding the student's cognitive, emotional, and physical strengths and limitations.

For adults who need vocational services, each state runs its own vocational services office. This office helps individuals with disabilities by sponsoring vocational evaluations, training and placement, and sometimes funding academic-related needs such as books, personal computers, and tape recorders. When referring brain injury survivors for vocational services, the rehabilitation case manager must work with the survivor and vocational counselor to ensure adequate follow-through. The rehabilitation facility will be asked to supply a copy of the records for each survivor. The case manager can assist the survivor in making sure that they are ready for the initial interview and that they understand the various steps in the process. The case manager should monitor the intake and evaluation process for problems. Survivors can get confused during the evaluation process, as it usually occurs over a several-week period. They may require much support and encouragement to persevere and complete the evaluation.

For survivors who are near retirement age or who are not going to be returning to work, it is critical for the case manager to help them establish a daily structure so they can maintain their functional skills and prevent regression. This can include referrals to social service agencies that offer leisure/recreational programs. Unfortunately, actual options can be limited due to barriers such as transportation, cost, or level of independence required. Nevertheless, case managers should acquaint themselves with various programs in the community. Alternative options such as adult education classes at local colleges or volunteer work may be more suitable for some survivors. Provision of information about local support groups for survivors and caregivers is essential.

Conclusion

Case management in the neuro-rehabilitation setting can be challenging and demanding. To be an effective rehabilitation case manager, a clinician must have excellent clinical, administrative and interpersonal skills. Knowledge of brain-injury-specific community resources, laws, and public benefit programs is vital. Rehabilitation case managers assist the survivor and family in navigating the different aspects of the neuro-rehabilitation program and help integrate the various components into a treatment plan that is well coordinated, collaborative and survivor-centered.

References and Resources

Abreu, B.C., Zhang, l., Seale, G., Primeau, L., Jones, J.S. (2002) Interdisciplinary meetings: Investigating the collaboration between persons with brain injury and treatment teams. *Brain Injury* 16(8):691–704.

Ahrendt, L. (2006) What is a case manager? http://birf.info/home/library/records/reccase_whatcase.html)

American Academy for the Certification of Brain Injury Specialists, www.aacbis.net.

Ashley, M.J., Lehr, R.P., Krych, D.K., Persel, C.S., Fledman, B. (1994) Postacute rehabilitation outcome: Relationship to case-management techniques and strategy. *Journal of Insurance Medicine* 26(3):348–354.

Brain Injury Association of America, www.biausa.org, 8201 Greensboro Drive, Suite 611, McLean VA 22102, Tel. 703-761-0750

Centers for Medicare and Medicaid Services. www.cms.hhs.gov/MedicaidStWaivProg DemoPGI/05_HCBSWaivers-Section1915(c).asp

Cesta, T.G. (2002) Close Up and Personal. *Case Management* 8(2):46.

Commission for Case Management Certification, www.ccmcertification.org

Commission on Rehabilitation Counselor Certification, http://www.crccertification.com/

Fitzsimmons, R.D. (2003) Brain injury case management: The potential and limitations of late stage intervention-a pilot study. *Brain Injury* 17(11):947–971.

Goodall, P., Dedrick, D., Zasler, N.D., Kreutzer, J.S. (1993, Sept–Oct) Survey of case manager training needs in traumatic brain injury. *Brain Injury* 7(5):455–461.

Kosciulek, J.F. (1994) Relationship of family coping with head injury to family adaptation. *Rehabilitation Psychology* 39:215–230.

Kreutzer, J.S., Sander, A.M., Fernendez, C.C. (1997) Misperceptions, mishaps, and pitfalls in working with families after traumatic brain injury. *Journal of Head Trauma Rehabilitation* 12(6):63–73.

Miller, W.R., Zweben, A., DiClemente, C.C., Rychtarik, R.G. (1999) *Motivational Enhancement Therapy Manual*, National Institute on Alcohol Abuse and Alcoholism, US Department of Health and Human Services.

Mozzoni, M.P., Bailey, J.S. (1996, 2) Improving training methods in brain injury rehabilitation, *Journal of Head Trauma Rehabilitation* 11(1):1–17.

National Institutes of Health (1998, October 26–28). Rehabilitation of persons with traumatic brain injury. *National Institutes of Health Consensus Statement* 16(1):1–41.

Prochaska J.O., DiClemente, C.C. Norcross, J.C. (1992) In search of how people change: Applications to addictive behaviors. *American Psychologist* 47(9):1102–1114.

Simpson, G., Mohr, R., Redman, A. (2000) Cultural variations in the understanding of traumatic brain injury and brain injury rehabilitation. *Brain Injury* 14(2):125–140.

Spearman, R.C., Stamm, B.H., Rosen, B.H., Kaylala, D.E., Zillinger, M., Breese, P., Wargo, L.M. (2001) The use of Medicaid waivers and their impact on services. *Journal of Head Trauma Rehabilitation* 16(1):47–60.

Thurman, O.J., Alverson, C., Dunn, K.A., Guerrero, J., Sncizek, J.E. (1999) Traumatic brain injury in the United States: A public health perspective. *Journal of Head Trauma Rehabilitation* 14(6):602–615.

Van der Broek, M.D. (2005) Why does neuro-rehabilitation fail? *Journal of Head Trauma Rehabilitation* 20(5):464–473.

Vaughn, S.L., King, A. (2001) A survey of state programs to finance rehabilitation and community services for individuals with brain injury. *Journal of Head trauma Rehabilitation* 16(1):20–33.

Webb, P.M., Glueckauf, R.L. (1994) The effects of direct involvement in goal setting on rehabilitation outcome for persons with traumatic brain injuries. *Rehabilitation Psychology* 39(3):185.

11
Balance and Vestibular Rehabilitation in the Patient with Acquired Brain Injury

James Megna

Introduction

Acquired and degenerative neurologic disorders are frequently associated with disequilibrium, dizziness, and vertigo. Conditions such as traumatic brain injury (TBI) and cerebrovascular accident (CVA) can present with varying degrees of motor, sensory, and central processing impairments that can dramatically impact daily life activities and increase the risk of injury due to falls. A majority of individuals who sustain brain injury complain of dizziness for up to 5 years following injury (Sataloff et al., 1993). Stroke survivors often have problems with balance, with a reported 40% experiencing a serious fall within the first year after the CVA (Health on the Net Foundation, 2003).

Falls and the fear of falling are associated with considerable mortality, morbidity, reduced functioning, and premature nursing home admission. A study of persons who fell at home reported a greater deterioration in mobility and independence in daily living than in age- and gender-matched controls (Wild et al., 1981). In addition to the impact falls can have on health and well-being, treating the resulting complications contribute to higher health care costs. Recurrent falls account for 40% of admissions to long-term care institutions (Centers for Disease Control and Prevention, 2003). Five percent of older people who fall require hospitalization and related injuries account for 6% of medical expenditures for this age group (Centers for Disease Control and Prevention, 2003). Medicare costs for hip fractures are estimated to be over 3 billion dollars per year (Centers for Disease Control and Prevention, 2003).

Each member of the brain injury rehabilitation team needs to be equipped to recognize persons who may be experiencing problems with the balance system. Physical therapists must be aware of the multifactorial nature of balance disorders and must be trained to uncover key underlying impairments that contribute to the symptoms of imbalance and dizziness. Other team members must recognize the value of their assessments in determining a patient's risk for disequilibrium and falls. Occupational therapists can provide an assessment of visual perceptual function and the potential contribution to the patient's imbalance. Similarly, the neuropsychologist can discuss observed cognitive deficits and coordinate team strategies to help mitigate them. Additionally, the attending physician can review current medications and manage them accordingly to minimize side effects, including dizziness. Once a balance deficit is identified, it is important for the team to refer the patient to the appropriate caregiver. Specialty physicians involved in diagnosing the origin of a balance disorder include neurologists, neurotologists (specialists in neurologic and inner ear disorders), and otolaryngologists (ear, nose, and throat specialists). Allied health personnel, such as audiologists and nurse practitioners, may also be involved in the diagnosis and treatment of disequilibrium. Finally, the nature of balance and vestibular rehabilitation requires that the therapist providing the intervention and management be specially trained and certified in vestibular rehabilitation. Rehabilitation of balance and vestibular problems involve technical skills that are not typically fully developed in general therapy education programs. This chapter seeks to provide the reader with an overview of balance and vestibular rehabilitation so that patients with symptoms of disequilibrium, dizziness, and vertigo are readily identified and well cared for.

Fall Risk Factors

Falls generally result from an interaction of multiple and diverse risk factors, many of which can be corrected. Risk factors for falls can be classified as intrinsic, extrinsic, and environmental in nature (American Geriatrics Society et al., 2001). **Intrinsic risk factors** include cognitive impairment, muscle weakness, poor visual acuity, presence of chronic illness, and balance disturbance. **Extrinsic factors** include the effects of medications on a person, such as the phenomenon of polypharmacy (multiple medications negatively interacting with one another). Many intrinsic (cognitive, visual, and balance problems) and extrinsic (multiple medications) factors are present after acquired brain injury. **Environmental risk factors** include environmental risks, such as lighting, tripping hazards, and lack of safety equipment in the home. As the number of risk factors increases, the risk for falls increases dramatically. This is known as **risk factor synergism**. Tinetti et al., (1988) found that older persons with less than two risk factors had a 27% chance of falling, where the risk for fall increased to 78% in persons with four or more factors. Unfortunately, these risks frequently become evident only after a fall-related injury.

Basics of Balance

Before specific rehabilitation techniques can be explored, a basic understanding of the balance system is necessary. Nashner (1989) defines the role of the balance system as maintaining the center of gravity over the base of support in a given sensory environment. The center of gravity (COG) is an imaginary point where all the forces acting on the body equals zero and is anatomically located in the pelvis anterior to the sacrum. A person is most stable when the COG is positioned midline within the base of support (BOS). The BOS in standing is the area contained within

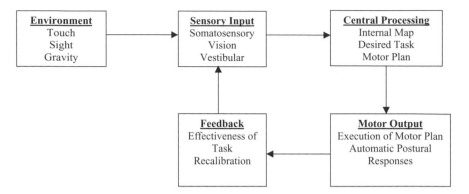

FIGURE 11.1. Example of an open system: Maintenance of equilibrium.

the perimeter of contact between the surface and the two feet. When the support area is small or irregular, the BOS is reduced. Control of the COG is maintained by the interaction of the components of the balance system. Human balance can be described as an open system with sensory inputs, central processing, motor outputs and a feedback mechanism (see Fig. 11.1).

Sensory Inputs for Balance

Nashner (1989) describes three sensory inputs that provide the balance system with information about the status of the COG and BOS. These senses are somatosensory (sense of touch, position and vibration), vision, and vestibular (senses pull of gravity and head movement). Each one of these senses provides unique information about the position of the COG and when this information is combined, it provides a complete "map" of the COG position over the BOS. Under normal surface conditions, somatosensory information is the dominant input. This means that an individual relies heavily on information related to the type of surface a person is standing on. If the surface conditions become unreliable (i.e., uneven or movable), the role of vision increases to compensate for the inaccurate somatosensory input. Vestibular input plays a minor role when useful somatosensory and visual inputs are available. However, the vestibular information becomes critical when somatosensory and visual information are unavailable or misleading. Additionally, the vestibular system is sensitive to head rotation and tilt and provides coordination of eye and head movements, maintaining accurate visual input when the head is moving rapidly (Shumway-Cook & Horak, 1990).

Central Processing of Balance Information

Central processing of balance information is located at many levels in the brain, including the brain stem, subcortical, and cortical regions (Nashner, 1989). Central processing is the link between sensory inputs and motor outputs. In general, central processing involves reception of information from the somatosensory, vestibular, and visual inputs (predominantly at the brain stem level); creation of an internal map of the current position of the COG (subcortical and cortical); comparing the current map to a desired task (subcortical and cortical); and creating a motor plan to execute the task while maintaining postural stability (subcortical, including basal ganglia). Additionally, the central mechanism (predominantly the cerebellum) provides feedback information related to the effectiveness of the balance task and provides recalibration of the system for future performance. The site of neurologic lesion determines the clinical presentation of the balance disorder. For example, lesions to the basal ganglia result in deficits in timing and sequencing (motor output), whereas cerebellar injuries present with the inability to regulate balance reactions (Fredericks & Saladin, 1996).

Motor Output

Motor responses for postural corrections need to be triggered rapidly to prevent a fall. The basic motor output for postural control is called an **automatic postural response (APR)**. An APR behaves in ways that are similar to short arc reflexes: there is a set latency, there is a unique stereotyped response, and they are triggered by external stimuli (Nashner, 1989). However, unlike reflexes, there is evidence to suggest that the amplitude (intensity) of APR's can be adapted with practice (Horak et al., 1986). There are two main APRs used for postural control: the ankle strategy and the hip strategy (Horak & Nashner, 1986). The **ankle strategy** is the predominant strategy in most day-to-day activities, and adequate ankle strength and range of motion is required for execution. Environmental conditions that favor the ankle strategy include firm support surfaces that are longer than the feet. The **hip strategy** acts as an "emergency backup" when the ankle strategy fails and a person has to make rapid COG adjustments to prevent a fall. Narrow or unstable surfaces favor the use of the hip strategy.

Diagnosis of Balance Disorders

The differential diagnosis for dizziness and disequilibrium can be elusive. Many times, standard "first line" tests such as blood tests, radiograms, CT scans, and MRIs fail to reveal underlying pathology. Common tests for balance disorders are videonystagmography (VNG) and computerized dynamic posturography (CDP). A VNG study is a test battery that examines the function of the inner ear (labyrinth) (Honrubia, 2000). Component tests stimulate the vestibulo-ocular reflex and the resulting eye movements are recorded and studied (see Table 11.1). Abnormal eye movements during testing can reveal underlying pathology in the vestibular system. In general, the VNG can determine hypofunction (weakness) in one or both ears, the side of the hypofunction, and can help determine if the problem is in the peripheral apparatus or within the central nervous system. Additionally, VNGs

TABLE 11.1. Common components of the videonystagmography (VNG) test battery

Fixation (ability to suppress spontaneous nystagmus)
Fixation inhibited (in darkness)
Gaze-holding nystagmus
Rapid and slow positional changes
Dix–Hallpike Maneuver
Saccades
Smooth pursuit
Optokinetic nystagmus
Bithermal caloric test

can detect an inner ear condition known as benign paroxysmal positional vertigo (BPPV). This problem can become apparent during positional testing that occurs during the VNG battery.

While the VNG can help localize *pathology* within the vestibular system, the CDP is able to reveal *impairments* related to postural control (Nashner, 1989). During a CDP study, the patient stands on a force plate that analyzes the amount of postural sway that occurs during manipulations of the patient's environment. Force-plate analysis of postural sway has demonstrated good test re-test reliability in patients with TBI (Lehmann et al., 1990). There are six testing conditions that determine how effectively the patient is utilizing each of the three input senses to maintain balance (see Table 11.2). Further analysis includes a determination of the predominant automatic postural strategy (ankle versus hip) and the motor response latency. The results of the CDP help to identify specific impairments within the feedback loop of the balance system, determine environmental conditions that may place the individual at risk for falling, and formulate an effective rehabilitation treatment plan.

Common Balance System Impairments

Impairments are abnormalities found in physiologic systems (i.e., the neuromuscular system) (American Physical Therapy Association, 2001) and typically follow

TABLE 11.2. Six sensory conditions included in computerized dynamic posturography

Condition 1	Measure of postural sway with eyes open while standing on firm surface
Condition 2	Measure of postural sway with eyes closed while standing on firm surface
Condition 3	Measure of postural sway with eyes open while standing on firm surface and movable visual environment
Condition 4	Measure of postural sway with eyes open while standing on movable surface
Condition 5	Measure of postural sway with eyes closed while standing on movable surface
Condition 6	Measure of postural sway with eyes open while standing on movable surface with moveable visual environment

pathology, such as an acquired brain injury. The following is a discussion of common impairments that are found in balance disorders.

Positional Vertigo and Dizziness

Benign paroxysmal positional vertigo (BPPV) is a condition of the inner ear. In BPPV, specific positions of the head can result in brief, severe bouts of vertigo. Displaced debris (calcium carbonate crystals called otoconia) in the semicircular canals of the vestibular labyrinth is believed to be the causative factor (Herdman, 1997). Bending, rolling over in bed, and tilting the head back in the shower can provoke the symptoms. People with BPPV may experience loss of balance during episodes of vertigo, and persons with coexisting TBI can experience disequilibrium even when spinning sensations are absent (Black & Nashner, 1984). BPPV can be caused by head trauma, infections of the inner ear, or can occur spontaneously. Symptoms can be alleviated with maneuvers designed to clear debris from the involved canal

An 83-year-old female fell down a flight of stairs and sustained a subdural hematoma. She was hospitalized for 3 weeks, including 5 days in ICU, and was subsequently transferred to the inpatient brain injury rehabilitation unit (BIU). During functional transfers out of bed, the occupational therapist noted that the patient experienced severe vertigo with loss of balance when she went from supine to sitting on the bedside. The attending physician was notified. Upon examination, the doctor noted bruising of the right mastoid process (battle sign) and ordered a CT of the skull. The CT revealed a transverse fracture of the temporal bone that was previously undetected. The doctor diagnoses the patient with BPPV secondary to trauma and the patient was referred to the balance and vestibular physical therapist. The therapist performed positional testing and observed nystagmus that dissipated after 10 seconds while the patient was in the right head hanging (Dix Hallpike) position. The therapist observed a right, upbeating, torsional nystagmus, concluded that there was free-floating debris within the right posterior semicircular canal and performed canal repositioning maneuvers. After several attempts, the Dix–Hallpike was negative and the patient's symptoms resolved.

Abnormal Dynamic Visual Acuity and Gaze Stability

One of the functions of the vestibular system is to coordinate eye and head movements when the head is moving rapidly (Shumway-Cook & Horak, 1990). Normally, the vestibulo-ocular reflex (VOR) is triggered when the head rotates. This enables the eyes to remain fixed in space (gaze stability) and maintain visual acuity during functional tasks (dynamic visual acuity). When the vestibular system is damaged, the VOR becomes impaired. As a result, the ability to stabilize the eyes during head movements is lost. Many patients with TBI will suffer from this type of eye-head dyscoordination (Pearson & Barber, 1973). Symptoms of impaired VOR function include complaints of dizziness, loss of balance, difficulty reading, and occasionally the sensation that the surrounding environment is moving (oscillopsia) (Shumway-Cook, 2000).

Abnormal Sensory Organization

Accurate input from the sensory systems for balance is critical in providing information about the environment and maintaining equilibrium during functional tasks (Shumway-Cook, 2000). Many neurological and vestibular disorders can result in abnormal processing and integration of somatosensory, visual, and vestibular inputs. Individuals experiencing abnormal sensory organization may have increased risk for falling in specific environmental circumstances. For example, a patient who may have sustained sensory loss due to a CVA may develop a decrease in the use of somatosensory inputs, forcing him or her to rely more heavily on visual cues. If this person were to try to walk around in his or her home in the dark, he or she would have a greater chance of falling. Both visual and somatosensory cues would be significantly reduced, leaving vestibular as the lone input into the system.

A 38-year-old female presented to the balance and vestibular clinic with complaints of nonspecific dizziness and loss of balance. She related a history of a mild CVA during labor and delivery that had occurred about 8 months prior. Upon examination she had no significant motor or range of motion deficits; however, she had difficulty maintaining balance with her eyes closed. A computerized dynamic posturography (CDP) was ordered to determine her ability to effectively organize her sensory inputs for balance. The CDP revealed decreased use of the hip response as well abnormal use of vestibular inputs with a preference for visual information (unusually high reliance on vision with significant instability when vision is absent). Additionally, she demonstrated abnormal dynamic visual acuity. She was placed on a therapy program that included tall kneel and balance beam exercises to facilitate hip strategies, sensory re-weigthing, such as standing on foam with head turns, keeping eyes open, and repeating with eyes closed to enhance vestibular inputs, and gaze stabilization exercises to improve eye and head coordination. She received therapy 2 times per week for 6 weeks and performed similar exercises at home on a daily basis. After 6 weeks, her hip responses and use of vestibular input were normal and dynamic visual acuity improved; however, a slight visual preference remained with occasional subjective symptoms.

Altered COG Position

Many impairments of the balance system can lead to faulty mapping of the COG. When the COG is offset from the midline position, it effectively decreases a person's **limits of stability**. Limits of stability (LOS) can be conceptualized as an imaginary cone that surrounds each person (Nashner, 1989). If the person moves within the confines of the cone, they can do so with confidence and stability. As they approach the limits of the cone, stability is reduced and the probability of loss of balance increases. When the COG deviates from its resting midline position, the limits of stability are decreased. Clinicians may observe an abnormally displaced COG position in patients following CVA and TBI with hemiplegia.

Abnormal Automatic Postural Responses

Impaired automatic postural responses (ankle and hip strategy) can result in ineffective maintenance of postural control. This can be caused by lower extremity weakness, restricted range of motion, delayed triggering of the response (Studenski et al., 1991), and abnormal sensory input into the system (Horak et al., 1990). A study by Horak et al. (1990) examined the role of somatosensory and vestibular information in the coordination of APRs. Results showed that neither vestibular nor somatosensory loss resulted in delayed or disorganized postural responses. However, both types of sensory deficits altered the type of postural response selected under a given set of conditions. Somatosensory loss resulted in an increased hip strategy, whereas vestibular loss resulted in normal ankle strategy, but lack of hip strategy. Alterations in APR selection can contribute to instability under certain environmental conditions and can increase risk for falls.

Lower Extremity Weakness and Restricted Range of Motion

Lower extremity weakness and restricted joint range of motion is frequently identified in the immobile neurologic patient. Frail, elderly patients with chronic neurologic dysfunction are particularly vulnerable (Espinoza & Walston, 2005). However, fear and anxiety related to disequilibrium may limit daily activity levels. Over time, this cycle of imbalance and immobility can cause weakness of key muscle groups, making further contributions to fall risk. It is important for clinicians to identify and address weakness and joint restrictions. It is equally important to perform a comprehensive evaluation that assesses *all* aspects of the balance system.

Evaluation of the Patient with Dizziness and Disequilibrium

History and Subjective Complaints

The examination of the patient with a balance disorder begins with the history. Appropriate questioning of the patient can effectively direct the focus of the examination and identification of underlying impairments. Questions related to dizziness need to be carefully constructed to clarify the differences among symptoms of vertigo, light-headedness, and disequilibrium. Reports of decreased activity level (long hours of sitting), "furniture surfing" (holding on to furniture when walking through the home), infrequent excursions into the community, and anxiety or depression may reveal that the person is experiencing disequilibrium. In addition to personal interviews, knowledge of underlying medical conditions can reveal the presence of a balance disorder. The presence of a neurologic condition increases the likelihood of impaired balance and mobility. Additionally, co-morbid conditions of the vestibular system (inner ear) such as labyrinthitis, Meniere's disease, acoustic neuroma, and ototoxicity can cause dizziness and falls. Subjective complaints can be quantified by using self-reporting questionnaires such as the Dizziness Handicap Inventory (DHI) and the Activity specific Balance Confidence (ABC) scale (Clendaniel, 2000). The results of the interview with the patient reveal the possible underlying impairments and become the foundation to an impairment-targeted approach to the evaluation and treatment of balance and vestibular disorders.

TABLE 11.3. Types of BPPV

Category	Behavior of nystagmus	Underlying problem
Canalithiasis	Delayed onset when placed in Dix–Hallpike position; becomes intense, then tapers off; dissipates within 60 seconds	Free-floating debris within the semicircular canals
Cupulolithiasis	Nystagmus begins once Dix-Hallpike position is assumed; persists for as long as head is in dependent position	Debris trapped in the cupula membrane of the semicircular canal

Positional Testing

Positional testing is indicated when vertigo or motion sensitivity is noted in the history. The Dix–Hallpike maneuver is the most common test used to detect BPPV (see Table 11.3) (Herdman, 1997). During the test, the clinician observes the eyes to detect stereotypical nystagmus. The presence of nystagmus confirms positional vertigo. The clinician notes the characteristics of the eye movements to help determine the type of BPPV, the involved side and the implicated semicircular canal. Many times BPPV is detected unintentionally and symptoms are provoked when a patient is put in the supine position for unrelated testing.

Oculomotor Exam

Several testing procedures are used to observe oculomotor function (Whitney & Herdman, 2000). These tests help determine the presence of vestibular hypofunction, the side of impairment and to help rule out peripheral versus central nervous system involvement. Oculomotor tests include the head thrust test, head shake test, and the observation of spontaneous and gaze evoked nystagmus (see Table 11.4). The head thrust test is used as a bedside exam to assist in detecting the side of the impairment. The gaze evoked and head shake test, performed under infrared video, help to confirm the findings of the head thrust test. The presence of spontaneous nystagmus may indicate an acute or neurologic condition, and may cause the clinician to seek a consultation with a physician.

Testing for Impairments of Postural Stability

There are many standardized measures for balance testing. When selecting tests to be included in the initial examination, the clinician needs to understand that his/her evaluation must be capable of detecting impairments in each component of the balance system. Traditional tests include the modified clinical test for sensory integration of balance (CTSIB) and Romberg (sensory component), and the timed up and functional reach tests (motor component) (Shumway-Cook, 2000). These procedures use objective metrics to quantify results; however, they lack the

TABLE 11.4. Components of the oculomotor exam

Test	Description	Interpretation
Spontaneous nystagmus	Patient is observed while looking straight ahead, with and without visual fixation	If vestibular nystagmus is present, suspect involved side opposite the beat of the nystagmus (i.e., right beating nystagmus implicates left side involvement); may be central in nature if unable to suppress
Gaze holding	Patient sustains eye position left, right, up, and down and observed for nystagmus in each plane	If vestibular nystagmus is present, suspect involved side opposite the beat of the nystagmus; may be central in nature if direction changing
Head shake	Patient's head is rapidly shaken left and right with head pitched 30 degrees; observed for nystagmus immediately after head is stopped	If vestibular nystagmus is present, suspect involved side opposite the beat of the nystagmus
Head thrust	Patient maintains eyes fixed on examiner's nose as head is rapidly thrust to each side	Inability to maintain eye fixation on nose suggests weakness to the side of the thrust

detail needed to illuminate underlying impairments fully. Advances in force plate technology have enabled rehabilitation specialists to obtain data specific to organization of somatosensory, vestibular, and visual inputs, predominance of ankle versus hip strategy, mapping of the COG and determination of limits of stability (Nashner, 1989). Data generated from testing protocols is automatically compared to age- and gender-matched normative data, bringing immediate attention to underlying problems. The ability to identify specific balance impairments allows the therapist to create an individualized treatment plan as well as make pre- and post therapy comparisons to monitor progress.

Lower Quarter Screen

Weakness and joint restriction of the lower extremities can make significant contributions to postural imbalance (Studenski et al., 1991). Screening of lower extremity strength and flexibility is an essential component of the overall balance evaluation. Abnormal findings in the lower quarter screen should be addressed in the overall balance treatment plan.

Functional Balance Tests

Many function-based balance scales have been developed and tested for their ability to predict the probability of falls in the community dwelling elderly. During these standardized tests, the patient is asked to perform specific tasks as the clinician scores his or her performance on a descriptive ordinal scale. Once all of the components of the test are completed, the scores for each task are summed to tally a final overall score. Many scales have fall-risk threshold scores that indicate that the risk for falling in the community is increased. If the patient's overall score falls below the threshold, he or she is identified as being at an increased fall-risk level. These tests can be repeated periodically to monitor changes during the therapy program and can also be used over the long term to assess changes in fall risk level. Examples of commonly used function-based tests are the Berg Balance Scale (Berg et al., 1995) and the Dynamic Gait Index (Wrisley et al., 2003).

Treatment of Balance and Vestibular Impairments

Once the evaluation process is complete, the clinician must formulate his or her assessment and develop a treatment plan. The assessment should include a listing of the identified impairments. Once the underlying impairments are clearly identified and documented, each impairment can be specifically targeted in the treatment plan.

Canal Repositioning and Liberatory Maneuvers

Herdman (1997) describes canal repositioning and liberatory maneuvers used to eliminate displaced otoconia in the semicircular canals. Canal repositioning is used to treat canalithiasis, a type of BPPV that involves free-floating debris in the involved semicircular canal. There are several repositioning techniques that are specific to the involved canal. During the repositioning, the head is moved through a series of positions to maneuver the otoconia crystals through the canal toward the common crus of the labyrinth. Once the otoconia reach this point, they drop out of the canal into the otolithic sacks, and the symptoms are relieved. Liberatory maneuvers are a more aggressive form of treatment and are utilized when it is believed that the debris is trapped on the cupula membrane of the semicircular canal (cupulolithiasis). Liberatory maneuvers are designed to dislodge the otoconia from the membrane and involve brisk and abrupt movements of the head. Once dislodged, the otoconia are maneuvered out of the canal using a repositioning technique. In many cases, the symptoms of BPPV can be alleviated in one or two treatment sessions.

Gaze Stabilization Exercises (Vestibular Adaptation)

Gaze stabilization exercises, also known as vestibular adaptation, are used to help recalibrate the vestibulo-ocular reflex (VOR) (Herdman, 1997). As stated earlier, the VOR is responsible for coordinating eye and head movements so that dynamic visual acuity is maintained. When the VOR is impaired, visual images are misaligned relative to the fovea, a phenomenon known as retinal slip (Whitney & Herdman, 2000). This triggers an error signal to the brain resulting in an adaptive recalibration of the VOR. Gaze stabilization exercises provide repeated stimulation of this system to realign the visual image on the fovea, thereby improving dynamic visual acuity. The exercise involves having the patient focus on a fixed visual target as they rotate the head in horizontal and vertical planes of movement. This is repeated at increasing speeds and with smaller targets over time. The patient is instructed to perform these exercises repeatedly, up to 6 times per day.

Vestibular Habituation and Substitution

Simply stated, habituation is a decreased response to a repeated stimulus. In the context of vestibular rehabilitation, patients are exposed to head positions that provoke their symptoms (Whitney & Herdman, 2000). When this is repeated frequently, the symptoms are dampened by the repair structures within the central nervous system. Patients are given exercises that reproduce the symptoms and are instructed to repeat the exercises daily for a finite period of time. The patient is monitored periodically to evaluate the effectiveness of the prescribed program. As habituation exercises tend to provoke symptoms of dizziness initially, the patient should be encouraged to work through these symptoms for a defined period of time, usually 7 to 14 days. When permanent impairment is suspected, vestibular substitution exercises are prescribed. These are exercises that enlist saccadic and smooth pursuit eye movements to help compensate for VOR loss.

Adaptation of Automatic Postural Responses and Motor Learning

Exercises emphasizing adaptation of APRs should be considered when developing the treatment plan. As stated earlier, APRs function to maintain the COG over the base of support. Ankle and hip strategies are the foundational APRs used for balance in humans. Theoretically, the use of each APR can be emphasized by manipulating the environment in which the balance task is performed. For example, facilitation of the ankle strategy is achieved by performing a task on a firm surface at slow speeds, such as forward reaching while standing on a tile floor. Alternatively, hip strategies are best elicited when a task is performed on an unstable surface or at more rapid speeds, such as balancing on a balance beam or rocker board. It is important for the therapist to know which response is desired and to alter the tasks accordingly. This approach is based on two principles: the amplitude of an APR can be adapted (scaled) when the response is anticipated; and there is a gradual habituation of the APR when a stimulus is presented repeatedly (Diener et al., 1988). Incorporation of motor learning principles can assist in the modulation of APRs. Three basic motor learning principles applied to balance retraining are the provision of feedback, knowledge of results, and ultimately, withdrawal of feedback (Fredericks & Saladin, 1996). As the patient performs a task, **feedback** is needed to ensure that the task is performed correctly and that the objective of the task is achieved. Once the task is completed the patient must receive **knowledge of results** related to the performance of the task. When the patient demonstrates an understanding of previous performance, a chance to repeat the performance with appropriate corrections should be given. Finally, as the performance of the task improves, **withdrawal of feedback** should be implemented to help the patient internalize the task.

Other Treatment Strategies

There are additional modalities that can be utilized in the neurologic patient who demonstrates disequilibrium. As always, weakness or restriction of lower extremity musculature (due to disuse or spasticity) must be addressed with traditional physical therapy modalities, such as stretching and therapeutic exercise, as well as home exercise programs. Other interventions include sensory re-weighting, training with assistive devices, and recommendations related to environmental modifications. **Sensory re-weighting** is a relatively new therapeutic concept that has been gaining attention since the commercial availability of dynamic force plate testing (Allison et al., 2003). The new technology has enabled clinicians to identify sensory impairments related to balance function. Additionally, the technology can be utilized to enhance an otherwise deficient sensory input. For example, a patient that demonstrates impaired vestibular function on force plate testing can be trained on an unstable surface with an unstable visual surround, essentially making the patient dependent on vestibular input for maintenance of balance. Theoretically, this re-weights the sensory system toward vestibular input, thereby enhancing the modality. When prolonged or permanent postural imbalance is evident, it is prudent to train and educate the neurologic patient in the use of **assistive devices**, such as canes, walkers, shower chairs, etc., in an attempt to reduce the risk for falls. In the same vein, education and instruction on **home modifications** for safety is crucial, including installation of grab bars and no slip surfaces in the shower, night time lighting, and remote emergency alert systems.

Conclusion

Disorders related to acquired brain injury are frequently associated with disequilibrium, dizziness, and vertigo. In many instances, the risk for additional injury due to falls is increased. Members of the neurorehabilitation team need to understand the complexity of the balance system and how their findings may contribute to the overall management of the balance disorder. Underlying impairments associated with disequilibrium can be identified and minimized through a targeted approach using diagnostic and therapeutic modalities that are available through recent technologic advances. As a result, specialized balance and vestibular oriented rehabilitation can help improve the quality of life and reduce the risk of secondary injury in patients with postural instability.

References

Allison, L., Kiemel, T., Kafoury-House, L. (2003) *Multisensory Reweighting in the Fall-Prone Elderly: Comparison to Healthy and Older Adults [abstract]*. Presented at the combined sections meeting of the American Physical Therapy Association, Tampa, Florida.

American Geriatrics Society, British Geriatrics Society and American Academy of Orthopedic Surgeons Panel on Fall Prevention (2001) Guideline for the Prevention of Falls in Older Persons. *Journal of the American Geriatrics Society*, 49:664–672.

American Physical Therapy Association (2001, January) Guide to Physical Therapist Practice, 2nd ed. *Physical Therapy* 81(1):S19–S42.

Berg, K., Wood-Dauphinee, S., Williams, J.I. (1995) The balance scale: Reliability assessment with elderly residents and patients with an acute stroke. *Scandinavian Journal of Rehabilitation Medicine* 27:27–36.

Black, F.O., Nashner, L.M. (1984) Postural disturbances in patients with benign paroxysmal positional nystagmus. *Annals of Otology, Rhinology, Laryngology* 93:595–599.

Centers for Disease Control and Prevention (2003) *Web-based Injury Statistics Query and Reporting System (WISQARS) [Online]*. National Center for Injury Prevention and Control, Accessed from: URL: http://www.cdc.gov/ncipc/wisqars.

Clendaniel, R.A. (2000) Outcome measures for assessment and treatment of the dizzy and balance disorder patient. *Otolaryngologic Clinics of North America* 33(3):519–533.

Dienci, H.C., Horak, F.B., Nashner, L.M. (1988). Influence of stimulus parameters on human postural responses. *Journal of Neurophysiology* 59:1888–1905.

Espinoza, S., Walston, J.D. (2005, December) Frailty in older adults: Insights and interventions. *Cleveland Clinic Journal of Medicine* 72(12):1105 1112.

Fredericks, C.M., Saladin, L.K. (1996) *Pathophysiology of the Motor Systems: Principles and Clinical Presentations*. Philadelphia, PA: FA Davis.

Health on the Net Foundation. *News: Strokes Can Strike at Balance*. http://www.hon.ch/news/HSN/511294.html. Accessed April 2006.

Herdman, S.J. (1997, June) Advances in the treatment of vestibular disorders. *Physical Therapy* 77(6):602–618.

Honrubia, V. (2000) In *Vestibular Rehabilitation*, 2nd ed. Philadelphia, PA: FA Davis.

Horak, F.B., Nashner, L.M. (1986) Central programming of postural movements: Adaptation to altered support surface configurations. *Journal of Neurophysiology* 55:1369–1381.

Horak, F.B., Nashner, L.M., Deiner, H.C. (1990, August) Postural strategies associated with somatosensory and vestibular loss. *Experimental Brain Research* 82(1):167–177.

Lehmann, J.F., Boswell, S., Price, R., Burliegh, A., deLateur, B.J., Jaffe, K.M., Hertling, D. (1990, November) Quantitative evaluation of sway as an indicator of functional balance in post-traumatic brain injury. *Archives of Physical Medicine Rehabilitation* 17:955–962.

Nashner, L.M. (1989) Sensory, neuromuscular, and biomechanical contributions to human balance. In *Balance: Proceedings of the APTA Forum*, Nashville, Tennessee.

Pearson, B.W., Barber, H.O. (1973) Head injury: Some otoneurologic sequelae. *Archives of Otolaryngology* 97:81.

Sataloff, R.T., Mandel, S., Schapiro, S.R. (eds.) (1993) *Minor Head Trauma-Assessment, Management, and Rehabilitation*. New York: Springer Verlag.

Shumway-Cook, A. (2000) In *Vestibular Rehabilitation*, 2nd ed. Philadelphia, PA: FA Davis.

Shumway-Cook, A., Horak, F.B. (1990) Rehabilitation strategies for patients with vestibular deficits. *Neurologic Clinics* 9(2):441–457.

Studenski, S., Duncan, P.W., Chandler, J. (1991, March) Postural responses and effector factors in persons with unexplained falls: Results and methodologic issues. *Journal of the American Geriatrics Society* 39(3):229–234.

Tinetti, M.E., Speechly, M., Ginter, S.F. (1988) Risk factors for falls among elderly persons living in the community. *The New England Journal of Medicine* 319:1701–1707.

Whitney, S.L., Herdman, S.J. (2000) In *Vestibular Rehabilitation*, 2nd ed. Philadelphia, PA: FA Davis.

Wild, D., Nayak, U.S.L., Isaacs, B. (1981) Prognosis of falls in old people at home. *Journal of Epidemiology Community Health* 35:200–204.

Wrisley, D.M., Walker, M.L., Echternach, J.L., Strasnick, B. (2003, October) Reliability of the dynamic gait index in people with vestibular disorders. *Archives of Physical Medicine Rehabilitation* 84(10):1528–1533.

12
The Role of the Occupational Therapist on the Neuro-Rehabilitation Team

PATRICIA KEARNEY, TAMI MCGOWAN, JENNIFER ANDERSON, AND DEBRA STROSAHL

Occupational Therapy

Occupational therapy is defined as "a health and rehabilitation profession that assists individuals of all ages who have had an injury, illness, cognitive impairment, mental illness, developmental, learning, or physical disability to maximize their independence" (AOTA). An occupational therapist's goal is to maximize a person's independence in all aspects of daily functioning. Various performance areas such as activities of daily living, work and productive activities, as well as play and leisure activities, guide the practice of occupational therapy. Treatment sessions focus on engaging individuals in meaningful and purposeful activities in order to assist them in achieving their goals so they reach their optimal level of independence, productivity, and satisfaction. This allows the individual to have a sense of increased self-efficacy, autonomy, purpose, competence, and especially wholeness.

Occupational Therapy and Acquired Brain Injury (ABI)

Occupational therapists play a pivotal role in the evaluation and treatment of an individual who has sustained a brain injury. The focus is to approach the individual's care in a holistic manner. This involves interviewing the individual as well as family, in order to thoroughly understand his or her medical, vocational, social, and emotional history. An occupational therapist will utilize the information obtained to guide the treatment program and more accurately evaluate the individual's level of impairment in the various performance areas.

Individuals with ABI may demonstrate various types of impairments that may or may not be consistent with their diagnosis. It is obvious when a person has a knee replacement that they will probably present with lower extremity weakness, pain, and impaired range of motion. When a person has sustained a brain injury, there may be various parts of the brain that were affected in a more subtle way, that were not reflected in the diagnosis. For example, when a person has hydrocephalus as a complication to an original focal injury, the pressure may exert a diffuse effect on the brain and produce functional impairments that were unexpected based on the primary diagnosis.

Occupational therapists that work with brain-injured individuals must be proficient in assessing how physical, cognitive, and behavioral impairments affect the various activities of daily living (ADLs). An activity analysis of each task is performed and is often used to guide the rehabilitation process.

Evaluation and Treatment

The evaluation is initiated by a thorough clinical interview, which should include open-ended questioning regarding social, medical, and vocational history, physical and social environment, as well as family and self-assessment of the individual's current level of functioning. The results will provide the therapist with a global picture of the person's former functioning, current insight, and awareness of limitations. It is extremely important to note the individual's level of insight (see Chapter 14). If it is impaired, safety may be of significant concern. For example, if an individual reports he has no physical deficits, yet through observation he or she clearly has a hemiparesis, this individual may attempt to stand without assistance. In order to assess the level of insight fully, the therapist will compare the individual's self-assessment of functioning with therapist observation, family report, and objective findings.

Following the interview, standardized assessments are utilized, in order to quantify deficits objectively. These include tests of motor, perceptual, attention, and executive functions. The interpretation of both the interview and formal test results facilitate the generation of a problem list. A treatment plan and short- and long-term goals are formulated with the survivor's input. When appropriate, the survivor's family will also participate in goal formation. In the brain injury arena, evaluation and treatment are closely connected. As the individual progresses, the therapist must continue to assess, analyze, and appropriately gauge the treatment plan. He/she does so by continually re-assessing an individual's insight and abilities across a hierarchy of tasks and by assessing the strategies that an individual uses when faced with a problem (Toglia, 1994). The next section will describe specific areas addressed by the occupational therapist in evaluating and treating an individual with acquired brain injury.

Upper Extremity Function

Evaluation of the upper extremity requires a comprehensive examination of an individual's range of motion, strength, tone, endurance, coordination (gross motor and fine motor), and sensation. The evaluation is completed through observation of an individual completing various tasks as well as through standardized testing, including goniometry and manual muscle testing. An accurate assessment of these areas is crucial in assisting the individual to develop the skills necessary to increase independence with all functional tasks. While traditional

TABLE 12.1. Recovery stages of the upper extremities

Arm	Hand
1. Flaccidity—no voluntary movement	1. Flaccidity
2. Synergies developing—flexion usually develops before extension (may be a weak associated reaction or voluntary contraction with or without joint motion); spasticity developing	2. Little or no active finger flexion
3. Beginning voluntary movement, but only in synergy; increased spasticity, which may become marked	3. Mass grasp or hook grasp; no voluntary finger extension or release
4. Some movements deviating from synergy: a. hand behind body b. arm to forward-horizontal position c. pronation-supination with elbow flexed to 90 degrees; spasticity decreasing	4. Lateral prehension with release by thumb movement; semivoluntary finger extension (small range of motion)
5. Independence from basic synergies: a. arm to side-horizontal position b. arm forward and overhead c. pronation-supination with elbow fully extended; spasticity waning	5. Palmar prehension; cylindrical and spherical grasp (awkward) Voluntary mass finger extension (variable range of motion)
6. Isolated joint movements freely performed with near normal coordination; spasticity minimal	6. All types of prehension (improved skill) Voluntary finger extension (full range of motion); individual finger movements

evaluation methods such as range of motion testing, manual muscle testing and dynamometer measurements can be helpful, it is often more appropriate and useful to utilize a qualitative, functional and descriptive approach to describing and assessing the hemiparetic upper extremity. Functional approaches for evaluating active range of motion (AROM) could include asking the individual to put on and button a shirt or to reach for items overhead. In addition, Brunnstrom (1970) provides a useful stepwise paradigm with which to describe the upper extremity (see Table 12.1).

Range of Motion (ROM) General

Scapular active and passive ROM (A/PROM) is the first area assessed. If limitations are present, then safe and functional movement of the entire limb will be affected. This is because the scapular-humeral rhythm is a 2:1 ratio. For example, if the individual's upper extremity moves to 180 degrees of shoulder flexion, the humerus moves through 120 degrees and the scapula 60 degrees (Davis, 1996). If this scapular-humeral rhythm is compromised, the individual is at risk for developing joint pain and trauma (i.e., bicep tendonitis). Treatment for limited scapular ROM involves the use of modalities, such as heat and ultrasound, and passive as well as active assistive range-of-motion exercises.

Passive and active goniometric measurements are taken for both upper extremities. If either passive or active ROM is not within functional limits, further evaluation is done in order to find the source of the problem. An example of a physical anomaly that causes both limited active and passive ROM with a hard-end feel is heterotopic ossification. This problem may require medical/surgical intervention and aggressive ranging of the extremity during treatment.

Glenohumeral subluxation is a common cause of pain in the hemiplegic shoulder that has low or mixed tone. With proper positioning and careful joint-approximated ROM, pain and/or impingement should not occur. It is the occupational therapist's responsibility to educate the individual, family, and other caregivers (e.g., nursing staff) about the precautions of ranging the upper extremity with a subluxed shoulder (Ikai et al., 1998; Shepherd & Carr, 1998). Slings can be used to support the affected upper extremity from soft tissue damage, or to allow for stability during ambulation and transfers. Other supportive methods include resting the hand in the individual's pocket, or on a handbag that is worn across the chest, or resting the arm on the tabletop surface or an armboard when seated. This support can be helpful, especially if the weight of the flaccid side appears to be affecting the individual's balance during ambulation. If a sling is used, caution should be taken to ensure that the individual does not remain in it for extended periods of time, as it positions the upper extremity in an internally rotated and flexed position. This positioning simulates the natural synergy pattern, and if the arm remains positioned as such, soft tissue contracture may result. Further, the sling should only be worn when in a standing position. Proper training in the use of a sling is needed to decrease the risk of improper application and contracture due to prolonged use (Zorowitz et al., 1995; Shepherd & Carr, 1998).

General

Muscle Strength and Tone

Manual muscle testing is used to assess the strength of both upper extremities. The OT utilizes this information to determine the areas that will cause limitations during performance of functional tasks, and the results will guide the treatment protocol for retraining the upper extremity. Specific treatment techniques derive from a variety of frames of reference, as summarized by Trombly (1997). The biomechanical model emphasizes educating the individual on various ROM and strengthening exercises, while utilizing equipment such as weight cuffs, dumbbells, and theraband. The neurodevelopmental-motor learning model focuses on utilizing normal movement patterns and other facilitatory and inhibitory techniques. The rehabilitative model stresses the use of compensatory strategy training and the use of adaptive equipment to improve the individual's ability to participate in functional tasks efficiently and without pain.

While each model presents its own theoretical framework regarding treatment, many therapists utilize dynamic and integrated approaches. Rood (as cited in Trombly, 1997a,b), for example, advocates the normalization of muscle tone by utilizing various sensory inputs (i.e., vibration, fast brushing, tapping, and prolonged stretch) to facilitate and inhibit motor responses and reflexes. The Neurodevelopmental Treatment (NDT) or Bobath (1990) treatment approach utilizes trunk stabilization and weight-bearing as building blocks for more distal action. Kabat's Proprioceptive Neuromuscular facilitation approach (1951) advocates the use of specific diagonal movements to facilitate the development of motor control.

The evaluation of muscle tone and tone management is another critical component for reeducating a hemiparetic upper extremity. Tone refers to the state of muscle contraction at rest and can be determined by its resistance to stretch (Jacobs & Jacobs, 2001). Most of the time, after the initial acute phase of the injury, a hemiparetic extremity has mixed tone. As the tone begins to return, it usually starts proximal to the body. For example, the scapula and the pectoralis muscles may be the first to increase in tone. When this is the case, the upper extremity will internally rotate and adduct from the force of the tone. If the individual is not positioned properly, this can lead to contractures, pain, and limited range of motion. The occupational therapist will identify and continually evaluate how increased tone and pain is limiting the individual's function (Gillen, 1998).

Once tone is identified more distally, the evaluation of splinting needs is completed. If a therapist has determined that a splint is required, a prescription from the physician will be requested. Splinting is done to assist in normalization of tone, decrease the risk of contractures, increase or maintain PROM, prevent skin breakdown, and keep the UE in a functional position. Some common splints used for this purpose are resting hand splint, stretch splint (i.e., dynasplint for the elbow), wrist cock-up and thumb opposition splint (Davis, 1996; Duncan, 1989). The splints are fabricated and then modified as the individual's functional movement and tone change, with the goal of totally removing the splint. Once the splint is fabricated, a splint-wearing schedule is provided for the individual and/or caregivers to ensure proper use of the splint. It is also important to note that if an individual's wrist and hand is flaccid (low tone), a splint will not ensure the integrity of the musculature in the hand. Without tone, the muscles will atrophy with or without a splint.

There is some question regarding the effectiveness of splinting the hemiplegic hand. Lanin (2003) performed a meta-analysis regarding the efficacy of splinting in adults following stroke. Based on this review of the literature, the author concluded that there was no difference between the conditions of providing an aggressive PROM program alone versus providing an aggressive PROM program in conjunction with splinting. However, it was noted that many of the clinical protocols included PROM programs which may be above and beyond the feasible constraints of clinical therapy programs. Thus, the evidence was inconclusive as to whether splinting might provide an adjunct when therapy time is limited.

Treatment for tone management focuses on regulation through the use of neuro-reeducation techniques such as facilitory or inhibitory techniques, proprioceptive neuromuscular facilitation techniques, and functional tasks to increase ROM, strength, and endurance. Both the individual and all of the individual's caregivers must be educated on the proper positioning and handling of the upper extremity. Incorporating weight bearing of the involved extremity while the individual performs self-care tasks will facilitate both the normalization of tone and promote awareness of the involved extremity. Communication between the physiatrist and the occupational therapist is also crucial in the area of tone management. The physician will utilize the feedback from the occupational therapist to assist in determining whether medications and/or injections should be used for decreasing the amount of tone in the involved extremity.

MA was a 18-year-old male involved in a rollover motor vehicle accident as an unrestrained passenger. His injuries included a right subarachnoid hemorrhage, left subdural hematoma with shearing injury. He also suffered bilateral pulmonary contusions with one reported seizure. He had a PEG tube placed for nutritional supplement, and required the support of a ventilator. He remained in a coma for approximately 6 weeks, and during that time developed severe contractures in bilateral upper and lower extremities. He was medically treated for the contractures and high tone with oral medications and responded well. The initial occupational therapy evaluation during his acute inpatient rehabilitation stay showed that all areas of self-care and functional mobility required maximal assistance of another person. The range of motion in his shoulders was within functional limits, but the range of motion in his elbows, wrists, and fingers was severely impaired and affected by his increased flexor tone.

Occupational therapy treatment sessions focused on increasing MA's independence with both self-care and functional mobility (transfer status). Passive range of motion with prolonged stretch was performed to maintain joint integrity and prevent soft tissue contracture. Resistive exercise was performed within the available range of motion. Adaptive equipment and techniques were taught, such as the use of built-up utensils for self-feeding and the use of enlarged grips for other self-care items such as combs and toothbrushes. In addition, naturalistic modifications in dressing were taught (such as the use of overhead versus button down shirts).

The occupational therapist collaborated with the physiatrist to monitor the effects of tone medications. Over time, the tone decreased in MA's lower extremities, which had a significant positive impact on his transfers. Over the course of months (encompassing acute, subacute, and outpatient rehabilitation) he became able to walk with supervision for safety and without the use of an assistive device. The range of motion increased in his upper extremities, which improved his self-care status. He was able to dress and groom himself with some adaptations (i.e., shoes that did not require tying).

Recently, a technique known as constraint induced movement therapy (CIMT; Taub & Uswatte, 2000) has received a great deal of clinical attention. This approach involves restraining the nonaffected upper extremity for distinct periods of time, thereby forcing the individual to use his/her paretic arm/hand for functional activities (e.g., reaching for a spoon). It is based on the principle of learned non-use; that is, the individual with hemiparesis instinctively learns to compensate for the impairment of the hemiparetic upper extremity by utilizing the non-affected hand. This non-use is adaptive in the sense that it allows for completion of ADLs in a one-handed manner. However non-use becomes maladaptive when the affected upper extremity begins to recover, but the habit of not using the affected arm (learned non-use) precludes the use of the affected arm during functional tasks. While early research protocols (reviewed by Taub & Uswatte, 2000) involved long hours of constraint (90% of waking hours) and therapy time (6 hours daily, 5 days per week), modified protocols more representative of clinically feasible conditions have been developed (e.g., 5 hours constraint daily, with 30 minutes of OT and PT, three times per week). Results of these modified protocols (Page et al., 2002a,b;

Ploughman & Corbett, 2004) have been shown to demonstrate positive results as well, including increased hand use and maintenance of these gains over time.

Coordination *General*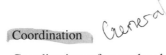

Coordination refers to the ability of muscle groups to complete a timely, smooth pattern and sequence of motion through proprioceptive sensory feedback. Ataxia is a specific type of coordination impairment, often caused by cerebellar lesions, which inhibits smooth or coordinated gross movements. Evaluation of gross and fine motor control is completed through naturalistic observation as well as standardized testing. Naturalistic evaluation may include observing the way the individual dons/doffs clothing, reaches for an object on a shelf or signs his/her name. Functional assessment of coordination is done using similar methods used to test range of motion, and specialized tests of fine motor coordination (e.g., Purdue Pegboard Test, 9-Hole Peg Test; as cited in Mathiowetz & Haugen, 1997). Treatment of coordination deficits should focus on the functional goals of the individual and can include remedial approaches such as therapeutic exercise, so that the strength of the muscles might overcome the intensity of the tremor or incoordination. Compensatory treatment strategies include bearing weight throughout the upper extremities during self-care and other functional tasks, or weighting the affected upper extremity or adaptive equipment (e.g., use of weighted utensils while eating). The weight increases proprioceptive feedback to the brain and can decrease the intensity of the resultant tremor. It is important to note that the type and amount of weight that is effective varies from individual to individual.

Sensation *General*

The evaluation and treatment of sensory deficits is important to ensure a person's safety while completing ADL tasks; sensation also plays an important role in coordination of movements (Gowland & Gambarotto, 1994). Touch, taste, smell, and vision are each evaluated by the occupational therapist (hearing is evaluated by the speech-language pathologist). The sense of touch (including ability to sense pain, pressure, and temperature) is often affected in a person with hemiplegia/hemiparesis, and can have a major impact on safety (e.g., individuals may not be able to sense the water temperature in the shower or feel pain if they get their affected arm wedged in a doorway while propelling their wheelchair). Taste and smell are senses that often get overlooked when evaluating an individual with acquired brain injury (Zasler et al., 1992), but changes in these sensations are important to identify, as they can impact other areas of functioning (e.g., appetite). Vision evaluation is discussed in detail in Chapter 8, and OTs often work collaboratively with neuro-optometrists in the treatment of individuals with visual impairments. Treatment sessions focus on normalizing an individual's sensation through sensory reeducation techniques and/or teaching adaptive techniques to ensure safety during completion of functional tasks.

Self-Care (general)

Self-care is the core component of basic activities of daily living (BADLs). The American Occupational Therapy Association lists self-care as one of its major performance areas. These activities include bathing, toileting, grooming, dressing, feeding, medication management and general hygiene. Naturalistic observation is the most appropriate method of evaluating independence in self-care. When performing an ADL evaluation, the therapist must carefully assess the level of assistance that the individual requires. In many traditional practice areas, the impediment to full participation in self-care is based on a physical deficit. When working in the brain injury arena, however, it is the interplay of physical, visual perceptual, behavioral, emotional, and cognitive deficits that truly impacts the performance of self-care (Mercier et al., 2001).

When initiating a self-care assessment, individuals may be asked to pick out their clothes and identify what items they need for bathing and grooming. It is noted whether or not they initiate this task immediately, require repeated cues, or need the task broken down into smaller components. Ability to sequence the task properly, time management, and initiation of compensatory strategies are also assessed. It is noted whether patients ignore one side of their body or forget how to use basic self-care items. Upon evaluation, it is important to play as passive a role as possible, in order to assess how an individual would perform each task as if the therapist was not there.

Retraining of self-care skills may involve the use of compensatory strategies such as one-handed dressing techniques. These techniques may need to be broken down into smaller components and/or explained with simple one-step commands. The level and type of compensatory strategy training must be matched to the specific cognitive deficits. This is one of the challenges of thorough functional neuro-rehabilitation. The therapist must consider the impact that each deficit has on the performance of each self-care task.

AJ is a 63-year old male who sustained a right-sided CVA. The CVA resulted in left-sided hemiparesis, and a marked left inattention. After hospital discharge and a 2-week stay in acute rehabilitation, AJ was transferred to a subacute brain injury unit for continued comprehensive rehabilitation. OT evaluated him in his room while performing his morning self-care. It was found that he needed maximal assistance transferring out of bed and into a wheelchair, onto a toilet and into the shower. He was only able to dress his strong side and was unable to dress the paretic side. He needed assistance with grooming and it was noted that when brushing his teeth, combing his hair, and shaving, he ignored his affected right side. Problems identified included left-side hemiparesis, decreased functional mobility (i.e., transfer skills), decreased attention to the left side, decreased basic self-care (i.e., dressing, grooming, etc). Short-term goals (to be achieved within 1–2 weeks) included being able to groom left side of face during oral care with minimum assistance and moderate verbal and visual cues, being able to don an overhead shirt using hemi-dressing techniques with moderate assistance and maximum cues, and being able to transfer from wheelchair to bed with moderate assistance. Long-term goals (to be achieved by discharge) included being able to perform all grooming tasks while seated at a sink with supervision for setup only, being able to don overhead shirt with supervision for setup only, being able to perform functional transfers (i.e., tub, bed, toilet) with contact guard assistance and being able to perform bathing with distant supervision for safety.

Treatment focused on upper and lower body dressing as well as grooming. AJ was seen in his room prior to the start of his day, in order to simulate his natural routine. He was trained on the use of compensatory strategies to effectively dress his hemiparetic side (e.g., dressing the weaker side first). Grooming tasks were performed at wheelchair level since decreased balance impacted his safety. One-handed techniques were taught for opening containers (such as toothpaste, shave cream). In order to improve his attention and awareness to his affected side, verbal and visual cues were utilized. The therapist first provided verbal cues (e.g., "did you get the left side" [of your face]), then progressed to visual cues as he was unable to internalize the strategy in order to self-cue. A sign reading, "Remember to check your left side" was placed on the mirror, which he was then able to follow in order to complete the task without assistance of another person.

After 5 weeks of comprehensive inpatient neuro-rehabilitation (including 2 weeks at an acute level followed by an additional 3 weeks on the subacute brain injury unit), AJ was independent enough to return home at a level of modified independence (extra time, visual cues) with his ADLs and began outpatient therapy to address home management and community re-integration skills.

Functional Mobility

The resultant hemiparesis and/or balance deficits that often accompany ABI affect not only a person's self-care ability, but also the individual's ability to move from place to place, or *functional mobility*. An individual's functional mobility must be thoroughly assessed in order to ensure proper wheelchair positioning, access to the environment, access to adaptive equipment, safety, and maximization of independence. This assessment includes evaluation of bed, toilet, and shower/tub transfers. Postural and trunk control, sitting and standing balance, and ability to navigate an environment with or without an assistive device will also be assessed. While evaluating functional mobility, the therapist will also take note of the automatic use or non-use of both appropriate and ineffective/unsafe compensatory strategies.

For wheelchair management, occupational therapists work with physical therapists and durable medical equipment providers to select an appropriate seating system. Because cognition is key to safety awareness, consideration of cognitive deficits plays a major role in the selection of a seating system. Evaluation of the individual's abilities and deficits determine whether a manual or electric wheelchair may be required, and a specialized wheelchair evaluation may be needed (Pesperin, 1998). The physical evaluation for wheelchair positioning begins proximally and progresses distally. The individual's physical height and weight determine the size of the wheelchair. The therapist should aim for a near 90-degree angle at the hips. This is achieved by adjusting a number of variables (Pesprin, 1998).

Cushion choice is based on an evaluation of the individual's weight, hip angle, and pelvic tilt, ability to weight-shift and relieve pressure, and any incontinence issues. Wedges may be used to assist in proper pelvic positioning. Placement of lateral supports may be needed to assist in maintaining proper trunk alignment because of decreased tone. The backrest will assist in hip angle and trunk alignment. Careful choice of armrests is especially important for the hemiparetic individual. Removable armrests assist in safety with transfers. Attaching a half-arm board or full lapboard to the armrest of the wheelchair promotes attention to the weaker side, as well as ensuring the arm does not get injured when the individual is not attending to it. Adjustable height armrests allow the therapist to position the elbow at ninety degrees and the scapula in a neutral position. This preventative measure may help the individual to avoid developing adhesive capsulitis and/or impingement syndromes. A wedge may also be placed on the lapboard to assist in edema management. Leg rests should be considered when one or both lower extremities are unable to assist in propulsion of the wheelchair. It is important that the supported leg(s) maintain a 90-degree angle at the ankle and the knee. Ideally, leg rests should be removable in order to increase safety with transfers, and should be able to elevate if the vascular system is compromised. The therapist may consider placement of a lap/seat belt, and/or chest and trunk straps for safety for individuals with impulsivity and/or decreased safety awareness. They can also be used to assist with the hip angle, and to prevent slipping out of the chair in individuals with poor postural control.

Once a seating system is chosen and properly fit to the individual, it is essential that the occupational therapist work with the individual on transfer training. Transferring refers to the ability to move from surface to surface (i.e., from wheelchair to bed or from bed to commode). The therapist takes into consideration the home setup and discharge environment, and ultimately focuses on transfers in the most naturalistic setup possible. Transfer options and/or devices include stand-pivot technique, use of a sliding board or mechanical (e.g., hoyer) lift. It is the goal of the OT to discharge the patient utilizing the least restrictive, yet safest transfer method.

Balance is another essential skill for safe mobility and ADL completion. It is affected by decreased trunk stability, strength, proprioceptive/kinesthetic awareness, and may also be affected by vestibular system dysfunction. It is imperative that the occupational and physical therapists collaborate when evaluating and treating balance dysfunction. It is often during ADL activity that deficits in balance are demonstrated and pose the greatest safety risk. The physical therapist, for example, might perform balance testing, and might challenge the individual by ambulating with him/her on a variety of surfaces. In this setting, the individual is often focused on his or her balance as the product of the treatment. However, when an individual is involved in an activity such as morning care, or in an IADL such as cooking, the individual's primary focus is often the activity, and not the component area of balance, and he/she may become less safe in terms of balance when involved in a functional activity. It is therefore the responsibility of the OT to help the individual recognize the functional impact of his or her balance deficits, and provide compensatory strategies in the natural environment. A comprehensive evaluation of the individual's static and dynamic balance while seated and standing helps to identify the supervision or assistance level that may be required during functional tasks (Gowland & Gabaretto, 1994; Alley, 2001; LePostollec, 2000). An individual may need an assistive device (e.g., cane) to help increase balance during ADLs. Some individuals may benefit from specialized vestibular retraining (see Chapter 11).

In summary, treatment of mobility deficits requires a multi-faceted approach including remedial techniques (e.g., strength, endurance training, tone management) and use of compensatory strategies and/or adaptive equipment (e.g., weight-bearing for ataxia, lapboards, sliding boards).

Cognitive Skills

ABI can lead to individuals experiencing a wide variety of cognitive deficits, as described below. While many disciplines evaluate and treat cognitive dysfunction (i.e., speech language pathology, neuropsychology), occupational therapy's unique role is in the interplay between cognition and activities of daily living. For example, it is the OT's role to assess memory in terms of how it is affecting the individual's daily functioning—Is the individual forgetting to take his medicine? Is he/she forgetting appointments? Is he/she forgetting to use the compensatory strategies that he/she learned in therapy the previous day? Correspondingly, the OT develops functional goals in reference to cognition. The individual might be taught to use a pill organizer or daily planner, or to use a set of written instructions and cues when performing new tasks.

Attention

Attention is a complex process that allows a person to take in and react to different stimuli and experiences (Zoltan, 1996). Attention deficits may result in problems with nearly any activity throughout an individual's day. There are five distinguishable levels of attention: focused, sustained, selective, alternating, or divided. Deficits in any of these areas can impact a brain injury survivor's ability to perform both basic and complex ADLs and can be a focus of OT treatment. Focused attention is the ability to perceive individual pieces of information. Sustained attention is a person's ability to concentrate while completing a task within a closed environment. A person experiencing difficulty with sustained attention may have problems with such activities as reading a book or having a conversation. Selective attention is a person's ability to concentrate despite the presence of distractions. Individuals demonstrating difficulties with selective attention may find they cannot concentrate with external distractions such as people walking in and out of a room or background noise (e.g., television or radio). An individual may also find it difficult to concentrate with internal distractions such as pain or anxiety. Alternating attention requires a person to shift focus or concentration from one thing to the next. For example, an individual may be preparing food in the kitchen when the phone rings. In order to answer the phone and participate in the conversation the individual must be able to shift attention to the new task at hand. Once the phone call is completed, the individual must successfully shift attention back to where he or she left off in meal preparation. Deficits in alternating attention may pose a safety risk. Finally, divided attention is the ability to multitask or devote attention to several different things at the same time. This is the most complex level of attention, but also the level that we use most frequently in life. For example, divided attention is required to drive a car. One must be able to accelerate or brake, while controlling the steering wheel, paying attention to the traffic, anticipating traffic lights or stop signs, using the rearview and side mirror, and perhaps even changing the radio station.

One evidence-based approach to the remediation of attention is a structured approach known as Attention Process Training (Sohlberg & Mateer, 1987). In this model, tasks are presented hierarchically, with more complex tasks presented only after the individual has mastered more basic levels/tasks. Stimuli can be presented auditorily or visually. Time-pressure management training (Fasotti et al., 2000), which teaches survivors to compensate for slowed processing speed and cognitive overload, is another technique that has been shown to improve attentional abilities. More functional approaches to improve attention include the use of structured tasks with a focus on challenging attention skills in order to facilitate generalization to ADLs (Novack et al., 1996). For example, a therapist might introduce the relearning of a self-care task such as upper body dressing in a quiet room with the curtain drawn and door closed, with the only stimulus being the individual's shirt. As the individual progresses, however, the therapist might introduce additional, more naturally occurring distractions, such as hallway noise, or sounds on television. To challenge the individual even further, the therapist might ask him/her to execute the dressing task while discussing discharge plans or verbally discussing his/her day's schedule with the therapist.

Executive Functions

Executive functions are high-level cortical skills that allow us to plan, organize, and execute complex activities. These skills include initiation, organization, sequencing, problem-solving, follow-through, self-monitoring, and time management. Impairments in executive functions are common, particularly in ABI survivors with frontal lobe injury, and affect performance with all productive activity including home, community, work, or school-based activities (Grafman & Litvan, 1999).

Initiation is the cognitive process of beginning any given task or action. Initiation deficits can range from mild to severe, but nonetheless require intervention. Severe deficits can manifest in even the simplest tasks like those seen in an individual's morning routine. Activities such as putting on one's shirt may require verbal and/or physical cues in order to begin the action of putting an arm through the sleeve. In other cases, poor initiation might itself manifest as the tendency to remain quiet and nonparticipatory in a group discussion unless asked a direct question. Once directly addressed or given prompts, the survivor with initiation deficits may be well able to engage in the conversation at hand.

Organization and follow-through require the individual to conceptualize the whole task and generate the appropriate sequence of steps necessary to complete it successfully. An example would be the common household task of cooking. In order to plan a hot meal with several dishes, one must plan, organize and prepare accordingly, correctly sequencing and anticipating how long each dish will take.

As with all OT treatment, executive function deficits are best treated from a holistic, person-centered, and performance-based approach. The therapist and individual will collaborate to identify a task, usually home- or community related, and determine, in a stepwise fashion, the components and sequence of the activity. The OT will provide structured cueing to help the individual to arrive at an appropriate plan. The therapist will also provide compensatory strategy training, such as list making, task segmentation, or the use of timers and calendars. There is evidence for the efficacy of various approaches to the rehabilitation of executive function deficits, including structured problem-solving training techniques such as goal management training (Levine et al., 2000).

Apraxia

Praxis is the conceiving and planning of a new motor act in response to environmental demands (Jacobs & Jacobs, 2001). A disorder in praxis, or apraxia, is the inability to perform purposeful movements in the absence of physical deficits (Zoltan 1996). *Ideomotor apraxia* is the inability to translate the idea of motion into an actual motor task. It presents as the inability to perform an action on command. The individual may be able to perform the task in a contextually relevant situation but be unable to perform the same task out of context and/or upon command. The individual's performance will improve when actual objects and visual cues are used (Zoltan, 1996). For example, the therapist might say, "Show me how to brush your teeth," and the individual would follow simply by lifting his arm, or with no action at all. However, the same individual, when given a toothbrush, would automatically and instinctively perform the act correctly.

Ideational apraxia is the inability to conceptualize a motor act. It presents as the inability to use tools and objects in appropriate sequence for the appropriate action. Individuals with ideational apraxia, without concurrent language deficits, may be able to articulate the appropriate use of familiar objects and tools, but be unable to produce the motor plan to reach out and grasp the tool. During self-care, this might present as an individual brushing his or her teeth after putting toothpaste on the wrong side of the toothbrush (Zoltan, 1996) or reaching to comb his hair with the toothbrush in hand. It is the job of the occupational therapist to facilitate the relearning of these once familiar tasks. The key to remediation of deficits as a result of apraxia is strategy use and repetition of each functional task until mastery is achieved. The specific steps can be demonstrated by using actual objects with hand-over-hand assistance, when necessary. Visual or verbal cues, or internal/external compensations can be individualized, based on the individual's needs. It has been found that strategy use for treatment of apraxia during ADL retraining is more effective that traditional ADL retraining (Donkervoort et al., 2001).

Visual Perceptual Skills

Vision is a key complex sensorimotor process that allows individuals to adapt successfully to their environment (Zoltan, 1996). Perception is the cognitive process of interpreting the images that the visual system registers. Inaccurate perception of the visual world leads to inaccurate interaction with the world. Because individuals rely so heavily on visual stimuli to learn and to interact with the world, visual perceptual deficits can lead to widespread functional implications, and often become evident when self-care tasks are observed in an unstructured manner. Common visual perceptual deficits include impaired figure ground and impaired spatial relations. Figure ground refers to the ability to recognize objects and forms in a competing background. Spatial relations refer to the ability to perceive and recognize the way objects relate in space, and to the individual. It includes the ability to recognize when objects are above, below, next to, or in front of other objects (Zoltan, 1996). Manifestations of visual perceptual deficits on ADL activities can include an inability to find the toothpaste in a visually cluttered medicine cabinet, or putting one's arm/leg into the wrong sleeve when donning clothing.

During an initial evaluation, the occupational therapist should identify gross visual and perceptual impairments, and areas which must be further explored. Consultation with the neuropsychologist and referral to a neuro-optometrist can also help identify and clarify the extent and nature of apparent visual perceptual deficits and guide treatment interventions. The observation of the individual during naturalistic, everyday activities (e.g., dressing, grooming) is an essential component of the OT assessment of visual perception.

Occupational therapists use the information from a vision screen and from a full neuro-optometric evaulation to help guide their treatment. For example, if a person is experiencing a visual field loss, treatment would focus on visual scanning techniques in order to help compensate and boost awareness of the full field of vision. A therapist can use a four-corner set up on a placemat or food tray, using stickers to cue the individual to view the entire field, thereby increasing independence with feeding (Hellerstein, 1997). Several recent studies have demonstrated the efficacy of visuospatial rehabilitation and visual scanning training in ABI survivors with visual neglect or other visuospatial deficits (Niemer, 1998; Bailey et al., 2002).

Instrumental Activities of Daily Living (IADLs)

IADLs (also known as work and productive activities) are those activities that are essential for one's full independence in society, beyond basic self-care abilities. The AOTA defines these as acts "oriented toward interacting with the environment that are often complex and generally optional in nature" (Dunn et al., 1994). They include activities such as meal preparation, money management, home management, care of others, and educational and vocational activities. IADLs are contextually and culturally specific and are integral to independent societal functioning. By their complex nature, IADLs involve a number of cognitive skills, including executive functioning.

Meal Preparation

The ability to prepare meals provides the individual with a sense of autonomy and will serve as a factor in discharge planning. Meal preparation requires a variety of skills, both physical and cognitive, in order to be carried out successfully. Adults with brain injury often demonstrate dysfunction in meal preparation, not only due to physical deficits, but also deficits in cognitive and perceptual skills (Niestadt, 1994). These can include hemiparesis, impaired bilateral arm coordination, impaired standing tolerance/balance, poor visual skills, or reduced sequencing, organizational skills, or safety awareness. It is the goal of the OT accurately to assess the primary limiting factors that prevent the individual from preparing meals and design a treatment plan that addresses these barriers and enables the individual to perform the task successfully. Successful meal preparation may require environment modifications to enhance accessibility. For example, because of reduced ROM, a therapist might put all equipment on easily accessible shelves. In individuals that are hemiparetic, their non-use or lack of use of one side of their body can be compensated for through the use of adaptive equipment, such as a rocker knife, dycem (which keeps objects such as plates from sliding) or plate guard to keep food from falling off a plate. Adaptive techniques are also instrumental for success with meal preparation. These include methods of energy conservation and work simplification. For example, a person can slide a heavy pot along the countertop rather than try to lift it; or do preparation such as chopping at a seated level instead of standing at the counter.

If cognition or visual perceptual skills are the primary deficit, alternative approaches would be used. If basic sequencing and memory are impaired, compensatory techniques such as task segmentation or writing a checklist could be helpful (Niestadt, 1994). For higher-level executive function deficits, treatment might focus on the planning, organization, and execution of a meal with multiple dishes, with treatment broken down across several sessions. One session might focus on choosing a menu, planning and organizing steps to cooking the meal, figuring out the recipe (altering measurements), problem solving through the supplies and equipment needed. A second session could be community-based, involving shopping to purchase required ingredients. A third session would then focus on execution of the meal, and subsequent clean-up. A therapist must consider the individual's level of function, grade the level of the cooking task accordingly, and assist the individual in transferring or generalizing the skills learned in the OT session to his or her home environment. Grading down would necessitate keeping the task simple, such as basic cold items, i.e., making a sandwich. If a therapist graded up, treatment might focus on a more complex hot meal with several dishes. A therapist must assess which level of meal preparation—basic cold snacks to complex hot meals—is appropriate and safe for the individual.

Money Management

Managing finances can be the key to independence for an individual who has sustained a brain injury. As in other areas, money management retraining should occur in a step-by-step, hierarchical fashion. The basis of all money management tasks is the ability to identify coins and currency, assign the appropriate value, and perform addition and subtraction. Once rote recognition and simple calculation is mastered, the therapist introduces the concept of simple purchasing and making change.

At higher levels, money management includes managing a checkbook, budgeting for household costs, calculating the cost of dining out in a restaurant, and budgeting for leisure/recreational events. As an individual's skills progress, it is important that the therapist grades the activity to meet the challenge of entering the community. Outings to local stores for simple purchases and organizing a bill management system are examples of treatment tasks, which can be used to facilitate the development of routines to assist individuals in performing money management tasks successfully.

Home Evaluations

Home evaluations are an important step for discharge planning from inpatient to home settings. They offer a broader, and sometimes different, insight as to how an individual is able to function/perform in a home and community-based setting. Following a brain injury, while an individual may be able to complete various tasks within the rehabilitation setting; when he or she returns to the home environment, the carryover of the training can be poor (Anemaet & Moffa-Trotter, 1999), or he/she may exhibit reduced safety awareness.

All areas of the home that the individual will be utilizing should be assessed (i.e., entrance to the home, bathroom, kitchen, bedroom, and living room). The evaluation begins with determining how the individual will enter the home. Considerations include whether the individual is able to enter the home safely without the use of adaptive equipment or is able to safely use the adaptive device that he/she has. It is noted if physical adaptations need to be made to the entryway (i.e., addition of a railing or the need for a ramp). The therapist will then observe how the individual performs various tasks within the home (i.e., transfer in and out of the tub/shower, with or without the use of a shower seat/bench, lie down in bed and/or get the milk out of the refrigerator). The therapist will assess the individual's overall safety within the home (i.e., safety while ambulating with an adaptive device; phone accessibility; if rugs should be removed). Cognitive/perceptual awareness (i.e., where the telephone is located) is also a determining factor regarding the level of supervision that will be recommended upon discharge. Physical measurements are taken in order to determine if each aspect of the home is accessible (i.e., measurements of door frames, if a three-in-one commode will fit in the bathroom space available and if the height of shelves and counters are accessible to an individual in a wheelchair). All of the above information enables the therapist to make recommendations for adaptive equipment that may be needed, rearrangement of items in the home, addition or removal of items, and whether or not the individual would be a safety risk for returning to the home environment. The social environment is also observed. The therapist will ideally have the caregiver or significant other present in order to take note of the dynamics between the individual and the person that will be providing assistance, if one is needed. This also facilitates training of the caregiver/family member while the individual is in the home environment.

The therapist may take into account the proximity of neighbors as well as layout and social supports of the community itself. A supportive community with nearby assistance (i.e., neighbors and friends) can be extremely helpful to the survivor as well as the caregiver. In addition, a simply organized neighborhood (e.g., streets with ascending numerical names) may facilitate an individual's independence in community mobility.

Driving Evaluations

For many brain injury survivors, driving is an essential part of their occupational performance (Hopewell, 2002). Occupational therapists contribute to the assessment of an individual's level of functioning and barriers to driving. The evaluation of driving includes a general medical and social history; driving history; assessment of motor, sensory, perceptual, and visual functions; balance; endurance; reaction time; various aspects of cognition; and general ADL and IADL level. Other disciplines assist in the evaluation process as well, such as the speech-language therapist regarding the individual's hearing and communication level and the neuropsychologist for determining the individual's cognitive and emotional functioning (Hawley, 2001). Once the neuro-rehabilitation team determines readiness, a referral can be made for an on-road- assessment.

The information obtained from the driving evaluation enables the occupational therapist to set up a specialized program for each individual. It has been shown that driver-retraining programs increase the ability of brain injury survivors to successfully return to on road driving (Giles, 1994). These programs may include educational sessions on traffic safety and road rules, how to read a map, give and receive directions, physical rehabilitation (strength and balance), visual/perceptual training (e.g., depth perception, peripheral vision), cognitive remediation (attention and memory training), and sensory training (proprioceptive and kinesthetic skills). Education on state laws/regulations re: driving following a change in health status, an on road evaluation and the steps to complete it can be provided (Hawley, 2001). Training sessions may be completed in a classroom setting using paper and pencil tasks, discussions, computer software, and use of a driving simulator, followed by on-road training (Galski et al., 1997). The goal is for the individual to complete the classroom and simulator training and then to complete the on road evaluation (Galski et al., 1992; Galski et al., 1993). Individuals may also require an adaptive equipment evaluation for changes to be made to their car or recommendation for an alternative vehicle (Strank, 1997).

For some ABI survivors, returning to safe driving is not possible. Because driving is often viewed as a strong measure of independence, it is imperative that the occupational therapist facilitates the individual's community independence by exploring additional travel options and engaging in travel training. These options may include various means of public transportation—buses, trains, or some community-based transportation available to individuals with disabilities. Transportation (which, while widespread in metropolitan areas, can be severely limited in more suburban or rural communities), county-subsidized bus service for seniors or individuals with disabilities, or local community agencies which may provide travel assistance. When appropriate travel options have been determined, travel training can proceed in a stepwise fashion, gradually fading cues and assistance to encourage independence. For example, maps/bus schedules would be obtained and reviewed; then the OT might accompany the individual on several short, routine trips, then shadow the individual, and ultimately progress to generalization of skills to novel, unfamiliar routes.

Community Reintegration

Community living skills are an essential component of being a productive participant in society. Successful community integration requires attention to all aspects of functioning, including physical, cognitive, and behavioral. Physically, the individual must demonstrate enough endurance to ambulate community distances, and be able to negotiate curbs and various types of terrain. Cognitively, they must demonstrate awareness of potential safety concerns (e.g., attention to traffic during street crossing) and the ability to self-direct, with or without cues (e.g., be able to follow a list of errands). Behaviorally, they must display the ability to interact appropriately with others (e.g., fellow shoppers, restaurant waiters).

Community-reintegration activities can provide a natural context in which to practice tasks learned or re-learned in the clinic. Occupational therapists will initially address these underlying skills in the clinic environment. However, while these skills might appear to be mastered in this controlled environment, with therapists available to assist and guide, the individual will encounter a very different reality in the community, where the expectations are for self-reliance and the responses of others are unpredictable.

Community reintegration training can be addressed via planning and carrying out of community-based activities. For example, the OT might work with an individual to plan an outing to a local store to purchase self-care items. While this might seem like a simple and straightforward task, it can pose many challenges to the individual with a brain injury. The individual might have to use the yellow pages or Internet to find a local store, and arrange transportation. They might need to prepare a list and create a budget for the items to be purchased. Once in the community, the individual would have to navigate an unfamiliar store, and locate items utilizing signage and other naturally occurring environmental cues. Finally the individual would have to perform the cash transaction ensuring proper change is given and received. All of these complex tasks must be performed in the context of a multi-sensory, highly distracting, often fast-paced environment.

After AJ (see page 222) completed his subacute stay, he continued on with comprehensive outpatient neuro-rehabilitation, including occupational therapy. Upon interview, AJ and his wife described that AJ had been retired, yet very independent and active prior to his stroke. He ran many errands outside of the home, managed his own medical appointments, and was active in several community organizations. He walked 3–4 miles daily, often stopping to purchase a newspaper and socialize with neighbors along his route. Following his stroke, AJ had not resumed these activities and wanted to do so. The neuropsychologist on the team also shared that AJ's self-esteem was reduced due to the loss of independence and social activity.

Following assessment, the OT identified the following concerns regarding AJ's safety and independence in the community:

1. *Topographical Orientation—did AJ know where he was in relation to his home—even when on previously familiar routes?*
2. *Money Management—Could AJ make simple community purchases ensuring the giving and receipt of proper change?*
3. *Emergency Management—Could AJ define an emergency situation, and did he know how to react in one?*

Treatment commenced in the clinic with the teaching of compensatory strategies for money management. This was done using a graded approach, starting with small dollar amounts. Thus, AJ learned to manage money in the context of purchasing a weekly newspaper.

In consultation with the physical therapist to determine AJ's walking endurance limitations, the OT, AJ, and his wife identified a local store which was both familiar and within a manageable distance. They determined a simple route which was safe, well-marked, and had crosswalks and signals. During clinic-based OT sessions, he practiced crossing streets, utilizing traffic signals and being attentive at corners. As treatment progressed, AJ learned to self-cue and use these safety strategies independently. This was observed both by the OT during treatment sessions, and AJ's wife during weekend activities.

Later, the OT arranged a community visit to AJ's home and community. During his walk to the store, the OT simply shadowed AJ. He completed his purchase and rested on a nearby bench before returning home. For safety, AJ had his mobile phone with him in case something unexpected should happen. Treatment focus then shifted to re-engagement in other community activities.

Pre-Vocational Training

Because vocational expectations for persons who have sustained a brain injury are extremely varied, it is imperative that the occupational therapist help individuals to develop a realistic view of their strengths/skills, weaknesses, and ultimate working potential. Occupational therapists can help individuals realize that a return to productive activity might not mean returning to former competitive employment status. The therapist might encourage individuals to resume or assume the role of homemaker or volunteer, or help develop a structured routine for leisure/avocational activities (e.g., participation in day program, regular exercise routine, and trips to museum/library). When considering an ABI survivor's potential to return to work, it is essential for an OT to develop a comprehensive understanding of the individual's job responsibilities as well as capabilities and limitations. This can be achieved by activity or task analysis (Creighton, 1992). Work simulations can then be developed to teach and reinforce the use of facilitatory/compensatory strategies. These can include using a daily planner to follow a schedule or using written checklists for sequencing and operation of equipment (e.g., computers). Environmental or task modifications (e.g., reorganization of the workspace, structuring/organizing the work day) can allow for successful completion of tasks which would otherwise be too challenging. Familiarity with vocational rehabilitation resources in the community is essential, and working with community-based vocational counselors, job coaches and employers is often required.

Once MA (see page 220) had met his primary ADL goals, OT treatment focus shifted to helping him develop meaningful participation in the community. Due to ongoing physical and cognitive challenges, MA was not ready to assume gainful employment. Consideration of his interests and residual strengths led to exploration of volunteer opportunities in the local community. Given the nature of his injury (he was a passenger in a motor vehicle operated by an intoxicated driver), MA wanted to share his experiences with his peers and educate them about the dangers of drinking and driving. His OT helped him organize a presentation and contact local schools at which he could speak. MA continues to do these presentations throughout his community, and has enrolled part-time at a community college.

OT as Interdisciplinary Team Players in Neuro-Rehabilitation

The occupational therapist is an integral member of the interdisciplinary team. Through collaboration with other team members, the OT is able to monitor the survivor's functional status from clinic to community. It is essential that close communication be maintained among the different disciplines to help reinforce carryover of learned strategies and to ensure that the individual's treatment plan is well coordinated. The OT focuses on functional abilities and meaningful activities, and incorporates an understanding of physical, cognitive, and behavioral deficits into development of a treatment plan. This plan will enable the brain injury survivor to maximize his/her ability to function during such meaningful activities, at home and in the community.

References

Alley, J. (2001) Regaining balance after neurological injury. *Advances for Occupational Therapy Practitioners* 17(23):8.

Anemaet, W., Moffa-Trotter, M. (1999) Promoting safety and function through home assessments. *Topics in Geriatric Rehabilitation* 15(1):26–55.

Bailey, M.J., Riddoch, M.J. Crome, P. (2002) Treatment of visual neglect in elderly patients with stroke: a single-subject series using either a scanning and cueing strategy or a left-limb activation strategy. *Physical Therapy* 82:782–797.

Bobath, B. (1990) *Adult hemiplegia: evaluation and treatment*, 3rd ed. London: William Heinemann Medical Books.

Brunnstrom, S. (1970) *Movement therapy in hemiplegia*. New York: Harper & Row.

Creighton, C. (1992) The Origin and Evolution of Activity Analysis. *The American Journal of Occupational Therapy* 46(1):45–48.

Davis, J. (1996) Neuro developmental treatment of adult hemiplegia: The Bobath approach. In Pedretti, L.W. (ed.): *Occupational Therapy: Practice Skills for Physical Dysfunction*, 4th ed. Saint Louis, MO: Mosby-Year Book, Inc., pp. 435–451

Donkervoort, M., Dekker, J., Stehmann-Saris, F. Deelman, B. (2001) Efficacy of strategy training in left hemisphere stroke patients with apraxia: A randomized clinical trial. *Neuropsychological Rehabilitation* 11(5):549–566.

Duncan, R. (1989) Basic principles of splinting of the hand. *Physical Therapy* 69(12):1104–1118.

Dunn, W., Foto, M., Hinojosa, J., Schell, B., Thomson, L.K., Hertfelder, S.D. (1994) Uniform Terminology for Occupational Therapy, 3rd ed. *American Journal of Occupational Therapy* 48(11):1047–1054.

Fasotti, L., Kovacs, F., Eling, P.A., Brouwer, W.H. (2000) Time pressure management as a compensatory strategy training after closed head injury. *Neuropsychological Rehabilitation* 10:47–65.

Galski, T., Bruno, R.L., Ehle, H.T. (1992) Driving after cerebral damage: A model with implications for evaluation. *The American Journal of Occupational Therapy* 46:324–332.

Galski, T., Bruno, R.L., Ehle, H.T. (1993) Prediction of behind-the-wheel driving performance in patients with cerebral brain damage: A discriminant function analysis. *The American Journal of Occupational Therapy* 47:391–396.

Galski, T., Ehle, H.T., Williams, J.B. (1997) Off-road evaluations for persons with cerebral injury: A factor analytic study of predriver and simulator testing. *The American Journal of Occupational Therapy* 51:352–359.

Gillen, G. (1998) Managing abnormal tone after brain injury. *OT Practice* 3(8):18–24.

Giles, G.M. (1994) Functional assessment and intervention. In Finlayson, M.A.J. & Garner S.H. (eds.): *Brain Injury Rehabilitation: Clinical considerations*. Philadelphia: Williams & Wilkens, pp. 124–156.

Gowland, C., Gambarotto, C. (1994) Assessment and treatment of physical impairments leading to disability after brain injury. In Finlayson, M.A.J. & Garner, S.H. (eds.): *Brain Injury Rehabilitation: Clinical Considerations*. Philadelphia: Williams & Wilkens, pp. 102–123.

Grafman, J. Litvan, I. (1999) Importance of deficits in executive functions. *The Lancet* 354:1921–1925.

Hawley, C. (2001) Return to driving after head injury. *Journal of Neurology, Neurosurgery and Psychiatry* 70(6):421–426.

Hellerstein, L.F. (1997) Visual Problems Associated with Brain Injury. In Mitchell, S. (ed): *Understanding and Managing Vision Deficits: A Guide for Occupational Therapists*. Thorofare, SLACK Inc., pp. 249–281.

Hopewell, C.A. (2002) Driving assessment issues for practicing clinicians. *Journal of Head Trauma Rehabilitation* 17(1):46–48.

Ikai, T., Tei, K., Yoshida, K., Miyano, S., Yonemoto, K. (1998) Evaluation and treatment of shoulder subluxation in hemiplegia: Relationship between subluxation and pain. *American Journal of Physical Medicine and Rehabilitation* 77(5):421–426.

Jacobs, K., Jacobs, L. (eds.) (2001) *Quick Reference Dictionary for Occupational Therapy*, 3rd ed. Thorofare, NJ: Slack Inc.

Kabat, H. (1951) Proprioceptive facilitation in therapeutic exercise. In Licht S. (ed.): *Therapeutic exercise*, 2nd ed. New Haven, CT: Elizabeth Licht, pp. 327–343.

Lanin, N.A. (2003) Is hand splinting effective for results following stroke? A systemic review and methodological critique of published literature. *Clinical Rehabilitation* 17:807–816.

LePostollec, M. (2000) Restoring balance post-TBI. *Advance for Occupational Therapy Practitioners* 19(19):25.

Levine, B., Roberson, I.H., Clare, L., Carter, G., Hong, J., Wilson, B.A., Ducane, J., Stuss, D.T. (2000) Rehabilitation of executive functioning: an experimental validation of goal management training. *Journal of International Neuropsychology & Sociology* 6:299–312.

Mathiowetz, V. Haugen, J.B. (1997) Evaluation of motor behavior: traditional and contemporary views. In Trombley, C. (ed.): *Occupational Therapy for Physical Dysfunction*, Baltimore, MD: Lippincott, Williams & Wilkins.

Mercier, L., Audet, T., Herbert, R., Rochette, A., Dubois, M.F. (2001) Impact of motor, cognitive and perceptual disorders on ability to perform activities of daily living after stroke. *Stroke* 32:2602–2608.

Niemer, J.P. (1998) The Lighthouse Strategy: use of visual imagery technique to treat visual inattention in stroke patients. *Brain Injury* 12:399–406.

Niestadt, M.E. (1994) A meal preparation treatment protocol for adults with brain injury. *American Journal of Occupational Therapy* 48:431–438.

Novack, T.A., Caldwell, S.G., Duke, L.W., Begquiset, Gage, R.J. (1996) Focused versus unstructured intervention for attention deficits after traumatic brain injury. *The Journal of Head Trauma Rehabilitation* 11:52–60.

Page, S.J., Sisto, S. Levine, P. (2002a) Modified constraint-induced therapy in chronic stroke. *American Journal of Physical Medicine and Rehabilitation* 81(11):870–875.

Page, S.J., Sisto, S., Johnston, M.V., Levine, P. Huges, M. (2002b) Modified constraint-induced therapy in subacute stroke: a case report. *Archives of Physical Medicine and Rehabilitation* 83(2):286–290.

Pesperin, J. (1988) Positioning: An adjunct to therapy. In Kovich, K.M. & Bermann, D.E. (eds.): *Head injury: A Guide to Functional Outcomes in Occupational Therapy*. Gaithersburg, MD: Aspen Publishers.

Ploughman, M. Corbett, D. (2004) Can forced-use therapy be clinically applied after stroke? An exploratory randomized controlled trial. *Archives of Physical Medicine and Rehabilitation* 85(9):1417–1423.

Shepherd, R. Carr, J. (1998) The shoulder following stroke: Preserving musculoskeletal integrity for function. *Topics in Stroke Rehabilitation* 4(4):35–53.

Sohlberg, M.M., Mateer, C.A. (1987) Effectiveness of an attentional training program. *Journal of Clinical and Experimental Neuropsychology* 9:117–130.

Strank, C. (1997) Physical disabilities and their implications on driving. *Work: A Journal of Prevention, Assessment and Rehabilitation* 8(3):261–266.

Taub, E., Uswatte, G. (2000) Constraint-induced movement therapy based on behavioral neuroscience. In Frank, R.G. & Elliot, T.R., (eds.): *Handbook of Rehabilitation Psychology*. Washington DC: American Psychological Association, pp. 475–496.

Toglia, J.P. (1994) Lesson 4: Attention and memory. In Royeen, C.B. (ed.): *AOTA Self-Study Series: Cognitive Rehabilitation*. Bethesda, MD: American Occupational Therapy Association.

Trombly, C. (1997a) Remediating motor control and performance through traditional therapeutic approaches. In Trombly, C.A. (ed.): *Occupational Therapy for Physical Dysfunction*, 4th ed. Philadelphia: Williams & Wilkins, pp. 437–446.

Trombly, C. (1997b) Theoretical foundations for practice. In Trombly, C.A. (ed.): *Occupational Therapy for Physical Dysfunction*, 4th ed. Philadelphia: Williams & Wilkins, pp. 15–27.

Zasler, N.D., McNeny, R., Heywood, P.G. (1992) Rehabilitative management of olfactory and gustatory dysfunction following brain injury. *Journal of Head Trauma Rehabilitation* 7(1):66–75.

Zorowitz, R., Idank, D., Ikai, T., Hughes, M., Johnston, M. (1995) Shoulder subluxation after stroke: A comparison of four supports. *Archives of Physical Medicine and Rehabilitation* 76:763–771.

Zoltan, B. (1996) *Vision, Perception and Cognition: A Manual for the Evaluation and Treatment of the Neurologically Impaired Adult*, 3rd ed. Thorofare, NJ: SLACK Inc.

13
Rehabilitation of Speech, Language and Swallowing Disorders

PEGGY KRAMER, DEENA SHEIN, AND JENNIFER NAPOLITANO

The speech-language pathology team is a dynamic component of the interdisciplinary neuro-rehabilitation team and is involved in many facets of care. The ultimate goal of this discipline is the restoration of communication competence, resolution of dysphagia, and improvement of oral motor function. The speech-language pathologist (SLP) works collaboratively with the acquired brain injury (ABI) survivor, family, and clinical team to create a comprehensive rehabilitation plan of care aimed at improving functional gains, independence, and quality of life.

Of critical importance in the neuro-rehabilitation process is the restoration of the survivor's communication competence. Without a means of communicating even the most basic needs, safety and well-being can be compromised, and the survivor's frustration can build very quickly, resulting in verbal outbursts or a shutting down of all attempts to communicate. Also of vital importance to the survivor is the restoration of swallowing function. Dysphagia, or disruption of swallowing, can compromise both the health and quality of life of individuals following an ABI and must be addressed early on in rehabilitation.

It is essential that the SLP be aware of evidence-based practice and best-practice recommendations when evaluating and treating survivors of ABI. As this is a rapidly advancing field, it is critical to remain up-to-date on research regarding effectiveness of treatment strategies (e.g., cognitive rehabilitation), and new technological developments (e.g., electrical stimulation, augmentative communication).

Evaluation

The evaluation process is initiated by a referral from the physician. SLPs begin their assessment when first greeting the survivor and his/her significant others. The combination of clinical interview, coupled with objective measures, will provide the foundation for a comprehensive evaluation. The interview includes obtaining information about social, educational, vocational, and medical history, as well as orientation status. Review of medical records is essential, as many ABI survivors are not able to report their history or current status accurately.

Interviewing family members is also important, as they can report observations regarding changes in communication which are not reflected in records, and of which the survivor may be unaware. Additional information is obtained regarding native language, handedness, need for eyeglasses, and present diet, including any restrictions or alternative consistencies for solids and liquids. Finally, eliciting comments from survivors related to their primary complaints regarding their communication competence provides information about their level of insight. The person's diagnosis, age, severity of impairment, and observations made during the interview, will determine which objective tests are chosen for the assessment.

An audiologic screening can help identify individuals that have hearing impairments that would interfere with their communication function. Pure tones are presented bilaterally via earphones at 1,000, 2,000, and 4,000 Hz at 25 dB for adults (ASHA, 2004). If the screening is failed, the individual can be referred for a comprehensive audiologic evaluation by an ear, nose, and throat (ENT) specialist or audiologist. Follow up testing will determine the severity of the hearing loss and the need for aural rehabilitation.

An oral peripheral examination is an essential part of the evaluation following an acquired brain injury. Movement and strength of structures including the tongue, jaw, and lips as well as velopharyngeal sufficiency need to be assessed. Taping a survivor's voice during the evaluation is helpful for assessing vocal quality, including pitch, volume, prosody, and speaking patterns, and can serve as a tool for providing feedback to the individual regarding his/her vocal quality. In survivors with known or suspected dysphagia, a swallowing evaluation will also be performed, as will be addressed in a later section of this chapter.

There are a number of evaluation tools that have been developed for the assessment of language/communication and cognition in the neurologically impaired individual. These include the Apraxia Battery for Adults, Second Edition (Dabul, 2000); Boston Diagnostic Aphasia Examination (Goodglass & Kaplan, 1983); Brief Test of Head Injury (Estabrooks & Hotz, 1991); Frenchay Dysarthria Assessment (Enderby, 1983); Measure of Cognitive-Linguistic Abilities (Ellmo et al., 1995); Minnesota Test for Differential Diagnosis of Aphasia (Schuell, 1965); Porch Index of Communicative Ability (Porch, 2001); Ross Information Processing Assessment, Second Edition (Ross-Swain, 1996); Scales of Cognitive Ability for Traumatic Brain Injury (Adamovich & Henderson, 1992); and Western Aphasia Battery (Kertesz, 1982). A complete listing of assessment tools can be found at the ASHA website (www.asha.org, "Directory of Speech-Language Pathology Assessment Instruments").

Communication/Language Deficits Following ABI

The results of the evaluation will lead to the formulation of the functional diagnosis, severity of the impairment, goals, and treatment plan. Communication deficits post-ABI can result from impairments in both the motor aspects of speech and/or the ability to use and understand language. The former include dysarthria and apraxia. The latter include various types of aphasia, cognitive impairments (e.g., memory, problem solving), and impairments in social communication (e.g., pragmatics).

Motor Speech Disorders

Motor speech disorders, apraxia and dysarthria, are caused by neurological impairments resulting in disorders of voice, resonance, articulation, and/or respiration. ASHA (2004) has identified a preferred practice pattern related to motor speech intervention in adults, which supports interventions including "improving accuracy, precision, timing and coordination of articulation." Apraxia is characterized by deficits in programming of sequential and volitional movement of the articulators (e.g., jaw, lips, tongue, cheeks) and is not caused by muscle weakness (Beukelman & Yorkson, 1991). Oral apraxia, where the survivor demonstrates groping behaviors, may be present (Gillis, 1996). Apraxia is not structurally related, as there is no weakness or slowness of movement or discoordination of articulators. The diagnosis of oral apraxia is most common in survivors with left-hemisphere cerebrovascular involvement and common among those diagnosed with aphasia (Beukelman & Yorkston, 1991).

Treatment approaches include rate modification, imitation of phoneme, and words and phrases of increasing length. As an example, using key words, such as "cook," facilitates the production of /k/ in initial and final position and aids in the kinesthetic awareness of tongue placement during phoneme production. Tapping of fingers or using pacing boards aids with establishing proper rate of speech. Prosody improvements can be targeted by drills using contrasting stress to improve variation of intonation and rhythm—for example, "*I* am hungry"; "I *AM* hungry"; "I am *HUNGRY!*" (Chapey, 2001).

Dysarthria refers to disruption of speech intelligibility due to "disturbances in muscle control over the speech mechanism due to damage of the central or peripheral nervous system" (Darley, et al. 1969). Diagnosing dysarthria is difficult in that the survivor's speech may be compromised by weakened muscle strength, reduced range of motion of the articulators, reduced speed of motion, and imprecise articulatory contact. In addition, acoustic changes may include reduced prosody, vocal quality, pitch, and volume due to respiratory insufficiency.

Treatment of dysarthria focuses on restoration, compensatory strategy implementation—or, in the event of poor prognosis for speech recovery—assessment and development of an augmentative communication system. Of paramount importance is education related to the disorder to aid with comprehension of the deficit, the rationale behind treatment, and counseling to help with adjustment to potential lifelong deficits. Goals include improving awareness of speaking habits, posturing, breathing patterns, rate of speech, and prosody. Yorkston (1996) reviewed the effectiveness of therapeutic intervention for dysarthria. Treatment may include prosthetic devices such as a palatal lift prosthesis to aid velopharyngeal closure, reduce hypernasality, and increase intraoral pressure. Pacing boards and metronomes can be utilized to slow speaking rate. Other strategies/techniques may include sitting, positioning, and pushing or bearing down to improve breath support; reducing rate of speech; and improving articulatory contact using oral motor exercises to strengthen and improve range of motion of articulators. Using audio and visual recordings is an excellent form of feedback and often useful in improving awareness of behaviors related to the disorder (Duffy, 1995). Word production drills, such as contrasting word pairs (e.g., bat, hat; map, lap; match, catch) and rapid changing word lists (e.g. may, me, my, mow, moo) are examples of additional treatments.

Augmentative/Alternative Communication (AAC)   General

According to ASHA's position statement (ASHA, 1991), AAC is an area of clinical research and educational practice for SLPs and audiologists that attempts to compensate and facilitate temporarily or permanently for the impairment and disability patterns of individuals with severe expressive and/or language comprehension disorders. AAC may be required for individuals demonstrating impairments in gestural, spoken and or written modes of communication. Acquired brain injury survivors may have severe communication impairments of this nature, and many could benefit from using AAC strategies (Glennen & DeCoste, 1997). These individuals exhibit significant difficulty effectively communicating with their families, friends, and co-workers. AAC is used when verbal expression is not considered to be a functional means of communication, and the ABI survivor is willing to consider alternative means of communicating. The goal of an AAC team working with an individual with an ABI is to provide communication assistance so that he or she is able to participate effectively in a rehabilitation program and be able to communicate ongoing needs (Beukelman & Mirenda, 1998).

Manual Systems vs. Electronic Systems

AAC devices can be divided into two general classifications, manual or electronic (see Table 13.1). Manual devices include object boards, single switch communicators, picture communication boards, wordbooks, and letter boards. By contrast, electronic devices employ the use of computerized software programs displayed on dynamic screens.

TABLE 13.1. Manual vs. Electronic Augmentative Communication Devices

Manual (light tech)	Electronic (high tech)
No technical problems	More independent
Customized/individualized	Accumulated Vocabulary to be used
Inexpensive	Societal perception that person is more intelligent
Ready for immediate use	Faster output/opportunities for more
Portable	communication partners

Major Features of AAC Devices

Mode of Access or Selection

Direct selection is a mode of access that requires the use of an upper extremity (hand, finger) or the head (eye gaze, optical pointer, mouth stick) to select the intended target. Indirect selection refers to the use of auditory or visual scanning to choose the intended target. Scanning involves the movement of a pointer or cursor that is automatic and continuous according to a present pattern. User indicates a selection by activating a switch to interrupt the cursor in order to make a selection (Cohen, 2004).

Language Characteristics

Most AAC devices operate via a symbol set or symbol system. Examples of typical symbol systems in hierarchical order from most to least concrete include: use of common objects, color photographs, line drawings, printed words or letters (Glennen & DeCoste, 1997; Cohen, 2004).

Output

Output refers to how the listener receives the message and can be in spoken or written form. Almost all currently available electronic AAC systems provide the user with the capability of producing spoken messages. Speech output allows the user to project voice and to communicate with many partners across distances. Two basic types are digitized (recorded human voice) and synthesized (speech is artificially produced). Some AAC devices have paper output consisting of small strip printers to keep the device small and portable. Computer-based AAC systems can use standard printers for output (Glennen & DeCoste, 1997). In addition, technologically advanced AAC devices have ways to enhance the rate of output (i.e., use of abbreviation, coding, word-prediction, and vocabulary storage).

Assessment

The AAC evaluation process should be performed as a team effort involving the patient, SLP, OT, PT, psychologist, and family member or caregiver (Glennen & DeCoste, 1997). Evaluation procedures range from naturalistic observations of the individual, to the use of formal and informal tests, including computerized assessment systems (Glennen & DeCoste, 1997). Naturalistic observation helps the SLP build a system based on the survivor's non-verbal communication strengths, which include gestures, facial expression, pointing, yes/no indication, and crying and/or laughing. Assessments include obtaining pertinent background information, speech, language and cognitive communication abilities, limitations of current system and communication needs, sensory function, postural and motor abilities, access selection techniques, symbol form, vocabulary storage, and rate-enhancement techniques (Cohen, 2004). The heterogeneous nature of this population requires the ongoing adjustment of evaluation and training procedures to meet the ultimate goal of communicative competence within a variety of functional contexts (Fletcher, 1997).

Acceptance

Individuals who receive an AAC system often follow a pattern of adoption and abandonment (Fletcher, 1997). It is vital that the individual be actively involved in the selection of an AAC system following a comprehensive evaluation process. Consequently, they will be more likely to use the system effectively, feel a greater sense of commitment, and be less likely to abandon the device. Training communicative partners (e.g., spouses, caregivers) is essential to facilitate carryover and may increase long-term acceptance of the AAC device (Fletcher, 1997). SLPs should educate the family/ caregiver on the benefits of AAC, to provide an outlet, reduce frustration, and facilitate communication rather than impede verbal communication. Survivors and families should also be counseled that the use of an AAC system might be temporary. While serving to increase immediate functional communication, it can be used as a bridge to the re-acquisition of speech.

Dysphagia

Historically, the assessment and treatment of dysphagia, or swallowing disorders, was not considered to be within the scope of practice of a speech-language pathologist (SLP). Today, however, dysphagia is in the forefront of the field and the management of swallowing disorders is considered to be a predominant aspect of the speech-language pathologist's role across neuro-rehabilitation settings.

Dysphagia and Its Causes

Dysphagia can be defined as when any one or more of the stages of swallowing becomes impaired due to changes in sensation, muscle strength, and coordination, whereby the patient can no longer safely or efficiently swallow (Logemann, 1998). Dysphagia can range from mild to severe and can be caused by physical and/or cognitive impairments with implications including malnutrition, dehydration, and aspiration pneumonia. There are many different diagnoses which can cause dysphagia, including cerebrovascular accident (CVA), traumatic brain injury (TBI), spinal cord injury, Guillian-Barre syndrome, tracheostomy and/or ventilator dependency, brain tumors, multiple sclerosis, Alzheimer's disease or other dementias, and movement disorders such as Parkinson's and Huntington's diseases.

When working in a neurological rehabilitation setting with patients who have concomitant diagnoses of an acquired brain injury (ABI) and dysphagia, impairments such as disorientation, agitation, impulsivity, decreased level of alertness, initiation, mood, attention, memory, problem solving skills, safety judgment, visual-perceptual deficits, insight, and poor motor planning can affect a patient's potential for carryover. According to Halper et al. (1999), the severity of the cognitive communicative deficits will determine the type of management program and its functional outcomes rather than the integrity of the physiological swallowing mechanism. Therefore, it is essential to involve the patient, his or her family, and the entire interdisciplinary rehabilitation team to enable a successful recovery.

Anatomy and Physiology of a Normal Swallow

A normal swallow includes four phases: the oral preparatory phase, the oral phase, the pharyngeal phase, and the esophageal phase. During the *oral prep phase* the lips, tongue, mandible, dentition, soft palate, and buccal cavity are engaged in order to arrange, chew, and mix with saliva to form and prepare the bolus of food that will eventually be swallowed. The *oral phase* is a transfer phase consisting of moving the cohesive bolus anterior to posterior using the tongue. The tongue propels the food posterior until the pharyngeal swallow is triggered. This phase is approximately 1 second in duration. The *pharyngeal phase* is an involuntary phase. During this phase the swallow reflex is triggered and the airway closes off at several levels (epiglottis, false and true vocal folds) to prevent a bolus from entering the airway. This phase is also approximately 1 second in duration. The final stage is the *esophageal phase.* This phase consists of the bolus continuing through the esophagus into the stomach via peristalsis. This phase is between 8 and 20 seconds in duration.

The normal swallow is an intricate dynamic process that involves sensation, range of motion (ROM), strength, and involuntary reflex response. In order to achieve normal swallow function, all of the phases must occur in a timely, coordinated manner. If there is a breakdown at any point along the mechanism during the swallow process, total swallow integrity may be compromised.

Dysphagia and Aspiration

Aspiration and aspiration pneumonia are major risks associated with dysphagia. Aspiration refers to a food or liquid bolus falling below the level of the vocal folds, into the airway. Breakdowns in the normal swallow process can result in bolus penetration into the larynx, which increases the risk of aspiration. Aspiration can occur before, during, or after the pharyngeal swallow (Lazarus, 1989). Saliva can also be aspirated; therefore proper oral hygiene is critical to reduce the risk of aspiration of oral bacteria. As a result of ABI, patients may have impaired sensation of the swallow mechanism. Therefore, signs and symptoms of aspiration may be delayed or silent. *Silent aspiration* refers to aspiration of a bolus with no overt behavioral signs or symptoms. According to estimates, silent aspiration may occur in up to 40% of patients with dysphagia, and it is not generally identifiable during the bedside swallow evaluation (Murray & Carrau, 2001).

Evaluation of Swallowing Disorders

Subjective Assessment Procedures

The bedside clinical evaluation assesses both structure and function of the swallow mechanism at the oral preparatory, oral, and pharyngeal phases of the swallow.

This involves assessing sensation, strength, and ROM (both volitional and reflexive responses) of the oral-pharyngeal structures. Assessment includes gathering a full medical history, noting pulmonary history, gastrointestinal history, nutrition and hydration status, current medications, and surgical history. A bedside evaluation also includes assessing the patient's cognitive-linguistic, voice, speech, and behavioral status as they impact current swallow function. During the bedside evaluation, the SLP may work with the occupational therapist to further assess a patient's positioning and self-feeding abilities.

Presentation of Food/Liquid During Bedside Evaluation

During the swallow assessment, the SLP assesses a variety of consistencies and textures with the aim of recommending the least restrictive safe and appropriate diet. The SLP assesses as many consistencies as possible given the patient's current level of alertness, cognitive, and physical impairment. Ideally, an evaluation should be conducted within the context of a full meal, as opposed to an isolated event, in order to simulate the patient's everyday naturalistic environment.

The following illustrates the signs and symptoms of dysphagia found during a bedside evaluation.

No technical

Bedside Findings: Signs and Symptoms of Dysphagia

General Findings

1. Facial asymmetry
2. Refusal/avoidance of specific foods
3. Abnormal head or body position
4. Reduced appetite or weight loss of unknown origin
5. Fever of unknown origin (possibly as result of aspiration)

Oral Findings

1. Hyper- or hypo-tonicity in oral facial structures
2. Decreased oral sensation (taste and smell)
3. Decreased lip, tongue, cheek ROM and strength
4. Food or liquid loss from mouth
5. Drooling
6. Slowed or inadequate chewing, biting, manipulation, transfer of bolus
7. Increased or decreased saliva production
8. Poor oral hygiene (gums, dentition)
9. Residue on tongue and/or pocketing in mouth
10. Expectorating/removing food from the mouth

Pharyngeal Findings

1. Delayed or absent swallow reflex
2. Decreased laryngeal elevation and excursion
3. Wet or gurgly vocal quality

4. Coughing before, during, after swallowing
5. Sneezing or watery eyes
6. Frequent throat clearing
7. Pharyngeal stridor
8. Regurgitation through the nose and/or mouth
9. Complaints of pain upon swallow or food getting "stuck"
10. Change in respiratory status

Objective Assessment Procedures   *General*

Modified Barium Swallow Study (MBS)

The SLP collaborates with a radiologist when performing a Modified Barium Swallow Study (also referred to as a Videofluorographic study). The MBS is a comprehensive, dynamic evaluation of all phases of swallowing requiring technical instrumentation and clinical expertise to interpret results. The recommendation of an MBS often follows the identification of dysphagia risk factors found during the clinical bedside evaluation (Murray & Carrau, 2001). The patient is presented with a variety of food and liquid consistencies, which have been impregnated with barium. The barium enables the pathway of the food and liquid to be visualized on a monitor through each stage of the swallow. "The modified barium swallow study is designed to assess not only whether the patient is aspirating, but also why, so appropriate treatment can be initiated" (Logemann, 1998). The study serves to identify abnormalities in the anatomy and physiology of the swallow mechanism, as well as the etiology and severity of potential aspiration. Furthermore, it helps to determine the safest diet texture as well as compensatory techniques to facilitate the safest most efficient swallow.

Flexible Endoscopic Evaluation of Swallowing (FEES) and Flexible Endoscopic Evaluation with Sensory Testing (FEESST)

In 1992, Flexible Endoscopic Evaluation of Swallowing (FEES) was put into ASHA's Scope of Practice and Policy Statement. Under the supervision of an otolaryngologist the SLP may perform a FEES, a test which involves a fiber optic endoscope that passes through the nasal cavity to a position above the epiglottis. It serves to examine the anatomy and physiology of the oral cavity and the pharynx from above, before and after the swallow (Aviv, 2000). Anatomical structures obstruct the camera's view during a brief period of airway closure, commonly referred to as the "white-out" phase.

The FEESST refers to the addition of sensory testing via an air pulse presented above the level of the vocal folds. This provides insight into the patient's ability to protect the airway and prevent aspiration.

Both the MBS and the FEES are used to gain objective information that cannot be obtained by the bedside evaluation alone, and serve to guide the SLP in appropriate diet progression. Both procedures are generally well tolerated, recorded on VCR or CD, begin with small graduated amounts and end with more challenging swallows

TABLE 13.2. Comparison of FEES vs. MBS

FEES	MBS
Regular food, actual meal tray (no barium)	Barium-impregnated foods
No radiation	Radiation
Can be used therapeutically	Limited therapeutic use
Portable	Radiology necessary
More cost effective	May view oral, pharyngeal and esophageal stages
View pharyngeal stage only	
Assess eating fatigue as risk factor	Time limited exam
Bedside or in chair	Videofluoroscopic imaging chair
More accessible	Not invasive
Can test patients difficult to transport (vent dependent, obese patients)	Indirect view
Direct view of surface anatomy, excellent view of larynx	Minimal risk factors
Useful for biofeedback	
Can be performed on cognitively impaired	
Patients do not have to follow directions	Cannot measure sensory threshold; however, silent aspiration/penetration is indicative of decreased sensation
No radiologist necessary, easier to schedule	

of each consistency (Aviv, 2000). In the field of speech-language pathology, MBS is seen as the gold standard and is most often recommended since it enables all phases of the swallow to be assessed. FEES is contraindicated for people who are on blood thinners, have uncontrolled seizure disorders, or acute cardiac problems (Aviv, 2000). However, FEES is useful in gaining direct information regarding vocal fold adduction (airway protection) during phonation and breath hold, which cannot be seen on the MBS. Table 13.2 highlights the primary differences between FEES and MBS.

The assessment of dysphagia is an ongoing, dynamic process, as patients demonstrate improvements and/or regressions in functioning, and may require frequent objective and/or subjective reevaluations on a case-by-case basis.

Treatment of Swallowing Disorders

A treatment plan can be developed and implemented following the completion of assessment procedures. A multidisciplinary approach is essential in order for the treatment plan to be carried out effectively. The team includes the SLP, occupational therapist, dietician, dentist, nurse, social worker, physician, family members, and/or caregivers. Patient and family education is an integral aspect of the treatment plan.

The SLP utilizes multiple approaches to swallow safety, including restorative therapy, compensatory techniques, and diet modification. An important decision needs to be made regarding whether to provide direct or indirect therapy. Direct therapy refers to the use of food and/or liquid during treatment, whereas indirect therapy restricts the use of food or liquid as a treatment modality. This decision is based on formal test results regarding both frank aspiration and the risk of aspiration.

Restorative Therapy Techniques

Oral-Pharyngeal Exercises

Oral-pharyngeal exercises are widely used to improve awareness, strength, movement, coordination, and volitional control of the lips, tongue, cheeks, mandible, larynx, and vocal folds. Vocal fold closure is a key factor in preventing aspiration; therefore vocal fold adduction exercises are important for patients whose vocal folds fail to close sufficiently. Bolus control and chewing exercises can also be used to improve fine motor coordination of the tongue. However, only limited data is available to demonstrate the efficacy of oral-pharyngeal exercises on positive clinical outcomes (i.e., weight gain, reduced aspiration), for patients with neurological impairments (Murray & Carrau, 2001).

Swallow Maneuvers

In addition to oral-pharyngeal exercises, the patient can be trained to perform specific maneuvers that are employed to improve volitional control over various aspects of the pharyngeal phase of the swallow. These include the following:

- Supraglottic—used to improve airway (vocal fold) closure and increase pharyngeal swallow reflex triggering
- Super-supraglottic—used to increase airway closure
- Effortful swallow—used to increase posterior movement of tongue base
- Mendelsohn—used to increase laryngeal movement and coordination of swallow

These maneuvers require alertness, physical effort, and the ability to follow specific complex directions. Therefore, they may not be a feasible treatment modality for patients who exhibit significant cognitive-linguistic impairments.

Thermal Stimulation

The purpose of this technique is to increase sensory awareness in the oral cavity prior to the swallow and to increase the timeliness of the pharyngeal swallow reflex response. Thermal stimulation requires the use of a laryngeal mirror, held in ice water for approximately 10 seconds, then used to stimulate the anterior faucial arches 4 or 5 times in rapid fashion. This is followed by a command to swallow saliva. Ideally, stimulation will be repeated 3–4 times a day for ten trials. It is theorized that touch with thermal stimulation provides heightened oral awareness and an alerting stimulus to the brainstem and brain to trigger the pharyngeal swallow faster than it would in the absence of stimulation (Rosenbek et al., 1998).

Deep Pharyngeal Neuromuscular Stimulation (DPNS)

Deep pharyngeal neuromuscular stimulation is defined as a systemized therapeutic method for pharyngeal dysphagia that utilizes direct neuromuscular stimulation to the pharyngeal musculature to restore muscle strength, endurance, reflex response, and reflex coordination for a restored, coordinated swallow. DPNS utilizes iced lemon glycerin swabs applied directly to eleven specific stimulation points in the oral-pharyngeal cavities. The interaction of cold temperature, sour taste, and deep pressure applied by the SLP works to elicit a motor response (i.e., tongue base retraction, velopharyngeal closure, laryngeal elevation, pharyngeal wall constriction, vocal fold closure, swallow reflex trigger, and saliva production) (Stefakanos, 1999, revised 2005).

Neuromuscular Electrical Stimulation for the Swallow (NMES)

Electrical stimulation is a restorative treatment modality that has traditionally been used by physical and occupational therapists. It has recently been gaining increased attention as a treatment for dysphagia and is currently being used in conjunction with traditional dysphagia therapy. NMES is the use of electrical stimulation for the activation of muscles via stimulation of intact peripheral motor nerves through a transcutaneous medium. The major treatment goals are to strengthen weak muscles, maintain or gain ROM, facilitate voluntary motor control, and increase sensory awareness (Wijting & Freed, 2003). The basic underlying principle of NMES is forced intervention, which refers to using an external source of energy, such as an NMES device, to move the muscles to a greater degree than a patient could on his own with traditional exercise, and dynamically simulate a total swallow. NMES begins by introducing a low-level stimulus to elicit a sensory response. The intensity of the stimulus is then increased in order to achieve a motor response (contraction). Over time the treatment aims to build patient's tolerance for increased intensity of contractions. Electrical stimulation may be paired with traditional therapy and food and/or liquid trials, as appropriate.

VitalStim® (Wijting & Freed, 2003) is an FDA-cleared method to promote swallowing through the application of neuromuscular electrical stimulation. Questions remain in the field regarding the type of electrical current used, manipulation of parameters within NMES devices, and electrode placement and size. Further research is needed to determine the efficacy of various NMES devices and methods in the treatment of dysphagia.

Compensatory Treatment Techniques

Two categories of compensatory techniques are used in conjunction with restorative dysphagia therapy as part of a holistic treatment plan.

Postural Techniques

A compensatory strategy such as the use of a head, neck, or body postural change generally requires less physical effort on the part of the patient and potentially

TABLE 13.3. Diet consistencies

Least restrictive to most restrictive consistencies	
Food	Liquid
Unrestricted diet	Thin
Mechanically altered	Nectar
Ground	Honey
Puree	
Therapeutic Feeding by SLP only	
NPO	

temporarily changes the dimensions of the pharynx and the direction of food flow. Postural changes have been shown to improve oral-pharyngeal transit times, reduce the risk of aspiration, and decrease the amount of residue after the swallow (Logemann, 1998). Widely used postures include chin tuck, head back, head rotation to the weaker side, and lying down on one side. In general practice, carryover of postural techniques may be compromised in patients with moderate–severe cognitive impairments. Further compensatory strategies for a patient with oral and pharyngeal deficits may include an SLP's recommendations to remain upright for 30 minutes post-meal to reduce risk of aspiration, take controlled bites and sips, alternate solids and liquids, cueing the patient to perform multiple swallows, and training the patient to clear or remove food pocketing in the mouth. These strategies also may help improve the patient's management of food orally and his or her ability to clear possible pharyngeal residue to reduce the risk of aspiration.

Diet Modifications

Diet modification is another component in the treatment of dysphagia; however, this should be considered as a last resort in treatment planning. Oral nutrition and hydration is the ultimate goal for patients with dysphagia. Currently there are attempts being made to develop a nationally recognized dysphagia diet (Murry & Carrau, 2001). However, at the present time, dysphagia diets vary across facilities. Even though there is variation, diets are typically developed in a stepwise progression of bolus consistencies. It is the goal of the SLP to improve the patient's swallow integrity in order to progress to the least restrictive, safe and appropriate diet. Table 13.3 demonstrates the progression of diet textures.

Quality of Life

Oral vs. Non-Oral Feeding

Since it is unsafe for certain patients to eat by mouth, it is determined that they must receive nutrition and hydration via alternative, non-oral means, a status known as NPO, or non-perioral. The decision of whether to have a feeding tube inserted for non-oral feeding is a crucial one for patients and families and they often do not understand that feeding tubes can be temporary. In these cases, counseling should clearly emphasize the benefits to the patient (i.e., good nutrition and hydration enabling them to do better in therapy) rather than the loss of oral feeding. It is important to note that aspiration does not always lead to aspiration pneumonia. A patient may evidence aspiration, however be tolerating a perioral (PO) diet that is against the recommendations of the rehabilitation team without developing aspiration pneumonia. Patients and families may choose to go against the recommendations for a specific dysphagia diet, and it is the SLP's responsibility to educate them regarding the potential health risks of aspiration.

HV is a 60-year-old male status post right-side CVA with left-sided weakness. Prior to the CVA, HV was independent and worked as a custodian. Moderate receptive and mild expressive language deficits included difficulty with auditory processing, word finding, and verbal fluency. Cognitive deficits were demonstrated in memory, attention, problem solving, and impulsivity. An MBS study done while in acute inpatient rehabilitation revealed decreased oral motor control, premature spillage, delayed swallow trigger with silent penetration on all liquid consistencies. Silent aspiration with delayed cough was noted on thin liquids. Head turn to the left eliminated aspiration. Upon admission to the subacute rehab unit, initial bedside evaluation results indicated moderate oro-pharyngeal dysphagia characterized by facial asymmetry and deficits in oral motor strength and ROM, mastication, bolus formation and transfer, and anterior food loss from lips on the left side. Pharyngeally, delayed swallow trigger, decreased laryngeal elevation, and audible swallow were noted. Wet vocal quality with cup sip trials of nectar and coughing on cup sip trials of thin liquid were evident. Honey thick liquids were tolerated without overt behavioral signs/symptoms of aspiration. Diet recommendations were for mechanical soft foods with honey thick liquids.

Compensatory strategies taught included remaining upright 30 minutes post-meal, small bites/sips, checking mouth for pocketing, and alternating solids/liquids. Restorative treatment goals included performing OMEs to improve oral motor strength and ROM, laryngeal elevation for airway protection, and NMES to improve swallow integrity. HV demonstrated difficulty isolating tongue/jaw movements. During therapy he required repetition, cues to decrease impulsivity, and increase attention. Carryover improved over time. Vital Stim® therapy was used for NMES. Over time, HV demonstrated increased tolerance for electrical stimulation, but continued to demonstrate decreased sensation on his left side. He tolerated NMES for 30–50 min a day, paired with an "effortful" swallow and head turn to the left with trials of thin liquids. Increased management of thin liquids was evident after 9–12 days of this therapy regimen. Repeat MBS revealed an improvement in swallow function, with mild oral-pharyngeal dysphagia characterized by decreased tongue base retraction and untimely swallow causing premature spillage; however, no penetration or aspiration was noted. Diet recommendations were regular foods cut up into small pieces, and cup sips of thin liquids. Recommendations for compensatory techniques were modified to include no straws, remaining upright 30 minutes post-meal, dry swallows to clear any residue in oro-pharynx, and monitoring for signs/symptoms of aspiration, pulmonary problems, and nutrition. HV was discharged to home with recommendations for outpatient ST.

Cognitive-Communication

According to Muma (cited in Chapey, 2001) there are three components of language: cognitive, linguistic, and communicative. The cognitive component refers to information processing, including recognition, comprehension, memory, convergent thinking, divergent thinking, and problem-solving. The linguistic component relates to the form (phonology, morphology and syntax) and content (topic, subject and meaning) of language. The purpose of using language refers to the communicative component of language (Chapey, 2001). All three components are interrelated. The American Speech Language Hearing Association (ASHA) has adopted the term "cognitive-communication" to describe deficits in communication. Coelho and DeRuyter (1996) note, "cognitive communicative impairments are the result of deficits in linguistic and nonlinguistic cognitive functions." There is an interdependent relationship between cognitive and communication skills, and it is important for an SLP to address cognitive deficits as these difficulties can interfere with the ability to use strategies to improve deficits in motor speech, swallowing or language.

The speech-language pathologist evaluates expressive (verbal and written) and receptive (verbal and written) language elements, as well as pragmatic (social) aspects of language. Cognitive-communication skills are also assessed, including attention, memory, planning, organizational skills, reasoning, and problem-solving (Gillis, 1996). Collaboration and sharing evaluation results between the neuropsychologist and occupational therapist helps to develop a comprehensive understanding of the ABI survivor's language, cognitive and functional impairments, and forms a basis for the development of a holistic treatment plan.

SLPs participate in the rehabilitation of cognitive deficits by assisting the ABI survivor to develop compensatory techniques and strategies to interact more effectively with those around them, and function more independently. For example, survivors can be taught to use aids or devices (e.g., daily planners, digital recorders/reminders) to facilitate the ability to organize and remember important information. There is evidence to support such strategy training (Cicerone et al., 2005) and that these can be beneficial to individuals many years post-brain injury (Ownsworth & McFarland, 1999).

CI, a 32-year-old married mother of a two young children status post aneurysm rupture, attended a neuro-rehabilitation inpatient program for 9 months and then received 3 months of home therapy. She was very friendly and social, calling everyone "girlfriend" (as she could not recall names) and would have two breakfasts (having forgotten she'd eaten) and call her family members numerous times between the hours of 8:00 and 9:00 A.M. looking for assurance that they would be there at dinnertime.

Each time she called, it was the same exact discussion. Her family was reluctant to give her feedback about her repetitiveness, as they didn't want to upset her. She was unaware of the severity of her memory difficulties, though she was putting on weight and constantly patting herself with powder because she couldn't recall whether she put on deodorant. Her family had recently moved to a new address and CI could only recall her former address. Her short-term memory was virtually nonexistent.

Using a memory book that contained highly structured sections including 12 hours to write specific tasks and activities (e.g., taking medication), places to keep track of incoming and outgoing phone calls, and calendars to aid with orientation were specifically designed for CI. Therapy included daily use of this book, including functional memory assignments, such as remembering to call her SLP at a certain day and time to tell her about the a story from the evening news. Through repetitive use of this book, CI began to demonstrate a greater ability to function independently. She became a very good compensator for a severe memory deficit.

Structured problem-solving training has been found to be an effective approach for rehabilitation of executive function deficits following ABI (Cicerone, 2005). Such training can be provided during individual or group sessions. When facilitated by a SLP, such sessions can address multiple goals, including receptive, expressive and social communication skills. Group feedback can also provide an opportunity to develop awareness and insight.

Aphasia

According to Holland et al. (1996), aphasia is defined as a language impairment associated primarily with focal brain damage, which usually involves the language-dominant cerebral hemisphere. In the large majority of individuals, this is the left hemisphere of the brain. Brain tumors, closed-head injuries, infection, and trauma may be causes of aphasia; however the predominant cause is stroke. According to the American Heart Association and the American Stroke Association's Fact sheet (2006) there are 700,000 strokes, new or recurrent, in America each year.

Aphasia disrupts a person's ability to communicate, both receptively (reading and listening) and expressively (writing and speaking), affecting not only words but numbers as well. Aphasic deficits are often accompanied by physical ramifications such as weakening or paralysis of upper and/or lower extremities. Chapey (2001) describes the aphasic survivor as having "lost functional, spontaneous language, or the ability to use connected language . . . " Aphasia affects the survivor and his or her caregivers. It can be extremely disruptive to one's social, vocational, and educational life, causing feelings of frustration, depression, and isolation.

Assessment of Aphasia

Assessment of aphasia begins with a thorough analysis of the survivor's ability to produce and understand language in all modalities: speaking, listening, reading, and writing. A language sample is a valuable tool to identify *paraphasias* that, according to Damasio (as cited in Chapey, 2001), refer to incorrect or unintended word or sound substitutions (e.g., "pea" instead of "peach"), or *neologisms* in which a novel word is substituted (e.g., "froxil" instead of "finger"). The term *jargon* is used to describe a condition in which most of the survivor's speech is filled with paraphasias. Proper diagnosis of type of aphasia is essential in order to determine appropriate treatment interventions. The general term "fluent aphasia" refers to a variety of specific conditions, including conduction aphasia, Wernicke's aphasia, and transcortical sensory aphasia. Conduction aphasics are described as fluent, with repetition of words more difficult in comparison to their spontaneous speech. According to Goodglass and Kaplan (as cited in Chapey, 2001), the primary impairment lies in the proper choice and sequencing of phonemes. Wernicke's aphasia is characterized by articulate speech with impaired comprehension; sound and word substitutions are typical, as are difficulties with writing, reading, and word finding. Transcortical aphasics are articulate with jargon and neologisms but have difficulty with auditory comprehension although they have intact repetition abilities.

The category of "nonfluent aphasias" includes Broca's, transcortical motor, and global aphasia. Goodglass and Kaplan (as cited in Chapey, 2001) describe Broca's aphasia as characterized by impaired articulation, restricted vocabulary, and grammar, but with relatively intact auditory comprehension. Transcortical motor aphasia is characterized by intact repetition, perseverativeness in behavior, poor auditory comprehension yet good confrontation naming (Goodglass and Kaplan, as cited in Chapey, 2001). In global aphasia, the survivor demonstrates limited verbalizations (that may only be automatized phrases or words) as well as impairments in comprehension (Wepman and Jones, as cited in Chapey 2001). This condition can be extremely disabling, as the individual has no communicative strengths on which to build.

Treatment of Aphasia

As outlined in Chapey (2001), treatment approaches for aphasia can be categorized as either stimulatory or compensatory. Stimulation approaches include auditory comprehension by matching pictures and/or eliciting responses (e.g., yes/no), while verbal expression targets "associating meaning with speech movements" (Chapey, 2001). Compensatory approaches include use of synonyms, word associations, and communication boards, designed to substitute for verbal responses for those individuals who are unable to communicate verbally (see Augmentative Communication section of this chapter).

Different types of language impairments require different treatment approaches. In Broca's aphasia, speech is typically halted, fragmented, and effortful; content is rich for nouns but limited for verbs, prepositions, and pronouns. Treatment methods include verbal cuing by providing initial phonemes and visual cuing such as presenting the object or a picture of the object in single words, phrases and sentences. Gestures can further facilitate word production. Melodic Intonation Therapy (MIT; Sparks et al., 1974) is a technique thought to access the uninvolved, non-dominant hemisphere by incorporating prosodic elements, and can enable the aphasic individual to express words/phrases that would otherwise not be possible.

BJ, a 55-year-old male s/p CVA 9 months ago was unable to state his address verbally. Numbers were particularly difficult for him to produce, so the therapist cued him to utter his house number ("thirty-nine") in a singsong voice. The therapist also used head motion to facilitate the retrieval of the house number, modeling for the survivor to move his head side-to-side. A combination of phonemic ("long.....") and gestural cues (drawing out the thumb and index finger across the air) helped him to produce the name of his town ("Longmont"), and he developed the ability to use the gesture independently to self-cue.

Global aphasia treatment targets basic functional communication strategies. Incorporating the family or other caregivers into treatment by having them provide background/biographical information, information on interests/hobbies, and photographs can make therapy more meaningful to the survivor. Multimodal communication is emphasized, including verbal (e.g., yes/no, carrier phrases), visual (pictures, drawings) and gestural (e.g., head nods/shakes, pointing) strategies.

The efficacy of therapeutic interventions for aphasia has been reviewed by Holland et al. (1996) and Cicerone et al. (2000, 2005). In their review, Holland et al. concluded that "generally, treatment for aphasia is efficacious," though noted that larger, more well-designed studies are needed. Based on their review, Cicerone et al. (2005) generated practice standards, including a recommendation that cognitive-linguistic therapies be included during acute and post-acute rehabilitation for individuals with language impairments secondary to left hemisphere stroke. Additionally, practice guidelines included cognitive interventions for specific language impairments (e.g., reading comprehension, language formulation) for individuals with left hemisphere stroke and TBI.

The effects of group treatment on linguistic and communicative performance in adults with chronic aphasia was studied by Elman and Bernstein-Ellis (1999). This study compared stroke survivors with aphasia receiving group communication treatment with age, education and severity-matched wait-listed control subjects. They found that those survivors receiving the group communication treatment had significantly higher scores on communicative and linguistic measures following treatment than those who did not receive the treatment. Finally, evidence supports the notion that greater intensity of treatment results in improved outcomes (Denes et al., cited in Cicerone, 2005).

Pragmatic Language

Pragmatic language involves the individual's use of language for communication purposes related to social interaction. The parameters of pragmatic language include topic choice, topic maintenance, and topic termination, turn taking, lexical selection, prosody, eye contact, body language and personal space. These interpersonal skills are interrelated during discourse and frequently disrupted in the ABI population. Survivors may go off on tangents, and anaphoric reference is frequently absent (e.g., when a speaker enters a conversation with pronoun reference that the listener has not had prior exposure to), causing confusion on the part of the listener. Perseveration, the repetition of the same idea or remark, is often demonstrated as well as difficulty "reading" the listener's facial expression and understanding nonverbal communication. Invasion of personal space may be demonstrated as self-regulation of behaviors is sometimes reduced or absent.

The primary goal of pragmatic language intervention is to heighten the speaker's awareness of inappropriate pragmatic language performance with gradual improvement secondary to feedback and training. Therapeutic intervention can be addressed within individual and/or group settings. One-on-one intervention, where there are fewer distractions and attention is more readily focused, is optimal in developing awareness of pragmatic language behaviors. This can be accomplished by role-playing of functional activities (e.g., a conversation at a picnic). Use of video and audiotaping can facilitate the survivor's ability to identify deficits and develop strategies to improve function. Group sessions, where education regarding appropriate pragmatic language function can be reviewed, provide the opportunity for the survivor to receive feedback from peers as well as the therapist. Specific goals can be addressed during each session with handouts provided related to terminology. A self-assessment tool can be utilized at the start of the session to determine the participant's self-awareness and serve as a basis for increasing insight. Each session can focus on a specific area such as nonverbal communication, topic maintenance, initiation, awareness of listener's comprehension, and cohesiveness of the message (Sohlberg & Mateer, 1990).

LK was 33 years old when an allergic reaction precipitated anaphylactic shock with a resulting diagnosis of anoxia. LK was fluent, but on initial testing, was judged to be severely impaired in both receptive and expressive language areas. Cognitively, LK was easily confused when presented with complex information, and had significant impairments in attention. When overwhelmed cognitively, she became easily agitated and verbally disruptive. Pragmatic language was severely impaired as well. She would perseverate, interrupt, and had great difficulty with both topic maintenance and set shifting. She required maximal cuing to follow and maintain the flow of conversation.

Treatment sessions focused on reducing perseveration, establishing appropriate distance when speaking with others, following one- to two-step verbal directions, and diminishing outbursts and inappropriate interruptions. As a result of individual and group communication sessions, LK learned to respond to verbal prompts (e.g., "focus") and visual cues (e.g., a raised finger) and began to self-monitor through improved awareness of appropriate vs. inappropriate behaviors.

Conclusion

As part of the comprehensive neuro-rehabilitation team, speech-language pathologists are responsible for evaluating, educating, and providing restorative or compensatory therapy for a broad spectrum of disorders including dysphagia, motor speech, cognitive-communication, and pragmatic language disorders. In each of these areas, it is essential to involve the family as partners in the therapy process, providing education and training to enable carryover into home and community-based settings. Maintaining an evidence-based practice approach is necessary in order to provide the best quality of care to the survivors of brain injury whom we serve.

References

Adamovich, B.B., Henderson, J. (1992) *Scales of Cognitive Ability for Traumatic Brain Injury (SCATBI)*. Austin, TX: Pro-Ed.

American Heart Association (©2001–06). CDC/NCHS. Available at http://www.americanheart.org

American Speech-Language Hearing Association. (1991) Report: Augmentative and alternative communication. *ASHA* 33(Suppl. 5):9–12.

American Speech-Language-Hearing Association. (2004) *Preferred Practice Patterns for the Profession of Speech-Language Pathology.* Available at http://www.asha.org/.

American Speech-Language-Hearing Association. (2006) *Directory of Speech-Language Pathology Assessment Instruments.* Available at www.asha.org.

Aviv, J.E. (2000) Prospective, randomized outcome study of endoscopy versus modified barrium swallow in patients with dysphagia. *Laryngoscope* 110:563–574.

Beukelman, D.R., Mirenda, P. (1998) *Augmentative and Alternative Communication: Management of Severe Communication Disorders in Children and Adults,* 2nd ed. Baltimore: Paul H. Brooks Publishing Co.

Beukelman, D.R., Yorkston, K.M. (1991) *Communication Disorders Following Traumatic Brain Injury: Management of Cognitive, Language and Motor Impairments.* Austin, TX: Pro-ed.

Chapey, R. (2001) *Language Intervention Strategies in Aphasia and Related Neurogenic Communication Disorders.* 4th ed. Baltimore: Williams & Wilkins.

Cicerone, K.D., Dahlberg, C., Kalmar, K., Langenbahn, D.M., Malec, J.F., Bergquist, T.F., Felicetti, T., Giacino, J.T., Harley, J.P., Harrington, D.E., Herzog, J., Kneipp, S., Laatsch, L., Morse, P.A. (2000) Evidence-based cognitive rehabilitation: Recommendations for clinical practice. *Archives of Physical Medicine & Rehabilitation* 81: 1596–1615.

Cicerone, K.D., Dahlberg, C., Malec, J.F., Langenbahn, D.M., Felicetti, T., Kneipp, S., Ellmo, W., Kalmar, K., Giacino, J.T., Harley, J.P., Laatsch, L., Morse, P.A., Catanese, J. (2005) Evidence-based cognitive rehabilitation: Updated review of the literature from 1998 through 2002. *Archives of Physical Medicine & Rehabilitation* 86:1681–1691.

Coelho, C.A., DeRuyter, F. (1996) Treatment efficacy: Cognitive-communicative disorders resulting from traumatic brain injury in adults. *Journal of Speech and Hearing Research* 39:S5–S17.

Cohen, C.S. (2004) *Augmentative and Alternative Communication: Assessment and Integration....the Basics and Beyond.* June 3–4, 2004. Hampton Cares, NY.

Dabul, B.L. (2000) *Apraxia Battery for Adults,* 2nd ed. Austin, TX: Pro-Ed.

Darley, F.L., Aronson, A.E., Brown, J.R. (1969) Differential diagnostic patterns of Dysarthria. *Journal of Speech and Hearing Research* 12:246.

Duffy, J.R. (1995) *Motor Speech Disorders Substrates, Differential Diagnosis and Management.* St. Louis: Mosby.

Ellmo, W., Graser, J., Krchnavek, B., Hauck, K., Calabrese, D. (1995) *Measure of Cognitive-Linguistic Abilities (MCLA).* Vero Beach: The Speech Bin.

Elman, R.J., Bernstein-Ellis, E. (1999) The efficacy of group communication treatment in adults with chronic Aphasia. *Journal of Speech, Language, and Hearing Research* 42:411–419.

Enerby, P. (1983) *Frenchay Dysarthria Assessment.* Austin, TX: Pro-Ed

Estabrooks, N., Hotz, G. (1991) *Brief Test of Head Injury (BTHI)* Austin, TX: Pro-Ed.

Fletcher, P.P. (1997) AAC and adults with acquired disabilities. In Glennen, S.L., DeCoste, D.C. (eds.): *Handbook of Augmentative and Alternative Communication: A Handbook of Principles and Practices.* Needham Heights, MA: Allyn and Bacon.

Gillis, R. (1996) *Traumatic Brain Injury Rehabilitation for Speech-Language Pathologists.* Boston: Butterworth-Heinemann.

Glennen, S.L., DeCoste, D.C. (1997) *Handbook of Augmentative and Alternative Communication: A Handbook of Principles and Practices.* Needham Heights, MA: Allyn and Bacon.

Goodglass, H., Kaplan, E. (1983) *Boston Diagnostic Aphasia Examination*. Philadelphia: Lea & Febiger.

Holland, A.L., Fromm, D.S., De Ruyter, F., Stein, M. (1996) Treatment efficacy: Aphasia. *Journal of Speech and Hearing Research* 39:S27–S36.

Halper, A.S., Cherney, L.R., Cichowski, K., Zhang, M. (1999) Dysphagia after head trauma: the effect of cognitive-communicative impairments on functional outcomes. *Journal of Head Trauma Rehabilitation* 14(5): 486–496.

Kertesz, A. (1982) *Western Aphasia Battery*. Austin, TX: Pro-Ed.

Lazarus, C.L. (1989) Swallowing disorders after traumatic brain injury. *Journal of Head Trauma Rehabilitation* 4(4):34–41.

Logemann, J.A. (1998) *Evaluation and Treatment of Swallowing Disorders*. Austin, TX: Pro-Ed.

Murry, T., Carrau, R.L. (2001) *Clinical Manual for Swallowing Disorders*. San Diego, CA: Singular.

Ownsworth, T.L., McFarland, K. (1999) Memory remediation in long-term acquired brain injury: Two approaches in diary training. *Brain Injury* 13:605–626.

Porch, B. E. (2001) *Porch Index of Communicative Ability–Revised (PICA-R) Albuquerque: PICA Programs*.

Ross-Swain, D.G. (1996) *Ross Information Processing Assessment*, 2nd ed. Austin, TX: Pro-Ed.

Schuell, N.M. (1965) *The Minnesota Test for Differential Diagnosis of Aphasia*. Minneapolis: University of Minnesota Press.

Sohlberg, M.M., Mateer, C.A. (1990) In Kreutzer, J.S., Wheman, P. (eds.): *Community Integration Following Traumatic Brain Injury*. Baltimore: Paul H. Brookes Publishing Co.

Sparks, R., Helm, N., Albert, M. (1974) Aphasia rehabilitation resulting from melodic intonation therapy. *Cortex* 10:303–316.

Stefakanos, K.H. (1999, revised 2005) *Comprehensive DPNS: A Dysphagia Workshop on Deep Pharyngeal Neuromuscular Stimulation. Resource text*. The Speech Team, Inc.

Wijting, Y., Freed, M.L. (2003) *VitalStim® Therapy Manual*. Hixson, TN: Chattanooga Group.

Yorkston, K.M. (1996) Treatment efficacy in Dysarthria. *Journal of Speech and Hearing Research* 39:S46–S57.

14
Counseling Individuals Post Acquired Brain Injury
Considerations and Objectives

JEAN ELBAUM

"I was just crossing the street, carrying bags full of presents to my friends for the holidays when I was hit by a car."

"I just got off the treadmill and I noticed that the right side of my body wasn't working right and I had trouble speaking."

"My partner and I fell 80 feet when our equipment broke. He died and I sustained a brain injury."

"I was on the way home from an Honor Society meeting in 12th grade and was hit by a car right near my school."

"I got into a car with a girl who had been drinking and taking pills and we drove right into a tree."

"I was working alone in my law office when someone came in and hit my head with a baseball bat several times."

"I lost oxygen to my brain after a heart attack I experienced when I was at the local library with my children."

"I started having headaches and experiencing these odd sensations where I would smell the scent of pine. I was diagnosed with a brain tumor."

"I was on vacation with my wife when our car was hit by a drunk driver, and as a result of the accident I totally lost my vision in addition to sustaining a brain injury."

"I told a lot of people that I fell down the stairs because I was carrying too much laundry, but my friends told me that I fell because I had been drinking too much."

These types of introductions are very familiar to members of the neuro-rehabilitation team. Although survivors generally don't remember their injury, they usually are able to describe what others told them occurred. Survivors of acquired brain injuries (ABIs) all need to cope with the suddenness of an unexpected, calamitous injury. In counseling brain injury survivors, the clinician encounters individuals whose characteristics vary across a multitude of dimensions, not limited to age, gender, cultural background, severity of trauma, or time since the injury. The clinician meets survivors whose educational backgrounds range from limited to extensive, whose personality styles range from private to demonstrative, whose coping skills are fragile to admirable, and whose support systems are uninvolved to overly involved. Whether employed as a firefighter, janitor, professor, ironworker,

259

physician, or fisherman at the moment of the injury, the individual abruptly becomes a brain injury survivor, trying to recapture as much of his or her pre-injury self as possible.

The exact nature of the injury will vary in terms of typicality, from the most common ABIs due to motor vehicle accidents, falls, or strokes to less common occurrences, such as unusual work accidents, random acts of violence, attempted suicides, and atypical encephalopathies, such as secondary to complications of anorexia or larium-induced toxicity. The exact nature of the injury will also vary in terms of causal factors, number of others injured or killed, the survivor's relationship to the others involved, and how responsibility is assigned. Survivors will vary in terms of severity of challenges, from subtle to very pronounced. The framework within which the survivor views the injury will also affect his or her emotional status. All these factors must be considered in understanding the survivor and facilitating an effective post-injury counseling experience.

Counseling Considerations and Goals

Emotional and social challenges following a brain injury may be the result of organic damage, reaction to the injury, or a combination of both. Pepping and Roueche (1990) summarized various psychosocial changes that are considered organically based, due primarily to fronto-temporal injuries. These include loss of ability to show empathy, disinhibition, childish behavior, apathy, emotional lability, irritability, and suspiciousness. Typical emotional reactions to ABI seen clinically include sadness and frustration due to factors such as loss of identity, change in status, lengthy setbacks, diminished control, lack of home or work support, and loss of hope regarding the future.

Very common counseling goals include improving insight, mood, frustration tolerance, stress management, self-esteem, and the active reintegration to meaningful roles. In some situations, the counselor is able to facilitate post-ABI growth, where unexpected positive changes occur consequent to the injury.

It is critical that the entire team be aware of the impact of emotional and psychosocial changes on a survivor's recovery. Referral for counseling and/or neuropsychiatric consultation (see Chapter 6) allows the survivor the opportunity to address emotional and behavioral challenges that may be interfering with recovery.

The clinician must always be sensitive to the uniqueness of each individual, provide education and encouragement, boost motivation, be knowledgeable about cultural differences, help differentiate short- and long-term goals, and assist in creatively finding ways to eliminate barriers towards progress. The counselor should also reinforce that survivors keep notes of sessions to aid recall and actively attempt to carryover counseling goals to the home and community.

Survivors need to be able to express fears and concerns in an arena that offers trust and respect. Once trust is established and a therapeutic alliance has developed, an individual becomes more receptive to feedback. Timing and sensitivity are very important in providing challenging feedback.

The survivor often needs assistance in shifting from obsession with post-injury changes to a more productive focus that involves reframing the injury in a manner that allows the acquisition of hope regarding the future. Whereas one-to-one counseling offers more individualized attention, group counseling helps alleviate feelings of isolation and difference. Peer support is also a powerful way for survivors to receive feedback about their behavior.

The Importance of Insight

Awareness of deficit after ABI is a fascinating topic that has been researched extensively (Prigatano & Schacter, 1991; Hart & Sherer, 2005). Survivors that have good awareness of their difficulties are often active partners in the recovery process. They are disturbed by their difficulties and eager to make progress. Individuals with poor insight have significant difficulty "seeing" post-brain-injury changes and how these difficulties affect daily living skills. Some survivors are totally unaware of very severe difficulties, and see themselves the way they were prior to the injury. These individuals can pose a very serious safety risk as they may insist upon returning to activities prematurely; e.g., return to work, school or driving. Prigatano and Schacter (1991) describe the "catastrophic consequences" that lack of insight can have on employment choice and interpersonal relationships. Other survivors may have partial awareness of their difficulties, with underestimation of how their difficulties affect their performance. Reduced awareness is associated with more severe injuries and a greater number of brain lesions (Sherer et al., 2005).

Kortte et al. (2003) discuss the challenge of differentiating organic lack of awareness from psychological denial. They describe how those in denial of their deficits show resistance when shown their difficulties, whereas those with organic lack of awareness are surprised when their difficulties are pointed out to them. They found that individuals who show a higher level of denial tend to use a greater number of coping strategies aimed at avoidance. They conclude that those who engage in avoidant coping strategies instead of actively processing the trauma are more at risk for depression.

Survivors who are unaware of their difficulties will vary in terms of receptivity to feedback. Some will be willing to follow clinical recommendations despite the fact they don't see their weaknesses. Crosson et al. (1989) provided a theoretical framework for self-awareness that consists of three levels: "intellectual awareness," "emergent awareness," and "anticipatory awareness." Intellectual awareness refers to the ability to recognize that particular difficulties exist secondary to an ABI. Emergent awareness refers to the ability to recognize the impact of these difficulties on everyday life. The model suggests that a person must possess some degree of both intellectual and emergent awareness before developing the third and highest level of anticipatory awareness. Anticipatory awareness refers to the ability to foresee difficulties in everyday life that could occur consequent to the injury and resultant impairments. For many, insight increases during the first few months post-injury, whereas for others it can take many years and repeated failure experiences to build awareness. Survivors ultimately need to establish a good level of insight so they can focus on ways to work around their deficits and become effective compensators.

LG was a 19-year-old college student status post a severe brain injury due to a pedestrian accident. Her insight into her difficulties was poor, and despite the fact that she had significant impairments in selective and divided attention, short-term memory, processing speed, visuoperceptual skills, fine motor coordination, and expressive and receptive language difficulties, she felt that she was "totally fine" and able to return to school. She had a negative attitude in all her therapy sessions, stating that she was exactly as she had been prior to the accident.

Before the injury, LG was an extremely good student, with a 3.8 GPA. At one year following her injury, the neuro-rehabilitation team felt that LG was ready to take one course at a local college with reasonable accommodations, such as extended testing in a private room and use of a note taker. LG was totally resistant to the idea of working with the Office of Disabilities and insisted that she take a minimum of four courses. Despite individual and group counseling efforts supported by her family and friends, and a meeting with another college student post-TBI who had successfully reintegrated to school on a gradual basis with reasonable accommodations, LG was uncooperative with recommendations. She thought that returning to school would mean a return to her former self.

At this point, the team and family agreed that it would be helpful for LG to return to school full-time so that she could see her true status. This was a major turning point in LG's awareness level. Her insight finally improved as she saw for herself that she could not perform academically as in the past. She did very poorly in her classes. LG went through a period of reduced mood and increased anger at her injury and altered capacities, which was followed by a gradual shift towards acceptance. She did return to school about one year later on a part-time basis, with accommodations. Prior to relocating to Florida a few years later with her parents, LG was instrumental in assisting several other clients with reduced insight in benefiting from her experience.

As illustrated above, lack of insight can compound the deleterious effects of brain injury. Not only can it waste a significant amount of clinical time, but it can also engender conflict between the survivor, family and therapy team. The sooner the impaired awareness is addressed, the better the ultimate outcome, as a recent study by Evans et al. (2005) found. According to this study, impaired self-awareness has an early, negative effect on prognosis, warranting early intervention.

Awareness is a high level integrative activity involving the frontal lobes (Stuss & Benson, 1986). When an individual has an impaired monitor, there is a defect in the feedback system preventing proper integration of information and monitoring of responses. Studies have shown that decreased awareness is associated with lack of compliance with rehabilitation, greater caregiver distress, decreased functional status at discharge, and reduced employment outcome (Sherer, 2005). Realistic self-appraisal is critical for positive therapeutic outcomes.

One effective way to build insight is through bombardment of the individual with feedback from many different sources, inclusive of significant others, therapists, and peers. Feedback from other survivors who overcame insight challenges can be very powerful in leading unaware survivors to a breakthrough in insight. Allowing survivors to view videotaped segments of their behavior can sometimes help improve awareness. Of course, it is clinically important to balance confrontation with support (Cicerone, 1989).

Educating survivors regarding frontal lobe insight difficulties can also be an effective insight-building tool. The survivor and primary team members can devise a list of current strengths and goal areas, to be reviewed and reinforced daily. Another way to improve insight is through performance feedback. Asking survivors to predict their performance on tasks and providing them with feedback regarding their actual performance can help improve awareness (Youngjohn & Altman, 1989).

As a final resort, some survivors, like LG, may need failure experiences in order to build insight. Another example was a legally blind client who believed firmly that he would be able to drive safely if he was put behind the wheel. He needed to take and fail numerous driving evaluations in order to be convinced that his vision precluded him from safe driving. Once a survivor becomes aware of his/her difficulties post-ABI, there is often a concomitant decline in mood (Sohlberg et al., 1998).

Mood Challenges

Lack of uniformity in defining depression has resulted in much variability in its reported frequency post-ABI. Estimates of the rate of post-TBI depression range from 14% to 77% (Cantor et al., 2005). Anxiety disorders, emotional lability, aggressive behavior, and substance abuse challenges are frequently associated with major depression post TBI, and their co-presence is a marker for negative cognitive and psychosocial outcomes (Jorge & Starkstein, 2005). There is evidence of a biphasic course in the prevalence of post-stroke depression, with one peak occurring within the first year of the stroke and the second occurring during the second year. Depressed patients are often less motivated to take part in rehabilitation, have longer hospital stays, lower functional outcome and decreased resumption of social activities following discharge from rehabilitation (Van de Meent et al., 2003).

Neurobiological and psychosocial factors lead to a unique presentation of mood challenges in each client. Alderfer et al. (2005) cite laterality of injury, dysfunction in dorsal frontal systems, and dysregulation of serotonergic activity as primary neuroanatomic factors affecting mood. They also discuss various psychosocial risk factors for post-TBI depression inclusive of poor pre-injury occupational status, poor pre-morbid social functioning, previous history of psychiatric diagnosis or alcohol abuse history, fewer years of formal education, and female gender. They report that the rate of depression is high in the first year post-injury, although clients are at increased risk for developing depression for many decades following their injury. These researchers suggest that biological factors have an increased role in acute-onset depression, with psychosocial factors having a more significant role in delayed onset depression.

The evaluation process for all survivors with ABI should include a clinical screening for depression, with recommendations made for individual and/or group counseling in addition to neuropsychiatric consultation, as needed. This is particularly important because a delay in treatment can negatively affect emotional and cognitive gains. Neuropsychiatric consultation is always indicated in cases of suicidal or aggressive ideation and in situations where non-pharmacological treatment has been insufficient. Scicutella (Chapter 6) discusses the differential diagnosis of apathy and pseudobular affect from mood disorders.

Even subtle changes in thinking or feeling can lead survivors to feel altered. Many express sadness and frustration due to loss of certain skills or functional abilities. They frequently describe their injury as a major marker in their lives, dividing their experiences into pre- and post-injury categories. Survivors who were high achievers prior to their injury tend to be especially frustrated by their inability to duplicate pre-injury roles. Those individuals who are able to return to work but at the cost of expending significantly more effort to achieve the same result often feel deeply saddened by this loss of efficiency. Loss of status can also occur due to an altered role at work or in the family.

Survivors frequently report decreased mood due to feeling out of control. Uncertainty about the future is particularly difficult to deal with, especially for those that were very control-oriented in the past. The enormous setback that can result from severe injuries can require many years of hard work and consistent use of compensatory strategies for success.

ABI can create a giant strain on relationships and place marriages at risk for "relationship breakdown" (Blais & Boisvert, 2005). Survivors who need to deal with divorce and separation from their children, in addition to their ABI, are at very high risk for depression.

Survivors with reduced mood post-ABI benefit most from emotional support, guidance with goal direction, and overall empowerment in their daily lives. They frequently describe the significant emotional boost they derive from success, such as doing well in a course or making active progress in therapy sessions. It is also important for the clinician to keep in regular contact with the survivor's significant others to monitor mood at home and in the community.

Cognitive-behavioral therapy (CBT) approaches (Beck, 1995) were designed to treat depression and anxiety in individuals without cognitive challenges. CBT has been adapted for use with individuals post-stroke (Hibbard et al., 1990). The efficacy of CBT has not been systematically examined in individuals with TBI (Gordon & Hibbard, 2005). A recent study (Tiersky et al., 2005) demonstrated that programming consisting of CBT and cognitive remediation showed promise in the treatment of depression and anxiety in individuals with mild to moderate TBI living in the community. Replacing cognitive distortions, such as, "I had a brain injury and am totally useless," with more accurate and adaptive interpretations has been found clinically useful in survivors of ABI. Mateer et al. (2005) highlighted the importance of integrating cognitive and emotional interventions in the treatment of individuals with ABI.

Prigatano (1999) emphasized the need for a set of guiding principles in psychotherapeutic work with ABI survivors. These include working within the survivor's subjective experience, addressing disorders of awareness, considering pre-injury characteristics as well as recognizing the interaction between cognition and personality. He advised clinicians to "focus on the present but with a sophisticated understanding of how the past may have contributed to patients' behaviors."

Couples counseling is often indicated post-ABI. Primary goals include assistance with adjustment to changes and redevelopment of trust, communication, and intimacy, as well as reinforcement of empathy, flexibility, mutual support, and respect.

Group counseling, in the form of an educational/support group, can provide clients with a sense of connection to others who have gone through similar experiences. Observing progress in peers can provide a boost in level of client hopefulness. Group counseling can also help improve social interactional skills and act as a forum for mastery of strategies to regulate emotions. Survivors report much benefit from group discussions regarding adaptive ways to cope with depression and frustration. Alumni can serve as role models and mentors for survivors receiving active rehabilitation as they can provide hope and encouragement based on their post injury successes.

Frustration, Anger, and Behavioral Challenges

Aggressive behaviors are considered common among brain injury survivors. Baguley et al. (2006) report that in the acute rehabilitation setting, aggression is associated with factors such as reduced communication skills, symptoms of post-traumatic stress disorder, frontal lobe injury, disorientation to place and time, and pre-morbid psychiatric and substance abuse history. They investigated the prevalence and predictors of aggressive behavior among clients with TBI up to 60 months post-discharge. Their primary findings were that both "depression" and a "younger age at time of injury" were the most significant predictors of aggression at 6, 24, and 60 months post-discharge, and that prevalence of aggression was at 25% following TBI at these different follow-up periods.

Survivors frequently report reduced frustration tolerance post-ABI, with over-reaction to minor triggers. This represents a decrease in tolerance for levels of stimulation that were tolerated effectively in the past. As preinjury characteristics are often amplified post-injury, it isn't surprising that those who were somewhat irritable before their injury may become significantly more so following their injury. Greatest sources of reported frustration are in relation to functional loss and restriction of autonomy.

Survivors frequently experience much anger at the source of the injury. Self-anger is noted in cases where the survivor was in some way responsible for his or her injury, such as due to a faulty suicide attempt, drug overdose, impulsivity, or negligent behavior. In cases where someone else caused the injury, the survivor's relationship to that person and the interpretation of events that led to the injury will influence the reaction. For example, a roommate who assaults an individual on the head numerous times with a flashlight will effect a different emotional reaction than a stranger who collides into a pedestrian due to a sudden heart attack behind the wheel. If the individual was a passenger in a car driven by a friend or family member who was driving recklessly, his or her reaction will be different than if the friend or family member was also a victim to a second driver who was intoxicated. In cases where a survivor experiences much anger related to the surrounding events of the injury, it may take several months or years to work through the anger and move forward. Although anger and self-pity are normal reactions to an ABI, when these emotions persist they can become toxic to the recovery process. Individual and group counseling can be very helpful in allowing the survivor an opportunity to ventilate anger and obtain feedback and support from others.

Reinforcement of adaptive coping strategies is critical in improving anger control and compensating for disinhibition. Impaired regulation of mood and behavior is a serious barrier to community reintegration. Survivors often need to relearn how to slow down and self-monitor during challenging interactions to prevent inappropriate outbursts or aggressive responses. It is helpful to reinforce the first-letter mnemonic COP to remind survivors of items to remember in their attempts at anger control. The C stands for communication of thoughts and feelings in a nonaggressive, constructive manner. Survivors are taught to try and remove themselves from situations where they feel they cannot communicate in an appropriate, nonhurtful manner. The O stands for constructive outlets used to help the individual handle frustration effectively, such as listening to music or relaxation tapes, physical exercise, or journaling. The P stands for preparation for dealing with triggers that evoke aggressive responses. In this way, the client can learn to both prevent escalation when triggered and to deescalate challenging situations that arise.

Medd and Tate (2000) studied the effectiveness of cognitive-behaviorally oriented anger management programs involving self-awareness and self-regulation training. Participants were trained to recognize and respond more effectively to their reactions to anger inducing situations. Results showed a significant decrease in the outward expression of anger by the treatment group, suggesting improved emotional self-regulation. Cicerone et al. (2005) reported that many studies have suggested, "behavioral improvement is not contingent on increased self-awareness."

Giles and Manchester (2006) discuss the value of both the operant neurobehavioral approach (ONA) and the relational neurobehavioral approach (RNA) to behavioral difficulties post-TBI. Both approaches focus on reducing disruptive behavior and reinforcing adaptive behavior. ONA involves teaching survivors to adapt to social norms within a structured environment with clear contingencies. The goal is to strengthen desirable behavior and extinguish undesirable behavior. Staff feedback is direct and authoritative. RNA targets the therapeutic relationship as a treatment variable, with the focus on promoting client motivation.

In cases where survivors are having difficulty controlling their behavior in therapy sessions, a behavioral rating scale can be very useful. The therapy team identifies the key areas interfering with the survivor's progress and those items are assessed on an hourly basis. At the end of each session, the treating therapist fills out the rating scale and gives feedback to the survivor, using a scale from 1 to 4, ranging from poor, fair, good to excellent. Common categories are "social appropriateness," "ability to focus on presented tasks," "awareness of social boundaries," and "promptness." In this way, survivors can receive regular quantitative feedback on their behavioral gains and can work towards a meaningful reward if they are successful.

Claudia Osborn (1998), a physician who sustained an ABI due to a motor vehicle accident, emphasizes the importance of acceptance in the recovery process. In her chapter entitled, "Not as I wish, but as I am," she discusses the critical steps of awareness, compensation, and ultimately acceptance "that some things about us cannot be restored." Once survivors reach some level of peace with the injury, their anger level usually significantly decreases, enabling increased productivity in their daily lives.

Anxiety and Stress Management

Anxiety is very common post-TBI and has been reported at rates as high as 70%, with 29% prevalence across all severity types of TBI. The most common symptoms of anxiety post-TBI are free-floating anxiety, fearfulness, intense worry, social withdrawal, and interpersonal sensitivity. Anxiety and depression have a high comorbidity rate (Moore et al. 2006).

Scicutella (Chapter 6) discusses the four subcategories of anxiety, including panic disorder, obsessive-compulsive disorder (OCD), post-traumatic stress disorder (PTSD), and generalized anxiety disorder. Gray and McNaughton (1996) present a model of a "behavioral inhibition system" in the brain that causes anxiety symptoms. They state that anxiety becomes a chronic problem when its correlating brain areas in the behavioral inhibition system malfunction and become overly sensitive to stimuli. They indicate that OCD arises when the septo-hippocampal system, which checks the environment for aversive or novel stimuli, reacts too frequently, resulting in persistent checking and searching. They explain that people who are vulnerable to anxiety have excessively reactive systems.

Brain injury survivors can experience an overwhelming amount of stress due to role changes and altered functional status. The life-threatening experiences they have undergone can create feelings of vulnerability and weakness. Moore et al. (2006) state that TBI is thought to break down psychological defenses and coping strategies, leaving the individual more vulnerable to previously experienced anxiety conditions.

Survivors experiencing significant anxiety will benefit most from individual sessions that reinforce the use of relaxation strategies and stress management techniques. Many survivors experiencing symptoms of anxiety will not be able to tolerate group counseling and will need more individualized attention. Individuals with PTSD benefit most from expressing and working through their emotions surrounding the injury, describing their memories associated with the trauma (such as being restrained in the hospital following the injury) and learning ways to gain control over their fears and concerns in a supportive, encouraging environment. A combination of strategies such as positive self-talk, breathing, imagery and relaxation exercises, as well as the use of constructive outlets such as music and physical exercise, can assist survivors in managing stress effectively.

Issues of Self-Concept

It is very common for survivors to report a reduction in self-confidence post-ABI. Most cited reasons include lessened mental acuity, a feeling of "brokenness," loss of autonomy, and decreased productivity in daily life. Additionally, survivors report reduced control over life decisions, the need to revise goals and expectations, as well as feeling devalued or stigmatized by others.

Survivors often need encouragement to avoid magnifying their errors and being overly critical of their weaknesses during the recovery process. Survivors report that gains in confidence are primarily linked to success in real-life activities and to the support and caring of significant others. Garske and Thomas (1992) found that ratings of self-esteem were most strongly related to satisfaction with family interactions, level of social contact, and positive emotional status.

Vickery et al. (2006) examined the impact of group therapy interventions on self-concept in brain injury survivors. They discussed past research that has shown how ratings of self-concept can improve following social skills training and participation in a physical conditioning exercise program and various recreational activities. Their research explored the effectiveness of a group intervention that focused on self-concept changes following ABI by expanding knowledge of the self and reinforcement of positive self-attributes, based on the concepts of self-complexity and importance differentiation. Self-complexity involves the recognition that there are many different aspects to the self and that a person need not be defined in narrow terms. Importance differentiation is the process of recognizing that certain aspects of the self may be more valuable than others. The authors were interested in seeing if challenging the importance of affected areas of self-concept could be curative. Their research evidenced that group members showed a significant increase in self-concept ratings at the end of the group intervention.

Tomberg et al. (2005) studied coping strategies and social support on quality of life post-TBI and found that individuals with TBI used task-oriented and emotional/social support strategies significantly less than control subjects and avoidance-oriented strategies significantly more than controls. They concluded that enhancing a survivor's well-being involves improving the quality and amount of the social support network. Anson and Ponsford (2006) found that coping strategies characterized as active, interpersonal and problem-focused are associated with higher self-esteem following TBI.

Counseling sessions to boost self-confidence include training in assertiveness, increasing awareness of strengths, providing praise and positive feedback, and assisting in the process of reintegration to meaningful roles. Pegg et al. (2005) studied the impact of person-centered information on patients' treatment satisfaction and outcomes post-TBI rehabilitation. They found that survivors with moderate to severe injuries who were given more personalized information about their treatment exerted greater effort in therapy sessions, made greater improvement in functional independence, and were more satisfied with the treatment. They concluded that moderately to severely impaired survivors can benefit from interventions designed to enhance their sense of control and empowerment over their care.

Reintegration to Meaningful Roles

ABI sequelae present a daunting challenge to survivors who are trying to reestablish their sense of work and personal identity. Discharge planning for all clients needs to involve reintegration to productive activities. Primary discharge options include return to work, school or vocational training, volunteer activities, active retirement, or structured day programming.

If a survivor's recovery allows for a return to a former position, appropriate timing and gradual reintegration are both critical to the success of the reentry. It is best to have a survivor start going back to work on a gradual basis, beginning with one to two days a week, and gradually increasing days and hours based on performance. It is important to coordinate efforts with the survivor's work supervisor, requesting reasonable accommodations as needed, and sharing best ways to facilitate the reintegration process. Supportive work supervisors are sometimes able to offer a survivor a modified position, either temporarily or permanently, to further aid the transition from rehabilitation to work.

Survivors who are high-school students receiving neuro-rehabilitation can benefit when they obtain both their tutoring and therapy sessions at the same location, so that tutors and therapists can coordinate efforts. Educating tutors about the best ways to work around the student's weaknesses and to utilize strengths is very helpful. Survivors returning to high school following an ABI may benefit from a gradual shift from the neuro rehabilitation program to part-time classes, with resource room as needed.

In working with a survivor returning to college or graduate school, it is best to coordinate efforts with the Office of Disabilities at the university. Reasonable accommodations most commonly recommended include extended time on tests in a private room and permission to tape lectures as well as to use the services of a note taker. Enlarging handouts and tests, as well as providing tests in multiple choice format, can be helpful for certain clients.

Volunteering is an excellent next step for many survivors who are not returning to school, work or homemaking responsibilities following rehabilitation. Within many hospital settings, there are many structured opportunities ranging from filing and basic clerical work to maintenance, paper delivery, food preparation, mail room responsibilities and gift shop work, to higher level positions, such as reading to children in pediatric wards or acting as a patient advocate. The clinical team and the coordinator of volunteer services can try to match a position to a survivor's abilities and interests.

For survivors who are unable to return to pre-injury work but are good candidates for reentry to competitive employment, coordination of efforts with a state or privately funded vocational program can sometimes lead survivors to appropriate career changes. For instance, survivors who cannot return to the physical work of construction may become trained in construction management or computer programming, or a survivor who was an Emergency Medical Technician (EMT) can be retrained as a lab technician.

Post-ABI Growth

CD was a 33-year-old electrician receiving neuro-rehabilitation subsequent to a cocaine-induced brain aneurysm. During the initial meeting, CD was agitated and devoid of insight, stating that he only used cocaine and alcohol infrequently "at weddings." He was in denial regarding his drug and alcohol problem and was totally unaware of neuro-cognitive changes following his injury. CD's only focus was on discharge and returning to his former life. Once a positive therapeutic alliance was gradually developed and insight grew, CD became more willing to explore and reevaluate his pre-injury life. He was able to see that his daily "partying" had hurt his self-esteem, career opportunities, financial status, interpersonal relationships, and finally his health and thinking abilities. The client had difficulties with attention, short-term memory, and processing speed, but was able to master compensatory strategies to work around his difficulties effectively.

CD spoke about the positive changes he wanted to institute in his life and the fact that his injury led him to personal growth. He ultimately used his injury and subsequent neuro-rehabilitation experience for the purpose of post-ABI growth. He began his own business, started a family, worked around his difficulties by consistent use of strategies, and stayed away from substances.

The concept of post-ABI growth developed as a result of working with hundreds of survivors like CD who demonstrated constructive life changes following an ABI. Post-ABI growth refers to any positive byproduct resulting from an ABI, such as an improvement in sense of self, an increase in appreciation of friends and family, a termination of destructive habits or introduction to new vocational or avocational pathways.

Substance Abuse Challenges

Coping with both ABI and substance abuse challenges result in "a multidimensional disability and presents a unique set of problems related to dual diagnosis." Alcohol is involved in the acquisition of 35–66 % of all TBIs (Dell Orto & Power, 2000). Once an individual has sustained an ABI, continued alcohol abuse is linked to increased likelihood of seizures, poor impulse control, and heightened cognitive deficits.

Some individuals may be predisposed to sustaining a TBI due to self-destructive behaviors as a result of depression or substance abuse. The higher the number of pre-injury vulnerabilities (such as a history of depression or substance abuse, lack of family support, or limited education), the more challenging the recovery process with a more guarded prognosis. Individuals with complex histories will require the collaboration of specialists in neuropsychiatry and substance abuse treatment to increase the likelihood of a favorable recovery.

Screening for alcohol and substance abuse during a survivor's initial intake to a neuro-rehabilitation program is critical. Findings suggest that CAGE (Cut down, Annoy, Guilty and Eye Opener) may be a useful screening tool for alcohol abuse and that the Substance Abuse Subtle Screening Inventory (SASSI-3) may be useful for assessing drug abuse in individuals with TBI (Ashman et al., 2004). CAGE is a four question-screening tool that addresses the drinking experience of the individual. Two or more positive responses are viewed as an indication of an alcohol problem (Ewing, 1984). Following screening, case management appears to have a beneficial effect on survivors with both TBI and substance abuse challenges (Heinemann et al., 2004).

Conclusion

The experience of counseling individuals post-ABI is always dynamic and demanding. The beginning challenges involve creating a favorable rapport, developing trust, establishing an environment where the survivor feels comfortable sharing personal issues, and assisting in empowerment of the individual in the process of recovery. Later challenges may involve effecting confrontation without alienation, keeping a goal-oriented approach, weaving significant others actively into the process, reinforcing strategies to improve mood and frustration tolerance, as well as ensuring that the survivor is on a productive path emotionally and socially. The final objectives are to keep the individual hopeful about the future despite awareness of residual weaknesses and to assist in the process of transitioning successfully to a next step that involves continued structure and stimulation, such as work, school or a volunteer role.

The counselor/psychotherapist is oftentimes the survivor's primary partner in the neuro-rehabilitation process, due to the clinician's awareness of the individual's fears, motivations, vulnerabilities, and triggers. It is highly important to integrate efforts with all other team members to assure that emotional and behavioral difficulties are not interfering with the survivor's progress in any domain. This type of close team communication and collaboration enables the survivor to receive consistent feedback from different team members and also highlights the fact that the team is working in concert, guiding the survivor towards goal achievement and reintegration to meaningful roles.

References

Alderfer, B., Arciniegas, D., Silver, J. (2005) Treatment of depression following traumatic brain injury. *The Journal of Head Trauma Rehabilitation* 20(6):544–562.

Anson, K., Ponsford, J. (2006) Evaluation of a coping skills group following traumatic brain injury. *Brain Injury* 20(2):167–178.

Ashman, T.A., Schwartz, M.E., Cantor, J.B., Hibbard, M.R., Gordon, W.A. (2004) Screening for substance abuse in individuals with traumatic brain injury. *Brain Injury* 18(2):191–202.

Baguley, I.J., Cooper, J., Felmingham, K. (2006) Aggressive behavior following traumatic brain injury. *Journal of Head Trauma Rehabilitation* 21(1):45–56.

Beck, J.S. (1995) *Cognitive Therapy: Basics and Beyond.* New York: Guilford Press.

Blais, M., Boisvert, J. (2005) Psychological and marital adjustment in couples following a traumatic brain injury: A critical review. *Brain Injury* 19(14):1223–1235.

Cantor, J.B., Ashman, T.A., Schwartz, M.E., Gordon, W.A., Hibbard, M.R., Brown, M., Spielman, L., Charatz, H.J., Cheng, Z. (2005) The role of self-discrepancy theory in understanding post-traumatic brain injury affective disorders. *Journal of Head Trauma Rehabilitation* 20(6):527–543.

Cicerone, K.D. (1989) Psychotherapy interventions with traumatic brain injury patients. *Rehabilitation Psychology* 34:105–114.

Cicerone, K.D., Dahlberg, C., Malec, J.F., Langenbahn, D.M., Felicetti, T., Kniepp, S., Ellmo, W., Kalmar, K., Giacino, J.T., Harley, J.P., Laatsch, L., Morse, P.A., Catanese, J. (2005) Evidence-based cognitive rehabilitation: Updated review of the literature from 1998 through 2002. *Archives of Physical Medicine and Rehabilitation* 86:1681–1691.

Crosson, B., Barco, P.P., Velozo, C.A., Bolesta, M.M., Cooper, P.V., Werts, D., Brobeck, T.C. (1989) Awareness and compensation in post-acute head injury rehabilitation. *Journal of Head Trauma Rehabilitation* 4(3):46–54.

Dell Orto, A.E., Power, P.W. (2000) *Brain Injury and the Family.* New York: CRC Press.

Dikman, S.S., Bombardier, C.H., Machamer, J.E., Fann, J.R., Temkin, N.R. (2004) Natural history of depression in traumatic brain injury. *Archives of Physical Medicine and Rehabilitation* 85:1457–1464.

Engberg, A.W., Teasdale, T.W. (2004) Psychosocial outcome following traumatic brain injury in adults: A long-term population-based follow-up. *Brain Injury* 18(6):533–545.

Evans, C., Sherer, M., Nick, T., Nakase-Richardson, R., Yablon, S. (2005) Early impaired self-awareness, depression, and subjective well-being following traumatic brain injury. *Journal of Head Trauma Rehabilitation* 20(6):488–500.

Ewing, J.A. (1984) Detecting alcoholism: The CAGE questionnaire. *Journal of the American Medical Association* (252):1905–1907.

Garske, G.G., Thomas, K.R. (1992) Self-reported self-esteem and depression: Indexes of psychosocial adjustment following severe traumatic brain injury. *Rehabilitation Counseling Bulletin* 36:44–52.

Giles, G.M., Manchester, D. (2006) Two approaches to behavior disorders after traumatic brain injury. *Journal of Head Trauma Rehabilitation* 21(2):168–178.

Gordon, W., Hibbard, M.R. (2005) Cognitive rehabilitation. In Silver, M., McAllister, T., Yudofsky, S. (eds.): *Textbook of Traumatic Brain Injury.* Virginia: American Psychiatric Publishing, Inc, pp. 655–660.

Gray, J.A., McNaughton, N. (1996) *The Neuropsychology of Anxiety.* Nebraska: University of Nebraska Press.

Hart, T., Sherer, M. (2005) Disorders of self-awareness. *The Journal of Head Trauma Rehabilitation* 20(4):287–367.

Heinemann, A.W., Corrigan, J.D., Moore, D. (2004) Case management for traumatic brain injury survivors with alcohol problems. *Rehabilitation Psychology* 49(2):156–166.

Hibbard, M.R., Grober, S.E., Gordan, W.A., Aletta, E.G., Freeman, A. (1990) Cognitive therapy and the treatment of post-stroke depression. *Topics in Geriatric Rehabilitation* 5:43–55.

Jorge, R.E., Starkstein, S.E. (2005) Pathophysiologic aspects of major depression following traumatic brain injury. *The Journal of Head Trauma Rehabilitation* 20(6):475–486.

Kortte, K.B., Wegener, S.T., Chwalisz, K. (2003) Anosognosia and denial: Their relationship to coping and depression in acquired brain injury. *Rehabilitation Psychology* 48(3):131–136.

Mateer, C.A., Sira, C.S., O'Connell, M.E. (2005) Putting humpty dumpty back together again: The importance of integrating cognitive and emotional interventions. *Journal of Head Trauma Rehabilitation* 20(1):62–75.

Medd, J., Tate, R.L. (2000) Evaluation of an anger management therapy program following acquired brain injury: A preliminary study. *Neuropsychological Rehabilitation* 10(2):185–201.

Moore, E.L., Terryberry-Spohr, L., Hope, D.A. (2006) Mild traumatic brain injury and anxiety sequelae: A review of the literature. *Brain Injury* 20(2):117–132.

Oppermann, J.D. (2004) Interpreting the meaning individuals ascribe to returning to work after traumatic brain injury: A qualitative approach. *Brain Injury* 18(9):941–955.

Osborn, C.L. (1998) *Over My Head*. Kansas City: Andrews McMeel Publishing.

Pegg, P.O., Auerbach, S.M., Seel, R.T., Buenaver, L.F., Kiesler, D.J., Plybon, L.E. (2005) The impact of patient-centered information on patients' treatment satisfaction and outcomes in traumatic brain injury rehabilitation. *Rehabilitation Psychology* 50(4):366–374.

Pepping, M., Roueche, J.R. (1990) Psychosocial consequences of significant brain injury. In Tupper, D.E., Cicerone, K.D. (eds.): *The Neuropsychology of Everyday Life Issues in Development and Rehabilitation*. Boston: Kluwer Academic.

Prigatano, G.P. (1999) *Principles of Neuropsychological Rehabilitation*. New York: Oxford University Press.

Prigatano, G.P., Schacter, D.L. (eds.). (1991) Awareness of Deficits After Brain Injury. New York: Oxford University Press.

Rath, J.R., Hennessy, J.J., Diller, L. (2003) Social problem solving and community integration in postacute rehabilitation outpatients with traumatic brain injury. *Rehabilitation Psychology* 48(3):137–144.

Sherer, M. (2005) Rehabilitation of impaired awareness. In High, W.M., Sander, A.M., Struchen, M.A., Hart, K.A. (eds.): Rehabilitation for Traumatic Brain Injury. New York: Oxford University Press, pp. 31–46.

Sohlberg, M.M., Mateer, C.A., Penkman, L., Glang, A., Todis, B. (1998) Awareness intervention: Who needs it? *Journal of Head Trauma Rehabilitation* 13(5):62–78.

Stuss, D.T., Benson, D.F. (1986) *The Frontal Lobes*. New York: Raven Press.

Tiersky, L.A., Anselmi, V., Johnston, M.V., Kurtyka, J., Roosen, E., Schwartz, T., DeLuca, J. (2005) A trial of neuropsychologic rehabilitation in mild-spectrum traumatic brain injury. *Archives of Physical Medicine and Rehabilitation* 86:1565–1574.

Tomberg, T., Toomela, A., Pulver, A., Tikk, A. (2005) Coping strategies, social support, life orientation and health related quality of life following traumatic brain injury. *Brain Injury* 19(14):1181–1190.

Van de Meent, H., Geurts, A.C.H., Limbeck J.V. (2003) Pharacologic treatment of post-stroke depression: A systematic review of the literature. *Topics in Stroke Rehabilitation* 10(1):79–92.

Vickery, C.D., Gontkovsky, S.T., Wallace, J.J., Caroselli, J.S. (2006) Group psychotherapy focusing on self-concept change following acquired brain injury: A pilot investigation. *Rehabilitation Psychology* 51(1):30–35.

Wood, R.L., Liossi, C., Wood, L. (2005) The impact of head injury neurobehavioral sequelae on personal relationships: Preliminary findings. *Brain Injury* 19(10):845–851.

Youngjohn, J.F., Altman, I.M. (1989) A performance-based group approach to the treatment of anosognosia and denial. *Rehabilitation Psychology* 34:217–222.

15
Acquired Brain Injury and the Family
Challenges and Interventions

JEAN ELBAUM

Introduction

In clinical practice, the neuro-rehabilitation team encounters families that have experienced trauma, turmoil, and significant losses. Injuries are generally ill-timed and families are frequently ill-prepared for the length, uncertainty, and challenges of the post-injury process. In the literature, much has been written about "caregiver burden" and the stressful impact an ABI can have on family systems. There is increasing awareness of the importance of identifying family needs and establishing effective and comprehensive interventions.

In some ways, families may actually experience more distress than the actual survivors of ABI. Crimmins (2000) described how accidents divide life into "the great Before and After." Survivors tend to have amnesia for the very time period that was most traumatic, whereas loved ones are clearly able to remember those unfortunate events. In the early months post-ABI, the entire family system tends to focus, almost exclusively, on the needs of the person who was injured. The amount of distress that a particular significant other will experience depends on a variety of variables, such as the quality of the relationship prior to the injury, the specific commitment to the injured loved one, the amount of time and extra responsibilities involved, other simultaneous life stressors, and the adaptiveness of coping skills. Each family subsystem confronts unique challenges, and each unit requires knowledge, partnership, and understanding from the team. In the best situations, the survivor has good insight, is hard-working, has a constructive attitude, makes very active gains, and can reintegrate to productive roles at home and in society. In the most challenging situations, the survivor has poor awareness, severe impairments, requires long-term care, and will not be able to integrate successfully to home or community settings.

Dell Orto and Power (2000) summarized various frustrations of primary caregivers such as trying to balance multiple roles, feeling overwhelmed due to the lack of assistance by other significant others, feeling restricted socially and dealing with the reality that their pre-morbid loved one may be permanently different.

Family Needs

Family members of individuals post-ABI are at increased risk for depression, anxiety, and physical illness (Oddy et al., 1978). Researchers have focused on the post-injury needs of families in an effort to identify appropriate treatment plans and interventions to effectively meet their needs. The Family Needs Questionnaire (FNQ) (Kreutzer et al., 1994) was developed to quantify the multiple needs of family members in order to identify families at high risk and target interventions appropriately. The six categories identified were needs for health information, emotional support, instrumental support (refers to the need for respite and practical everyday assistance), professional support, community support, and involvement in care. The scale was developed based on extensive family interviewing and a comprehensive literature review (Serio et al., 1997). Research has shown that medical needs are perceived to be most important as well as most frequently met. In contrast, emotional needs were most often perceived as unmet (Serio et al., 1995). Witol et al. (1996) reported that families are generally satisfied with the information and support provided by professionals at early and late post-injury intervals. However, family members have difficulty getting their emotional and instrumental support needs met, a situation worsening over time in the case of emotional support.

Preliminary data, involving comparison of FNQ results in three different settings, reflected more unmet needs in families attending a long-term stroke support group than in families of survivors in outpatient or inpatient neuro-rehabilitation programs (unpublished data). The low percentage of needs being met in families of individuals in the long-term stroke support group may be due to a selection factor, as the stroke group participants are not representative of all people post-stroke. The stroke group is a social/recreational program that meets on a weekly basis for survivors and caregivers. The families studied had been caregiving for an average of 7 years.

Serio et al. (1995) reviewed the predictors of family outcome by studying injury, patient, and family characteristics. They concluded that time since injury influences family reactions as caregivers report more unmet needs over time, consistent with our unpublished data. These authors also reported that patients' emotional and behavioral problems correlated with increased caregiver stress. Family members' perceptions of patients' problems are more important predictors of needs than test results. In terms of family characteristics, they found that spouses had more difficulty adjusting to the injury of a loved one than parents, reporting more depression, anxiety, isolation, and distress.

Family Coping

Families are the neuro-rehabilitation team's primary partners in facilitating survivor progress, and they play a major role in client recovery. The high level of stress they experience, resulting often in long-term use of tranquilizers and sleeping pills as a palliative, compromises their effectiveness. Consequently, meeting caregivers' needs and reinforcing positive coping skills is critical (Serio et al., 1997).

The literature on family coping post-ABI includes many references to Kubler-Ross's (1983) stages of denial, anger, depression, and adjustment following a major loss. Each member of the family as well as the entire family unit as a whole goes through an adjustment period following the ABI of a loved one. In clinical practice, many survivors and families have rebelled against the terms "adjustment" and "acceptance" of an injury, assuming that that these words denote "giving in" to the injury instead of overcoming it. In reality, these terms refer to the ability of the client and family to go forward in a productive manner despite the sequelae of the injury.

Lezak's classic article (1978) "Living with the Characterologically Altered Brain Injured Patient" describes the qualitative challenges that families face in dealing with loved ones who have behavioral difficulties following an ABI. She discusses several categories of behavioral alterations that create the greatest adjustment challenges for families: reduced empathy and self-centered behavior, reduced self-regulation, increased impulsivity and silliness, reduced executive functioning abilities such as difficulties with initiation and planning, increased or reduced sexual interest, and difficulty with social learning. Over time, there has been more emphasis on quantitative measures of family needs and coping styles.

Nabors et al. (2002) described various factors that are powerful predictors of family adjustment, such as pre-injury family functioning, level of financial stress, perceived level of burden, coping mechanisms used, and availability of social support systems. They highlighted the importance of ongoing assessments of family needs.

Man (2002) identified several types of adaptive coping strategies used by families of ABI survivors, inclusive of positive appraisal, resource requisition, family tension management, and acquisition of social support.

Although there are meaningful and rewarding aspects of being a primary caregiver, at times the role can be very overwhelming, lonely and thankless. It is not uncommon for survivors to unfairly direct a significant amount of post-injury frustration and anger toward their loved ones, by verbal attacks or disrespectful behavior. Caregivers usually have to bear the brunt of their loved one's frustration. It is important for significant others to learn how to deescalate stressful encounters and how to cope constructively with a loved one's unreasonable behavior. Without proper training to handle these challenging situations, many caregivers can turn towards destructive coping strategies.

Cameron et al. (2006) found that caregivers experience more symptoms of depression when they care for survivors of stroke who exhibit memory and comprehension symptoms. Their study demonstrated that 45% of caregivers reported elevated levels of symptoms of depression. They emphasized the importance of addressing the needs of caregivers by providing needed information and resources on how to handle neuro-cognitive difficulties.

Family Subsystems

Spouses, parents, siblings, and children are frequently the caregivers that are involved in the recovery process as primary caregivers.

Individuals who are dealing with the ABI of a marital partner are often dealing with financial, social, and personal stressors in addition to adjusting to the particular physical, cognitive, and psychosocial changes in their spouse. A spouse whose loved one has been severely injured may lose a confidante, sexual partner, household co-manager, and childrearing assistant all at once (Serio et al. 1995).

Kreutzer et al. (1994) stated that caregiving spouses reported greater family dysfunction and increased likelihood of depression compared to parents who acted as primary caregivers. Spouses of individuals post-ABI face a loss of peer-based, reciprocal relationships when they take on caregiving roles, compared to parents who return to roles familiar from child-rearing years (Wood et al. 2005). The concept of social limbo experienced by spouses after the ABI of their partner refers to the fact that spouses may not only lose the equal partnership with their loved one but they also lose the ability to maintain friendships outside of the marriage. This is the case because of lack of time or rejection by peers due to the survivor's neurobehavioral changes (Lezak, 1978). Wood et al. (2005) found that unpredictable behavior on the part of the survivor imposed the greatest burden on marital relationships and contributed to relationship breakdown.

Blais and Boisvert (2005) examined the factors associated with marital adjustment following ABI. They found that frequent use of problem-solving skills and positive reinterpretation of problems encountered, in addition to low use of avoidant coping skills were associated with higher adjustment levels.

Katz et al. (2005) researched the impact of wives' "coping flexibility" and duration of time since the husband's traumatic brain injury (TBI) on perceived burden. They focused on wives in particular because their literature review demonstrated that TBI creates more difficulties for wives than for other family members. These authors defined coping flexibility as the ability to modify an ineffective coping approach and to seek a more appropriate and adaptive coping strategy. They found that only in cases of wives that had reduced coping flexibility did perceived burden increase with time since injury.

Each survivor's particular combination of neurobehavioral, cognitive, and physical difficulties in addition to the effects of medications can pose unique challenges to intimacy. Problems with focused and sustained attention can interfere with both social and physical aspects of sexual activity. Frontal lobe disinhibition can lead to socially inappropriate sexual behavior. At the other extreme are survivors who are very withdrawn or passive following their ABI and who demonstrate a very decreased libido. Functional deficits such as communication problems, mobility loss, perceptual problems, loss of sense of smell, reduced sensation and tremor can all contribute to intimacy challenges. As survivors with ABI may no longer have the full capacity for empathy and interpersonal sensitivity, they may no longer be able to satisfy their partner's need for affection or intimacy (Lezak, 1978).

Spouses may struggle with shifting from caregiver to sexual partner, especially in cases where the injured spouse has become very childlike.

Screening survivors and families for concerns regarding changes in intimacy should be part of the initial clinical interview, so that difficulties can be identified and addressed early on.

When parents are the primary caregivers, the role shift is different from that of a spouse. In cases where there are two parents, both can help each other assist their child. There is some familiarity in caring for a grown child as parents once did in the past, in contrast to a spouse who has always been an equal with his or her marital partner. Additionally, parents generally feel unconditional love and responsibility towards their child regardless of the level of challenge presented. In the case of a marriage partner, there is always the option of divorce. Testa et al. (2006) reported that caregivers had more complaints at 2 years post-injury than at 6 months, which they speculate may underlie the high rate of divorce, up to two-thirds, at 2 years post-injury. Their study noted a strong relationship between neurobehavioral problems and impaired family functioning.

Benn and McColl (2004) stated that parents that viewed the ABI of their child as a manageable family challenge instead of a catastrophe were able to adapt more successfully. These researchers discussed the process of redefinition of stressful events to make them more meaningful. They emphasized that coping strategies that allowed parents to reframe stressors and to obtain social support helped to reduce stress.

MS sustained a severe TBI due to a fall at age 27. He had a substance abuse history and had preinjury challenges relating to self-esteem, anxiety, and depression. D, his mother, was his only significant other and primary caregiver. D was bright, highly educated, and very eager to help her son improve. She suffered post-traumatic stress disorder (PTSD), activated by the events that started when she received the frightening phone call from the police department on the night of her son's injury. Each time MS had a setback, D's PTSD was reactivated. MS's lack of insight, anger control problems, and poor attitude in addition to physical and cognitive difficulties were very upsetting to his mother, who was hopeful that the injury could bring about post-ABI growth (Chapter 14).

D attended counseling sessions aimed at reducing symptoms of post-traumatic stress disorder and teaching strategies to set limits with her son, communicate her thoughts in a constructive fashion, and improve her sense of control and use of adaptive outlets for frustration. Fortunately, MS gradually made remarkable gains in his insight, attitude, and functional status. D also recovered from the emotional trauma and was able to foster her son's continued growth and reintegration to school and work.

Parents of young children or adolescents post-ABI frequently report significant distress and fears regarding their child's altered skills and their recovery. The family unit can become more cohesive or more at risk for breakdown following a child's injury, depending on the family unit's preinjury closeness and the amount of support and guidance they receive. Their primary challenges include making certain that their child receives the appropriate neuro-rehabilitation programming and that he or she is reintegrated successfully to school at the appropriate time. Preventing social isolation and boosting self-esteem are usually important goals for children post-ABI that the clinical team can help address. Parents of young children are usually very eager to help the team by carrying over goals to the home setting and reinforcing home exercise programs. It isn't uncommon for parents to be in conflict relating to how to discipline their child with ABI, and how lenient or strict to be in rule setting and expectations. It is helpful for the clinician to train both parents in providing the same message to their child so as to increase clarity about parental expectations. Family counseling with the emphasis on parents working together as a team for the benefit of the family unit is usually very productive.

Parents of grown, married children who sustain an ABI can be very helpful to the survivor's spouse, who is usually exhausted by the demands of caregiving in addition to his or her other usual responsibilities. It is in everyone's best interest when different families members come together to best meet the needs of an injured loved one. In families where there is much tension or lack of cohesiveness, the survivor will ultimately suffer. Frequently, competition arises between the parents of the injured individual and his or her spouse regarding decision-making and treatment planning. A counselor can be very helpful in assisting different family members in working together for the survivor's benefit despite different viewpoints.

Elderly parents who become the primary caregivers of an adult child status post an ABI are in a particularly difficult situation. They suddenly have increased pressures and responsibilities instead of fewer daily activities and the pleasures of retirement. In cases where their child will need long-term programming, parents usually gain greater peace of mind if they are able to locate a long-term residential program during their life time, thereby reassured that their loved one is being taken care of properly. It is important that elderly parents be encouraged to secure the assistance of an aide or other support services to ensure some respite.

Young children of a parent with an ABI often deal with the challenge of receiving less attention than they did prior to their parent's injury, as one parent suddenly has increased needs and the other parent consequently has less time. The child may feel an internal void due to the lack of attention and parental support. Additionally, in cases where the survivor has become childlike or attention seeking after the injury, competition may arise between the child and the injured parent for the other parent's time. Also, the child may be saddened or embarrassed by the fact that the parent is acting silly or inappropriate. Young children whose parent was injured frequently express guilt relating to somehow contributing to their parent's injury, and often require reassurance that they were not responsible. Additionally, children tend to express fear that their uninjured parent will get hurt, as they tend to feel more vulnerable following their other parent's injury. It is important to alert the child's principal, teachers, and school psychologist about the parent's injury and the need for the child to be given extra support and attention. It is also important for the child to be educated, based on his or her age level, on ABI sequelae, for better understanding of the parent's injury. This type of training should be offered through the neuro-rehabilitation program that the parent attends.

It is very difficult for a parent who sustained an ABI to reestablish his or her status at home after a lengthy post-injury absence due to hospitalization and acute rehabilitation. Oftentimes, the household developed new norms while the survivor was away and it's very common for children to have become accustomed to having all their needs met by the uninjured parent. The injured parent usually is frustrated by his or her loss of power and may feel unimportant or excluded from the rest of the family. He or she may have particular difficulty setting limits and demonstrating good frustration tolerance. Hyper-sensitivity to noise and motion may also negatively affect parent–child interactions. Confidence may be very reduced as the parent post-injury is dealing with the loss of status at home in addition to other post-ABI changes.

Adult children tend to become the significant other for their parent in cases where the other parent is deceased, disabled or not involved. As grown children usually are in the process of developing their career and busy with their own family needs, time management usually becomes exceedingly difficult. These family members will require substantial support and training from the neuro-rehabilitation team to facilitate positive coping.

Siblings become the primary caregiver in cases where the injured brother or sister was single and their parents are either deceased, in another state, or don't speak English. Clinically, it has been noted that siblings tend to be very devoted significant others and usually stricter and less protective than parents. It is emotionally very draining for siblings to try to care for their injured loved one while trying to manage their own daily responsibilities, and they will require a lot of team support and guidance.

Young siblings whose brother or sister was injured have to deal with reduced attention by parents, increased tension at home, change in the quality of the relationship with the injured sibling, and embarrassment in cases where the injured brother or sister display neuro-behavioral difficulties. It is important to alert the school about the challenges that the sibling is experiencing so increased attention and support can be offered.

Family Training

One of the significant benefits of educating families on the repercussions of ABI is the reduction in number of common errors or misunderstandings. For instance, families tend to confuse a survivor's reduced initiation and executive functioning skills with laziness. Also, families tend to misinterpret a survivor's lability with depression, and they confuse organic lack of awareness with psychological denial.

Lezak (1988) found that families cope more effectively with a loved one's injury when they have knowledge about the nature of the emotional changes associated with ABI.

Reinforcement of adaptive coping skills and positive problem-solving abilities is very important during family training. Grant et al. (2004) found that a negative orientation toward problem-solving and a lack of preparedness for the caregiver role were variables that were associated with a higher risk of depression in caregivers of stroke survivors.

Family-based psychosocial intervention after stroke has been shown to increase efficacy and control, optimize social support, improve family cohesion, and promote effective problem-solving (Glass et al. 2000).

Palmer et al. (2004) discussed the value of educating survivors and families about depression post-injury and reviewing ways to adaptively solve psychosocial challenges that can contribute to depression. They also reviewed ways to recognize, identify, and manage symptoms of depression.

Dell Orto and Power (2000) highlight the value of group counseling for families by describing it as a "counterforce to helplessness, isolation, and desperation." Group counseling provides a forum for families to learn from each other's successes and failures and obtain training regarding productive ways to respond to survivor's behaviors and needs. Families can also benefit from being paired with other families who are further along in the process, who can act as mentors based on their first hand experience with similar challenges.

"Rehabilitation is an equalizing process. No one much cares what you did before; they're focused on what you can do now and how you can learn to live independently again." (Crimmins, 2000). In running family groups, the equalizing process that Crimmins refers to becomes very apparent. For example, an unexpectedly close kinship developed between two women that were members of a family educational/support group. One was a pediatrician and the other was a toll-booth operator. Prior to their husbands' injuries, the two would likely not have become friends due to differences in age as well as cultural and educational backgrounds. However within the group they were equals and they shared strategies and resources in a supportive manner. Their husbands who also had little in common except their ABIs were also group equals in their attempts to regain their autonomy and proceed to the next step of the process.

No one can understand and relate to a family whose loved one was injured the way another family in a similar situation can. Group counseling can be a great source of peer and professional support.

SL sustained a stroke about 10 years ago, ending his career as a college professor. His primary difficulties included expressive aphasia and rigid thinking. He and his wife, J, were both in their sixties and were struggling to keep their relationship intact despite post-injury challenges.

In a stroke caregiver's group, J shared her plan to sell the family home of many years due to her own physical difficulties that made the upkeep of the house too cumbersome. Her husband was very against the move, due to his desire to remain in a familiar setting and exert some level of control over his life. He also was experiencing post-injury rigidity of thinking and difficulty with change. Despite J's attempts to reason with her husband and have others, including professionals and family members, try to convince him of the merits of the move, he remained uncompromising and hostile. J was very emotionally distraught by her husband's lack of support of her needs since she had always been very dedicated and supportive of him. J benefited greatly from ventilating her mixed emotions to the group, who could relate to her challenging situation and provide reassurance, emotional support, understanding and helpful advice. Over time, J felt empowered by the support and advice of the group to go forward with the sale of the house.

How Families Can Help

To begin with, families need to know that it is a priority that they address their own physical and emotional health so that can successfully persist in caregiving. The following suggestions can optimize their effectiveness.

1. Reinforce carryover of learned strategies to the home setting to help survivors generalize progress to real life situations.
2. Praise survivors on progress and provide only constructive criticism to help rebuild self-confidence.
3. Help provide structure for survivors when they are not in rehabilitation so as to facilitate continued gains.
4. Keep survivors stimulated and active to help prevent regression.
5. Be in regular contact with the neuro-rehabilitation team to exchange relevant information. Find out about available resources. Come to meetings prepared with questions.
6. Find an appropriate balance between over- and under-protectiveness to assure that the survivor is safe but also not prohibited from making gradual gains in autonomy and feelings of self-worth.
7. Encourage survivors to do home exercises.
8. Be flexible in creating a useful and realistic role for the survivor in the family.
9. Learn how to de escalate stressful situations so that the home is an environment of peace instead of chaos.
10. Participate in a family support group to obtain continued support and information.
11. Keep hopeful about continued progress.

The primary value of structured educational/support groups for families is that they provide knowledge about ABI and reinforce best practices for facilitating a loved one's recovery. It is comforting for families to meet others who can truly relate to the daily challenges they experience. Exchanging helpful ideas about how to handle difficult situations that arise can provide much support and reassurance to significant others. An agenda that is structured, facilitated by different team members each week and that provides information about medical, physical, cognitive, and neurobehavioral sequelae of ABI is well received. A sample agenda includes—

1. Introduction—Review of the role of all team members and what to expect from rehabilitation.
2. Questions and answers with the team physician—The neurologist or physiatrist discuss concerns regarding medications, seizures, headaches, and pain management.
3. Discussion regarding emotional and social changes post-ABI.
4. Discussion regarding neuro-cognitive changes post-ABI.
5. Discussion regarding the specialized roles of the physical therapist, speech/language pathologist and occupational therapist.

6. Stress management training.
7. Problem solving challenging situations that arise.

Conclusion

A primary mission of the neuro-rehabilitation team is to alleviate family distress by providing information and support in a clear and sensitive manner. The team needs to aid and never impede a caregiver's attempts to cope constructively with the injury of a loved one. When the team is ineffective in meeting family needs, caregiver stress and frustration will be increased.

It is important for neuro-rehabilitation team members to be aware of the effects of prolonged caretaking on caregivers. The long-term implications of ABI can generate severe strain and tension on the survivor's family unit. Knowledge of the specific challenges that each family is dealing with and their particular strengths and vulnerabilities will help guide recommendations. All team members are responsible for prevention of caregiver breakdown and in providing families with skills, knowledge, support, and a sense of mastery.

References

Benn, K., McColl, M. (2004) Parental coping following childhood acquired brain injury. *Brain Injury* 18(3):239–255.

Blais, M., Boisvert, J. (2005) Psychological and marital adjustment in couples following a traumatic brain injury: A critical review. *Brain Injury* 19(14):1223–1235.

Cameron, J.I., Cheung, A.M., Streiner, D.L., Coyte, P.C., Stewart, D.E. (2006) Stroke survivors' behavioral and psychologic symptoms are associated with informal caregivers' experiences of depression. Archives of Physical Medicine and Rehabilitation 87(2):177–183.

Crimmins, C. (2000) *Where is the Mango Princess.* New York: Vintage Books.

Dell Orto, A.E., Power, P.W. (2000) *Brain Injury and the Family.* New York: CRC Press.

Glass, T., Dym, B., Greenberg, S., Rintell, D., Roesch, C., Berkman, L. (2000) Psychosocial intervention in stroke: The families in recovery from stroke trial. *American Journal of Orthopsychiatry* 70(2):169–181.

Grant, J.S., Weaver, M., Elliot, T.R., Bartolucci, A.A., Giger, J.N. (2004) Family caregivers of stroke survivors: Characteristics of caregivers at risk for depression. *Rehabilitation Psychology* 49(2):172–179.

Katz, S., Kravetz, S., Grynbaum, F. (2005) Wives coping flexibility, time since husbands' injury and the perceived burden of wives of men with traumatic brain injury. *Brain Injury* 19(1):59–66.

Kreutzer, J.S., Gervasio, A.H., Camplair, P.S. (1994) Primary caregiver's psychological status and family functioning after traumatic brain injury. *Brain Injury* 8:197–210.

Kreutzer, J.S., Serio, C.D., Bergquist, S. (1994) Family needs after brain injury: A quantitative analysis. *Journal of Head Trauma Rehabilitation* 9(3):104–115.

Kubler-Ross, E. (1983) *On Children and Death.* New York: Macmillan.

Lezak, M.D. (1988) Brain damage is a family affair. *Journal of Clinical Experimental Neuropsychology* 10:111–123.

Lezak, M.D. (1978) Living with the characterologically altered brain injured patient. *Journal of Clinical Psychiatry* 39(7):592–598.

Man, D. (2002) Family caregivers' reactions and coping. *Brain Injury* 16(12):1025–1037.

Nabors, N., Seacat, J., Rosenthal, M. (2002) Predictors of caregiver burden following traumatic brain injury. *Brain Injury* 16(12):1039–1050.

Oddy, M., Humphrey, M., Uttley, D. (1978) Stress upon the relatives of head injured patients. *British Journal of Psychiatry* 133:507–513.

Palmer, S., Glass, T.A., Palmer, J., Loo, S., Wegener, S.T. (2004) Crisis intervention with individuals and their families following stroke: A model for psychosocial service during inpatient rehabilitation. *Rehabilitation Psychology* 49(4):338–343.

Serio, C.D., Kreutzer, J.S., Gervasio, A.H. (1995) Predicting family needs after brain injury: Implications for intervention. Journal of Head Trauma Rehabilitation 10(2):32–45.

Serio, C.D., Kreutzer, J.S., Witol, A.D. (1997) Family needs after traumatic brain injury: A factor analytic study of the Family Needs Questionnaire. *Brain Injury* 11(1):1–9.

Testa, J.A., Malec, J.F., Moessner, A.M., Brown, A.W. (2006) Predicting family functioning after TBI: Impact of neurobehavioral factors. *The Journal of Head Trauma Rehabilitation* 21(3):236–247.

Tooth, L., McKenna, K., Barnett, A., Prescott, C., Murphy, S. (2005) Caregiver burden, time spent caring and health status in the first 12 months following stroke. *Brain Injury* 19(12):963–974.

Williams, J.M., Kay, T. (1991) *Head Injury. A Family Matter*. Maryland. Paul H. Brookes Publishing Co.

Witol, A.D., Sander, A.M., Kreutzer, J.S. (1996) A longitudinal analysis of family needs following traumatic brain injury. *NeuroRehabilitation* 7:175–187.

Wood, R., Liossi, C., Wood, L. (2005) The impact of head injury neurobehavioral sequelae on personal relationships: Preliminary findings. *Brain Injury* 19(10):845–851.

16
Long-Term Challenges

DEBORAH M. BENSON AND JEAN ELBAUM

As triumphant as the survivor, family, and neuro-rehabilitation team may be on the day of a successful discharge, it is premature to forecast continued growth or even stability at a later date. Numerous studies suggest ongoing challenges experienced by both survivors and caregivers, which can persist years after the injury, and long after rehabilitation ends, as is illustrated by the case of LV, below.

The accident struck me like a lightning bolt. A speeding motorist rear-ended my car, fracturing my skull, causing a severe brain injury. I was comatose for 35 days. I would not be returning to my previous life. My eyes crossed. I lost my sense of smell. I experienced severe coordination and balance difficulties. I had major visual challenges as well as cognitive and emotional difficulties.

Before the accident, I balanced my family (husband and two young sons) and career as a dentist successfully. I was just 49 years old, youthful and dynamic.

Post-injury, following the prolonged coma, I started the neuro-rehabilitation journey, which has been my primary job since the accident. I followed all the steps from acute to post-acute inpatient programming, shifting to daily, intensive outpatient therapies, and gradually reducing to part-time outpatient rehabilitation as my condition improved and my needs changed. It took 21 months to finally return home and become an outpatient.

I had corrective surgery to reposition both eyes for accident-induced esotropia and diplopia. Esotropia was eliminated but diplopia persists to this day. My double vision has been corrected through the use of prismatic lens eyeglasses. The improvement in my vision has also helped to increase my balance. I have been struggling to be cleared to return to driving and was recently re-authorized to drive again, eight years following my injury.

I was in a wheelchair for approximately 3 years followed by 2 years of using a walker. For the past few years, I have been using a cane to help me ambulate due to residual balance difficulties. I have made enormous gains in all areas, including my thinking skills, especially memory, emotional status, and in the use of compensatory strategies to work around my weaknesses.

Identified long-term challenges include a high incidence of perceived needs and ongoing barriers (Corrigan et al., 2004; Powell et al., 2001); frequent re-hospitalizations (Cifu et al., 1999; Marwitz et al., 2001), persistent cognitive and

286

emotional difficulties (Pagulayan et al., 2006), and social isolation (Dikmen et al., 1993; Oddy et al., 1985; Weddell et al., 1980).

In addition to being persistent, many of these changes/challenges worsen with age (Brooks et al., 1987; Felicetti et al., 2005) and the development of a variety of health-related problems as brain injury survivors age has been noted (Hibbard et al. 1998; Felicetti et al., 2005). Correlations have been found between traumatic brain injury (TBI) and early cognitive decline (Houx et al., 1991), and Alzheimer's disease (Starkstein & Jorge, 2005).

The long-term effects of brain injury are not only on survivors. Caregivers report high levels of stress/burden (Verhaeghe et al., 2005), and have been shown to have a high incidence of accidents/injuries themselves, particularly those experiencing greater levels of stress (Hartke et al., 2006).

In his study of community integration following TBI, Corrigan (1994) noted that an ideal outcome occurs when the survivor is satisfied with his/her life, is contributing more to society's shared efforts than he/she is dependent on them, and is able to sustain a state of physical and mental health that also contributes to the health of others in his/her life. Thus, success is a multifaceted concept, and must be measured not only by clients having met identified discharge goals, but by their being able to participate actively in home, community, work, and/or school settings; their emotional and physical health; the quality of their relationships; and the stability of these activities, states and relationships over time. Following this tripartite model, Sherwin et al. (2006) proposed a minimal data set by which to standardize the measurement of community integration outcomes following TBI, to facilitate program comparison and evaluation.

Given the above considerations, it is clear that responsibilities of the neuro-rehabilitation team do not end on the day of discharge from rehabilitation. Our goal must be not only to achieve successful short-term outcomes of our interventions, but to have these outcomes extend beyond the rehabilitation phase, so that the survivor and family are able to maintain their achievements and successes, and continue to grow and thrive throughout the remainder of their lives. How do we achieve this "extended" level of support?

Preparing for Discharge

It is commonly said among rehabilitationists that discharge planning begins upon the day of admission. While some survivors and families may be taken aback by discussion of discharge planning so soon upon entering the rehabilitation program, this focus is critical to facilitate a smooth transition from one phase of recovery and rehabilitation to the next, maximizing the potential for success and preventing setbacks. It is essential for the neuro-rehabilitation team to project survivor/family needs beyond their current status, and begin to lay the groundwork for the next step(s). For example, the acute rehabilitation team should work with the client/family to identify post-acute-rehabilitation needs (e.g., after acute-inpatient care and home or outpatient therapies), and locate appropriate programs/services from which the family can then visit and choose. The outpatient team must identify community/work re-integration options (e.g., competitive employment, vocational training, volunteerism), and begin working toward those goals while the client is still in rehabilitation. Post-discharge medical and psychosocial supports must be identified and discussed with the survivor/family, along with education regarding the importance of developing community-based support structures/systems, in order to maintain health and wellness once formal rehabilitation services have ended.

Specific Post-Discharge Challenges

Return to Work

As acquired brain injuries (ABIs) occur to individuals from every possible profession, the neuro-rehabilitation team has the challenge of assisting clients in returning to a wide variety of careers. These professions include various fields in medicine, law, business, and accounting as well as police work, maintenance, office work, and housekeeping. Clients who were unemployed pre-injury pose a different type of challenge, many having pre-injury vocational issues which need to be addressed along with the post-injury challenges.

There are six primary challenges noted clinically that hinder return to work post-ABI: lack of readiness, suitability, support, stability, insight, and incentives. Lack of readiness refers to inappropriate timing. Survivors who return to work prematurely are at high risk for failure. Lack of suitability refers to the fact that a survivor's pre-injury work may no longer match his or her post-injury level of functioning. Clinical examples include a cab driver that became legally blind, a construction worker with balance problems, a teacher with aphasia who no longer can communicate functionally, or an accountant who struggles to perform basic calculations. Loss of work identity presents a radical challenge to an individual's self-definition. Once the survivor is emotionally ready to accept a new role, he or she may choose vocational retraining, meaningful volunteer work, as in the continued case of LV below, or a more active role at home.

As a result of some of my residual difficulties, a return to my profession wasn't possible. Since I loved my profession but could no longer practice, I worked hard to obtain an appointment as a clinical assistant professor at a school of dental medicine. I have spent the last 6 years as a volunteer faculty member at the dental school, where I've instructed students in correct radiography techniques and interpretation.

Lack of support refers to an employer's creation of barriers to a survivor's re-integration to work. Clinical experience has shown that many supervisors have difficulty accepting an employee's post-injury changes, such as reduced speed on tasks, the need for compensatory strategies to aid memory and learning, behavioral differences, reduced attention to grooming or hygiene, and difficulty understanding humor. These variations may be quite subtle and even within normal limits but are less acceptable when compared to pre-injury performance standards. Despite protection provided by the Americans with Disabilities Act (ADA) of 1990, an unsupportive employer can sabotage a survivor's successful reentry. Providing education and counsel to supervisors can be very helpful in developing empathy and understanding. Lack of emotional or medical stability will prevent a successful return to work for numerous reasons. Challenges with alcohol or substance abuse have also been linked to failure in community reintegration (Dell Orto & Power, 2000). Lack of insight challenges were reviewed in Chapter 14. Survivors with awareness deficits believe they can return to work prior to their actual readiness, and often return pre-maturely, resulting in failure. There can be various disincentives to return to work which surface during the rehabilitation period. These include financial (e.g., potential to jeopardize social security/disability benefits), legal (e.g., pending lawsuit), and emotional/psychosocial disincentives (e.g., adoption of the "sick" role).

In order to optimize a survivor's reintegration to work, it is strongly recommended that the appropriate steps be followed (Malec & Moessner, 2006). Firstly, it is important to integrate vocational rehabilitation goals with general interdisciplinary therapy goals while the survivor is in the neuro-rehabilitation program. Simulating work responsibilities is critical in assessing survivor readiness. Once the client is doing consistently well in the neuro-rehabilitation program and is successful on all simulated tasks or work trials, the time is appropriate to coordinate with the individual's work supervisor to begin discussion regarding a gradual return to work and any needed reasonable accommodations. The work supervisor will need input on the survivor's current strengths and weaknesses and the most effective ways to best facilitate his or her return to work.

In cases where survivors are no longer well suited for their former careers, various options are possible. They may choose to retrain through state or privately funded vocational agencies/programs for individuals with disabilities so that they can begin a new career based on their current strengths. They may be able to find competitive or volunteer work in their field in a modified position. Survivors who were physical laborers prior to their injuries may choose to become caretakers for their children or homemakers for their families, especially in cases where they are not able to return to physical work and are not interested in returning to school or pursuing a different career. Additionally, given the wide range of volunteer opportunities in major hospitals, nursing homes, public schools, university settings and libraries, many clients are able to find a suitable position that can be both fulfilling and flexible, in terms of hours/days.

In cases where survivors are not appropriately supported by their employers in their efforts to return to work, it is critical that support be provided by either a job coach (funded by state, county, or paid for privately) or by a primary therapist/ counselor assisting the transition to work by maintaining regular contact and exchange of information with the employer. If the survivor is able to perform his/her essential job functions and the employer is not willing to provide reasonable accommodations, legal action may be necessary.

In terms of medical stability challenges in returning to work, it is critical that survivors have ongoing medical follow-up, especially in cases of seizure disorders or pain syndromes. The degree of control that a survivor has on medical challenges will greatly influence his/her attempts to successfully reintegrate to work. Continued counseling during the reintegration process can significantly assist the survivor in maintaining emotional stability and coping with difficulties that arise. Follow-up counseling sessions can also assist survivors in improving their awareness level as well as coping with mood challenges that may emerge once insight increases. Counseling/psychotherapy can also help survivors overcome various disincentive barriers.

School Re-Integration

A comprehensive review of challenges and strategies to facilitate school re-integration following brain injury is beyond the scope of this chapter. While some school districts are very supportive and welcoming of recommendations for students reintegrating back to school, others have great difficulty adjusting their policies or standard procedures in order to provide the necessary accommodations. Some survivors are able to easily return to school with accommodations and resource room help. Others may need a more specialized school setting that offers more individualized attention and flexibility. Due to severe emotional or behavioral difficulties, certain students may need one to one tutoring in place of a classroom setting until they are ready for, or can tolerate, group interaction. The neuro-rehabilitation team must partner with the school system (which becomes part of the care team for the survivor), serving as advocates, educators, and advisors, in order to ensure the student receives all of the supports that he/she needs in order to achieve a successful return. Taking advantage of supports available through county/state agencies or advocacy groups can also be of assistance.

Social/Leisure Involvement

Persistent difficulties in areas such as executive function, communication, vision, and balance will pose particular challenges with regard to maintaining or redeveloping an active social life following brain injury. Barriers toward social reintegration typically include a lack of transportation, withdrawal of pre-injury friends, and financial limitations. Lower-cost, accessible transportation options (e.g., county/state para-transit services for persons with disabilities) for those survivors unable to return to driving, afford taxis/car service, or manage the complexities of using the public transportation services must be explored and facilitated by the rehabilitation team prior to discharge, so they are available when the survivor will need them. Information about community-based advocacy and support services (e.g., local, regional advocacy associations, support groups) should be given, as well as information/support available in the home (e.g., internet-based support groups, websites, and long-term home and community-based support services).

The neuro-rehabilitation program itself can and should develop a mechanism for providing post-discharge support services, which can extend the neuro-rehabilitation continuum of care, offered at low to no cost to survivors and families following discharge from formal rehabilitation. These can include alumni and care-giver support groups, which can provide an opportunity for continued education, networking and validation of feelings and experiences. Other post-discharge support services can include educational (e.g., wellness) programs, exercise programs, weekend activities, volunteer opportunities, and peer mentoring. Telephone follow-ups can help to identify barriers or challenges, allowing proactive interventions to be made in order to avoid crises. Bell et al. (2005) have demonstrated the effectiveness of such telephone interventions in producing positive outcomes. These types of post-discharge services can offer a sense of security, ongoing support, and connectedness/community that is often lacking in the post-injury lives of survivors and families.

For many, the onset or experience of an acquired brain injury is a life-changing event, with lifelong consequences, affecting not only the injured person, but also their families and communities. The period of rehabilitation following such an event becomes a critical, though not exclusive, component of the rebuilding of the life that has been altered, and the healing that must take place, as is demonstrated by the continued story of LV.

I believe that my excellent recovery so far has been due to the combination of the intensive, integrative therapies I received as well as my strong determination. My gains would have been impossible without either component.

What lies ahead? I hope that I can continue to establish new pathways in the unused portions of my brain to help further boost my walking, talking, vision, fine and gross motor skills, as well as balance. These days my cognitive and emotional/social statuses are at pretty good levels.

My greatest challenge over the past 8 years has been to stop bemoaning my losses and get on with my life as fully as possible. I know I will always bear some scars from the brain injury, but I am hopeful about the future. I expect to continue to get stronger and better able to function. I hope to continue to be an example of fortitude and perseverance in the face of the unexpected. I've learned that you always have to be prepared because you never know how life's rudders will twist and turn your pathways.

The neuro-rehabilitation team has an enormous responsibility; not only to ensure the excellence and effectiveness of formal rehabilitation services provided, but the coordination of such services to meet the holistic needs of the survivor and family, and the extension of services beyond the period of formal rehabilitation, to facilitate the maintenance of function and quality of life, and continued health of those whom we serve.

References

Bell, K.R., Temkin, N.R., Esselman, P.C., Doctor, J.N., Bombardier, C.H., Fraser, R.T., Hoffman, J.M., Powell, J.M., Dikmen S. (2005) The effect of a scheduled telephone intervention on outcome after moderate to severe traumatic brain injury: A randomized trial. *Archives of Physical Medicine and Rehabilitation* 86(5):851–856.

Brooks, N., McKinlay, W., Symington, C., Beattie, A., Campsie, L. (1987) Return to work within the first seven years of severe head injury. *Brain Injury* 1(1):5–19.

Cifu, D.X., Kreutzer, J.S., Marwitz, J.H., Miller, M., Hsu, G., Seel, R.T., Englander, J., High, W., Zafonte, R. (1999) Etiology and incidence of rehospitalizations after traumatic brain injury: A multi-center analysis. *Archives of Physical Medicine and Rehabilitation* 80:85–90.

Corrigan, J.D. (1994) Community integration following traumatic brain injury. *Neuro Rehabilitation* 4:109–121.

Corrigan, J.D., Whiteneck, G., Mellick, D. (2004) Perceived needs following traumatic brain injury. *Journal of Head Trauma Rehabilitation* 19(3):205–216.

Dell Orto, A.E., Power, P.W. (2000) *Brain Injury and the Family*. New York: CRC Press.

Dikmen, S.S., Machamer, J.E., Temkin, N.R. (1993) Psychosocial outcome in patients with moderate to severe head injury: A 2-year follow up. *Brain Injury* 7:113–124.

Felicetti, T., Trudel, T., Mozzoni, M. (2005) Health, aging and traumatic brain injury: Four years of investigation. *Lippincotts Case Management* 10(5):264–265.

Hartke, R.J., King, R.B., Heinemann, A.W., Semik, P. (2006) Accidents in older caregivers of persons surviving stroke and their relation to caregiver stress. *Rehabilitation Psychology* 51(2):150–156.

Hibbard, M.R., Uysal, S., Sliwinski, M., Gordon, W.A. (1998) Undiagnosed health issues in individuals with traumatic brain injury living in the community. *Journal of Head Trauma Rehabilitation* 13(4):47–57.

Houx, P.J., Vreeling, F.W., Jolles, J. (1991) Rigorous health screening reduces age effect on memory scanning task. *Brain and Cognition* 15(2):246–260.

Malec, J.F., Moessner, A.M. (2006) Replicated positive results for the VCC model of vocational intervention after ABI within the social model of disability. *Brain Injury* 20(3):227–236.

Marwitz, J.H., Cifu, D.X., Englander, J.E., High, W.M. (2001) A multi-center analysis of rehospitalizations five years after brain injury. *Journal of Head Trauma Rehabilitation* 16:307–317.

Oddy, M., Coughlan, T., Tyerman, A., Jenkins, D. (1985) Social adjustment after closed head injury: A further follow-up seven years after injury. *Journal of Neurology, Neurosurgery and Psychiatry* 48:564–568.

Pagulayan, K.F., Temkin, N.R., Machamer, J., Dikmen, S.S. (2006) A longitudinal study of health-related quality of life after traumatic brain injury. *Archives of Physical Medicine and Rehabilitation* 87:611–618.

Powell, J.M., Machamer, J.E., Temkin, N.R., Dikmen, S.S. (2001) Self-report of extent of recovery and barriers to recovery after traumatic brain injury: A longitudinal study. *Archives of Physical Medicine and Rehabilitation* 82:1025–1030.

Sherwin, E., Whiteneck, G., Corrigan, J., Bedell, G., Brown, M., Abreu, B., Depompei, R., Gordon, W., Kreutzer, J. (2006) Domains of a TBI minimal data set: Community reintegration phase. *Brain Injury* 20(4):383–389.

Starkstein, S.E., Jorge, R. (2005) Dementia after traumatic brain injury. *International Psychogeriatrics* 17(Suppl. 1):S93–S107.

Verhaeghe, S., Defloor, T., Grypdonck, M. (2005) Stress and coping among families of patients with traumatic brain injury: A review of the literature. *Journal of Clinical Nursing* 14(8):1004–1012.

Weddell, R., Oddy, M., Jenkins, D. (1980) Social adjustment after rehabilitation: A two year follow-up of patients with severe head injury. *Psychological Medicine* 10(2):257–263.

Index

294 Index

Printed in the United States of America.